OSTEONECROSIS

OSTEONECROSIS

Sudhir Babhulkar MS (Orth) D (Orth) PhD (Orth) DSc (Orth) FAMS
Professor Emeritus
Indira Gandhi Medical College and Mayo General Hospital, Nagpur, Maharashtra, India
Director
Sushrut Hospital, Research Center and
Postgraduate Institute of Orthopedics
Nagpur, Maharashtra, India
sudhirbabhulkar@gmail.com

Foreword
DP Bakshi

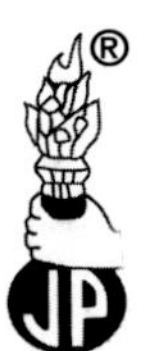

JAYPEE BROTHERS MEDICAL PUBLISHERS (P) LTD

New Delhi • London • Philadelphia • Panama

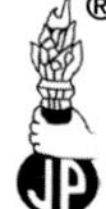 **Jaypee Brothers Medical Publishers (P) Ltd.**

Headquarters
Jaypee Brothers Medical Publishers (P) Ltd.
4838/24, Ansari Road, Daryaganj
New Delhi 110 002, India
Phone: +91-11-43574357
Fax: +91-11-43574314
Email: jaypee@jaypeebrothers.com

Overseas Offices

J.P. Medical Ltd.
83, Victoria Street, London
SW1H 0HW (UK)
Phone: +44-2031708910
Fax: +02-03-0086180
Email: info@jpmedpub.com

Jaypee-Highlights Medical Publishers Inc.
City of Knowledge, Bld. 237, Clayton
Panama City, Panama
Phone: + 507-301-0496
Fax: + 507-301-0499
Email: cservice@jphmedical.com

Jaypee Brothers Medical Publishers Ltd.
The Bourse
111, South Independence Mall East
Suite 835, Philadelphia, PA 19106, USA
Phone: + 267-519-9789
Email: joe.rusko@jaypeebrothers.com

Jaypee Brothers Medical Publishers (P) Ltd.
17/1-B, Babar Road, Block-B, Shaymali
Mohammadpur, Dhaka-1207
Bangladesh
Mobile: +08801912003485
Email: jaypeedhaka@gmail.com

Jaypee Brothers Medical Publishers (P) Ltd.
Shorakhute, Kathmandu
Nepal
Phone: +00977-9841528578
Email: jaypee.nepal@gmail.com

Website: www.jaypeebrothers.com
Website: www.jaypeedigital.com

Osteonecrosis

First Edition: **2013**

ISBN: 978-93-5090-407-7

Printed at Sanat Printers, Kundli.

Dedicated to

A perfect wife is the one who does not expect a perfect husband

My dear wife, Aruna, for her unconditional love and support…

FOREWORD

I have had the privilege of being acquainted with Professor Sudhir Babhulkar since 1980. Over the last 30 years, we have met and interacted in various regional, national and international meetings. I have always been impressed by his scientific clinical work, excellent documentation and dedication to research activities. I am personally aware of his extensive clinical work on osteonecrosis carried out over a period of four decades. This particular monogram is a culmination of the vast experience and knowledge gained over such a long period.

The book is a comprehensive guide on the subject of osteonecrosis encompassing the entire spectrum from etiopathology to various surgical treatments. The importance of early diagnosis and timely intervention is aptly stressed upon in order to ensure a pain free and active life of young adults who are the victims commonly of this debilitating disease.

The association of sickle cell disease with osteonecrosis is well documented. Osteonecrosis of hip prevalent around the world is well known, knee, ankle, talus, shoulder, hands, feet and spine, are described in great details.

I am convinced that the book will serve as a complete guide on osteonecrosis to all my orthopedic colleagues.

DP Bakshi
Retired Professor and Head
Department of Orthopedics
Calcutta Medical College and Hospitals
Kolkata, West Bengal, India
Past President of
Indian Orthopedic Association

PREFACE

Aseptic necrosis occurs when there is loss of blood supply to bone causing bone death. This disease attacks people in their late 30s and 40s, i.e. young adults; and if left untreated, results in total joint destruction with joint replacement remaining the only treatment option. It is an extremely debilitating condition though not life-threatening. The incidence of osteonecrosis is increasing globally mostly due to the use of high dose of steroids for certain medical conditions and increasing alcohol abuse. Sickle cell disease remains a common cause of osteonecrosis.

Since the beginning of my practice in 1970, we have managed a large number of patients with osteonecrosis. In 1994, our institute had the privilege of hosting an international symposium on osteonecrosis, which was attended by two giants in this field, Professor Y Sugioka from Japan and Dr JP Jones Jr from USA. Infact, these two pioneers in the field of osteonecrosis inspired me to maintain meticulous records of my patients, collect scientific data and focus my research on this topic. The book is a culmination of over four decades of dedicated clinical work, research and knowledge gained through various national and international meetings, especially on osteonecrosis.

The book covers the etiopathology of the disease including the research studies done on the different conditions associated with osteonecrosis. It will discuss in detail the various diagnostic tools including X-rays, CT scan, MRI and bone scan. Classification and staging are described at length with reference to importance in planning the treatment and correlation to prognosis. Various mimics of osteonecrosis are covered in the differential diagnosis. Association of sickle cell disease with osteonecrosis is covered in great details. Numerous illustrations have been included to ensure easy understanding of the disease. Surgical procedures are described with attention to details to ensure maximum benefit to the reader.

The book attempts to cover the entire spectrum of osteonecrosis with special emphasis on femoral head necrosis, this being the most common bone being affected.

I would like to thank my colleagues in the Department of Orthopedics, Indira Gandhi Medical College and Mayo General Hospital, Nagpur, Maharashtra, India, for their support, help and encouragement in bringing together the book. I would also like to thank our publisher, M/s Jaypee Brothers Medical Publishers (P) Ltd, New Delhi, India, for the support and encouragement.

I sincerely wish that the book will serve as a concise guide to all the students and practicing orthopedic surgeons all over.

Sudhir Babhulkar

CONTENTS

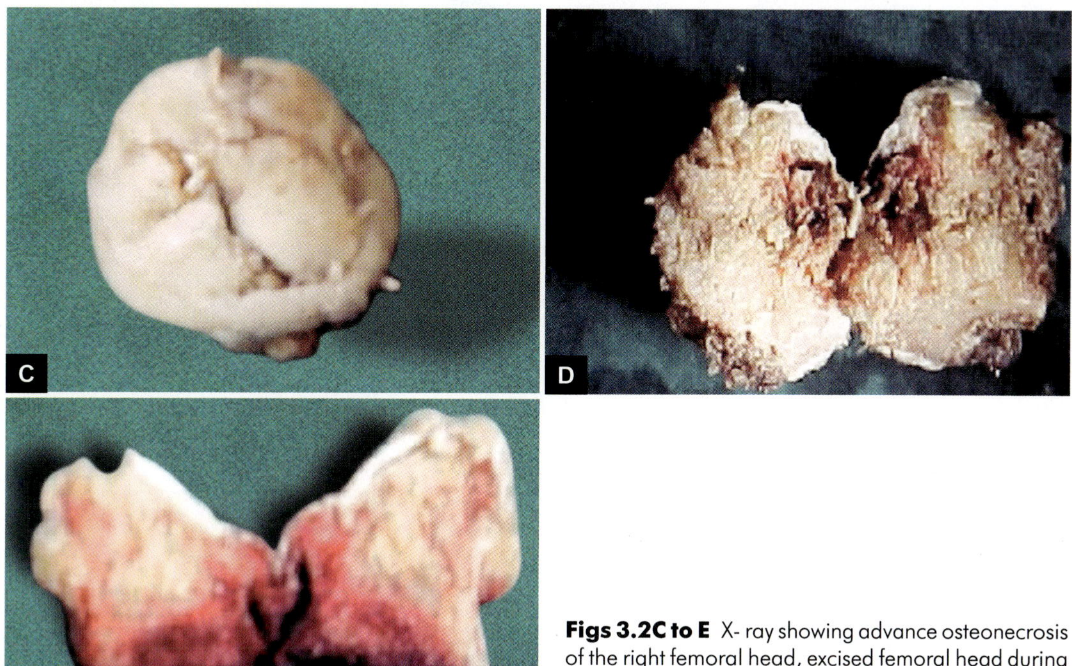

Figs 3.2C to E X- ray showing advance osteonecrosis of the right femoral head, excised femoral head during surgery, and the cut section of the femoral head which is sent for histopathology

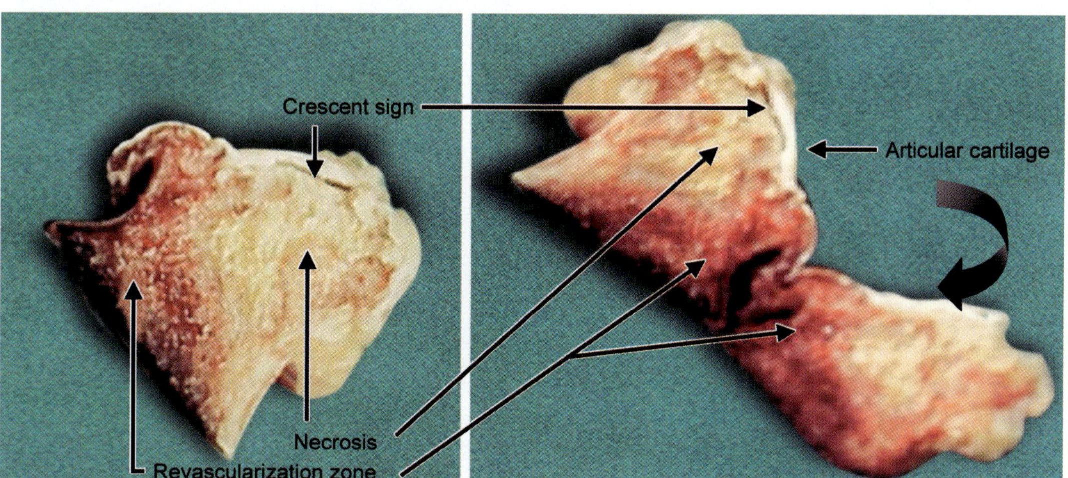

Fig. 3.5 Specimen of excised femoral head during replacement arthroplasty, showing gross appearance of the femoral head right hip

Plate 2

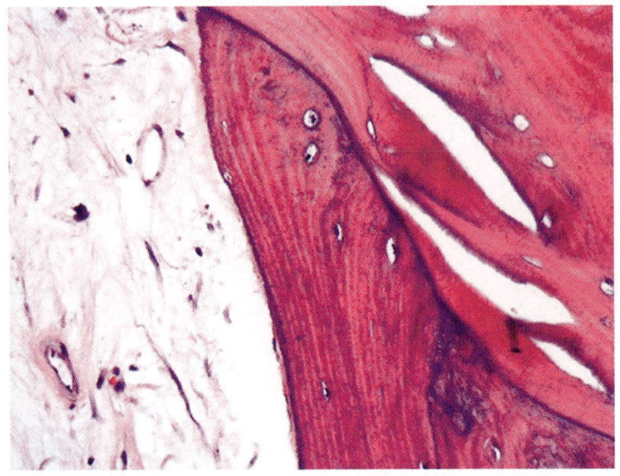

Fig. 3.6 Histopathology slide showing—Normal bone trabeculae with lacunae showing osteocytes

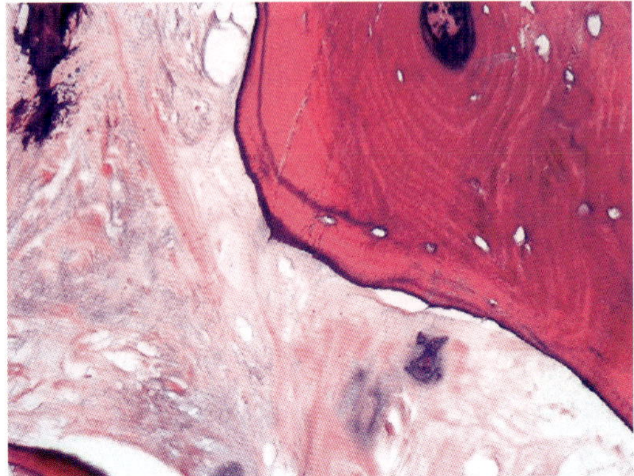

Fig. 3.7 Calcium deposit in necrotic marrow with nonviable trabeculae without osteophytes in lacunae

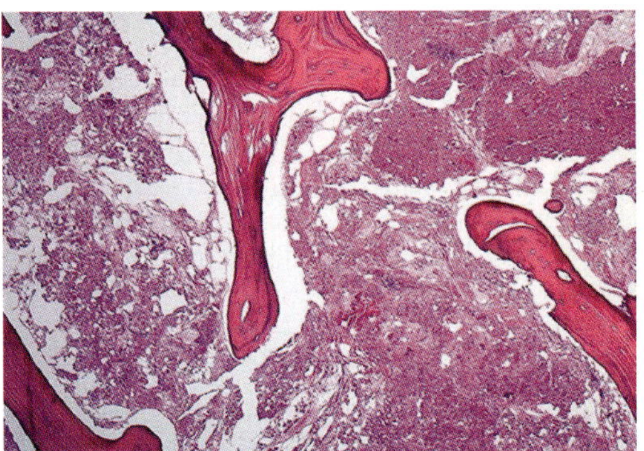

Fig. 3.8 Histopathology slide showing infarcted marrow

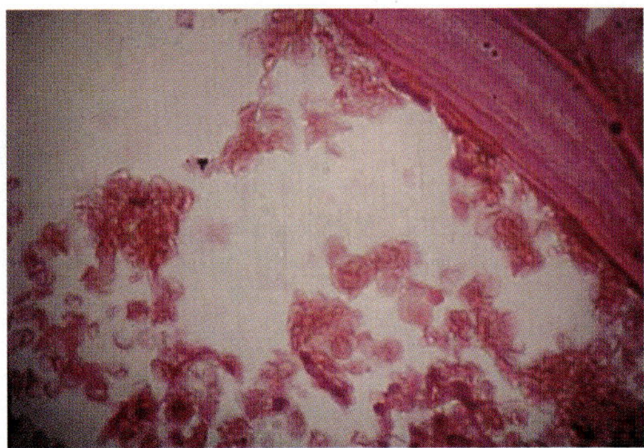

Fig. 3.9 Infarcted marrow with ghost cells in background

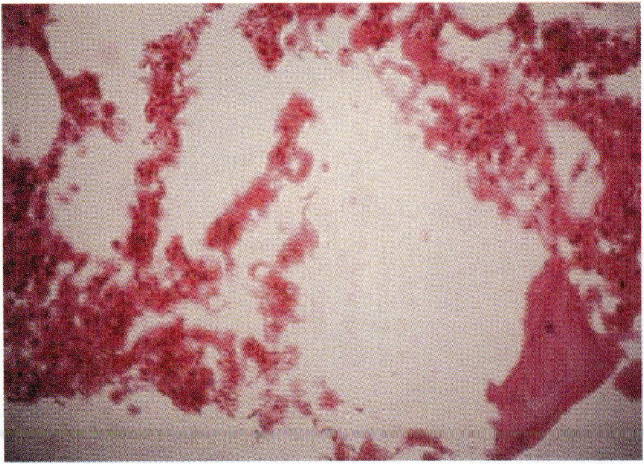

Fig. 3.10 Histopathology slide showing sickled RBCs with necrotic bone

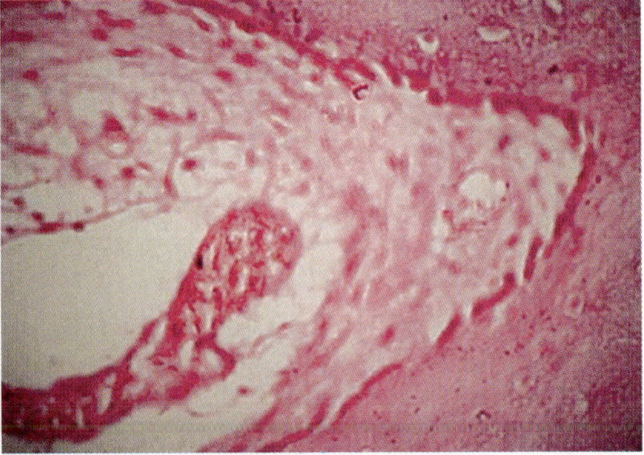

Fig. 3.11 Collagenized connective tissue at periphery

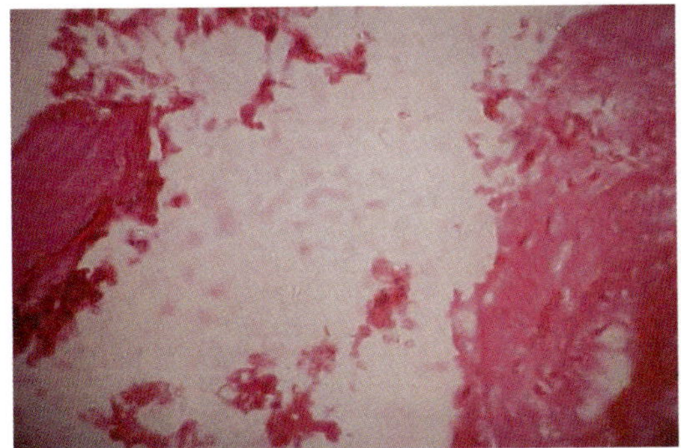

Fig. 3.12 Histopathology slide sickled RBCs with necrotic bone

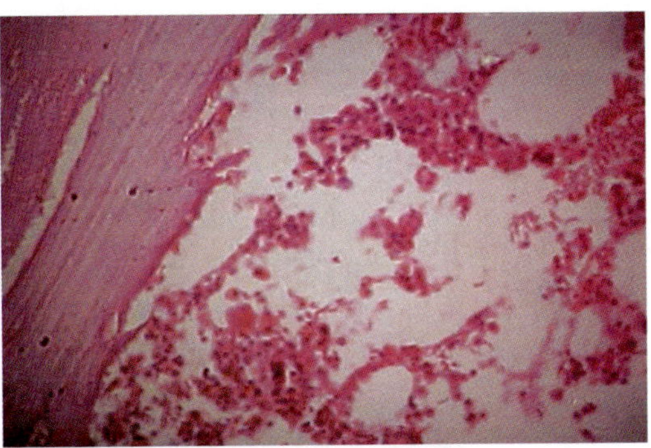

Fig. 3.13 Infarcted marrow with ghost cells in background

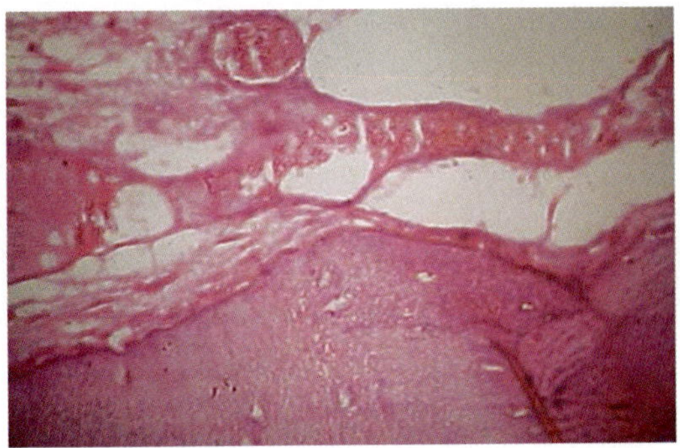

Fig. 3.14 Histopathology slide showing sickled RBC thrombus

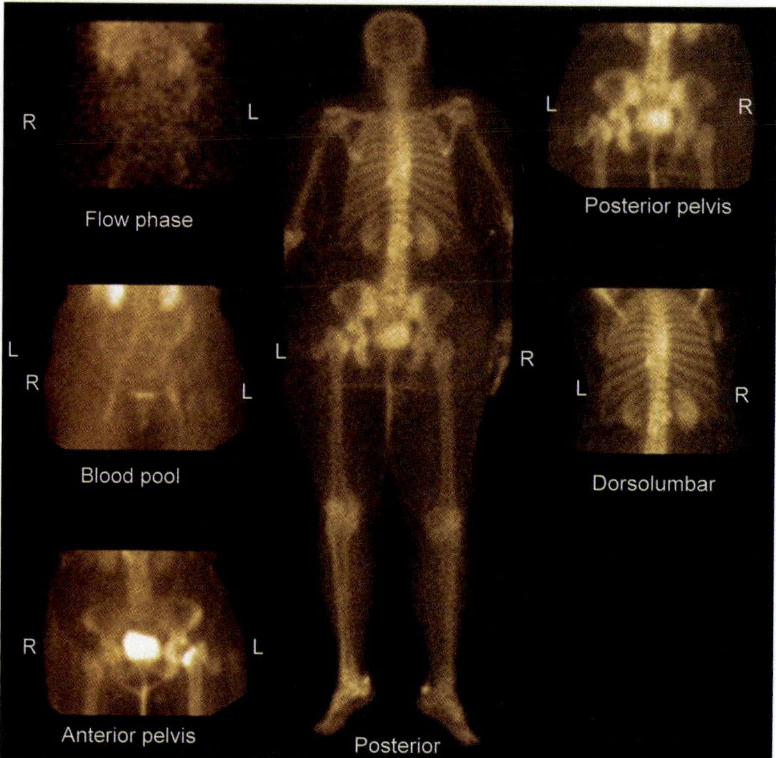

Fig. 7.13 Radioisotope bone scan showing normal flow phase. Blood pool not showing any abnormal soft tissue uptake. Anterior pelvis shows increased tracer uptake in obliquely linear fashion involving the neck of left femur with photopenic (Cold) area involving superomedial aspect of femoral head with a hot rim of activity suggesting early case of stage I osteonecrosis of the femoral head

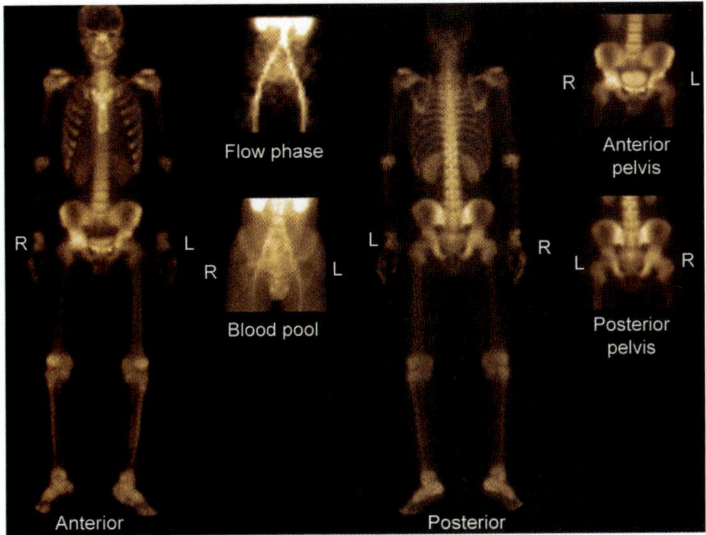

Fig. 7.14 The delayed anterior pelvis shows abnormal diffusely increased tracer uptake by the entire right femoral head suggestive of delayed or revascularization phase of osteonecrosis—stage III of right femoral head

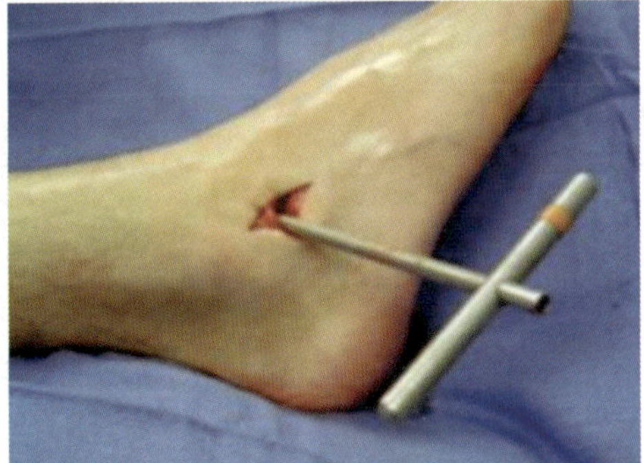

Fig. 22.14 Operating room picture showing a large bore for decompression

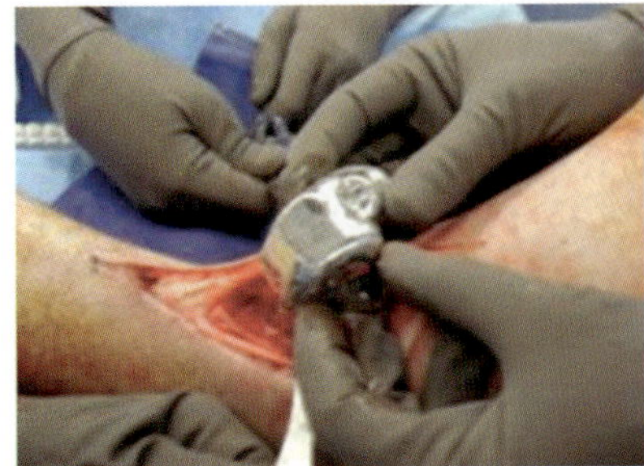

Fig. 22.16B Clinical picture showing talar prosthesis

1 INTRODUCTION

Osteonecrosis is a disease, which can lead to the collapse of bone and is caused by an inadequate supply of blood to the specific bone tissue involved. As a living tissue, bone is continuously remodeling and requires a certain amount of blood in order to function properly. Without an adequate blood supply, in the stage of insufficiency, serious cases of avascular necrosis can develop that leads to the death of bone tissue. Commonly, it affects young patients between the age of 30 to 60 years. Osteonecrosis is often referred to as an ischemic necrosis of bone, aseptic or avascular necrosis (AVN) or idiopathic avascular necrosis. It is an irreversible state of bone disorder that can be excruciatingly painful, disfiguring and disabling. Although osteonecrosis can be an extremely painful and debilitating disease, it is not considered to be fatal. In fact, there are hundreds of thousands of patients suffering from osteonecrosis, living with the disease throughout the world.

Osteonecrosis is divided into two categories: post-traumatic osteonecrosis and non-traumatic osteonecrosis.

Post-traumatic osteonecrosis refers to the onset of the bone disorder after experiencing a significant trauma. This is associated with mechanical interruption of the circulation to the femoral head. A severely broken bone or dislocated joint is typically the underlying cause behind the development of osteonecrosis.

Non-traumatic osteonecrosis refers to the onset of the bone disorder for reasons unrelated to a physical trauma. Several pathologies have been reported to be associated with this type of osteonecrosis. People may be more susceptible to development of bone disorder, if they have a history of diseases or activities known to disrupt blood supply, such as alcoholism, smoking, blood clotting disorders, hepato-renal disease, connective tissue disease, lupus erythromatosis, or have undergone treatment with high levels of corticosteroids and organ transplantation. More recently, a family of drugs called bisphosphonates has been linked with the development of non-traumatic osteonecrosis.

The signs and symptoms in early stages of osteonecrosis are similar to those associated with arthritis. During activity, osteonecrosis patients may experience pain and aching of the limbs and joints affected. The discomfort is often sporadic and short-lived, holding many osteonecrosis sufferers back from consulting physician with regards to the issue. As such, osteonecrosis often goes undiagnosed for a period of time until the occurrence of increasingly disabling painful symptoms causing severe arthritic changes, restricting the activities of daily living. The earlier an osteonecrosis diagnosis can be made, the better the chances are of limiting the severe and long-term effects of the painful bone disorder. If a case of osteonecrosis goes untreated, it can eventually culminate in bone collapse and arthritic changes (Figs 1.1A and B).

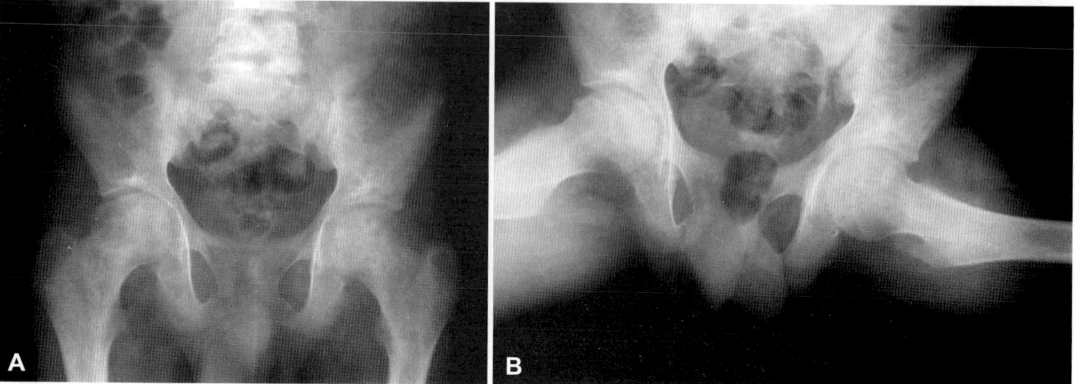

Figs 1.1A and B X-ray of pelvis showing changes of osteonecrosis of both femoral heads with deformation of right femoral head in a young 20 years, sickle cell disease patient

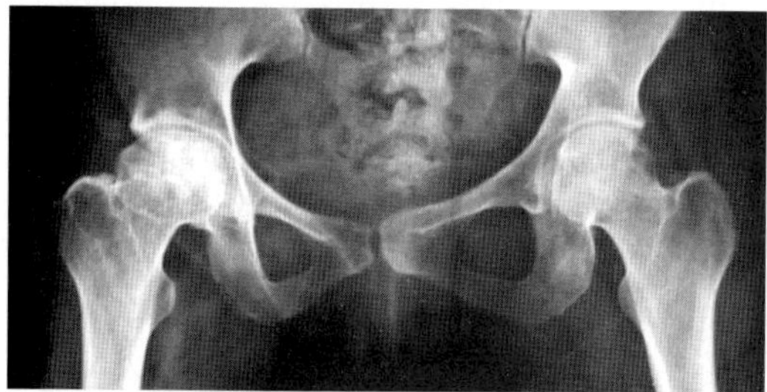

Fig. 1.2 X-ray pelvis showing classical radiological changes of osteonecrosis of right femoral head in a young female 24 years with lupus erythematosus

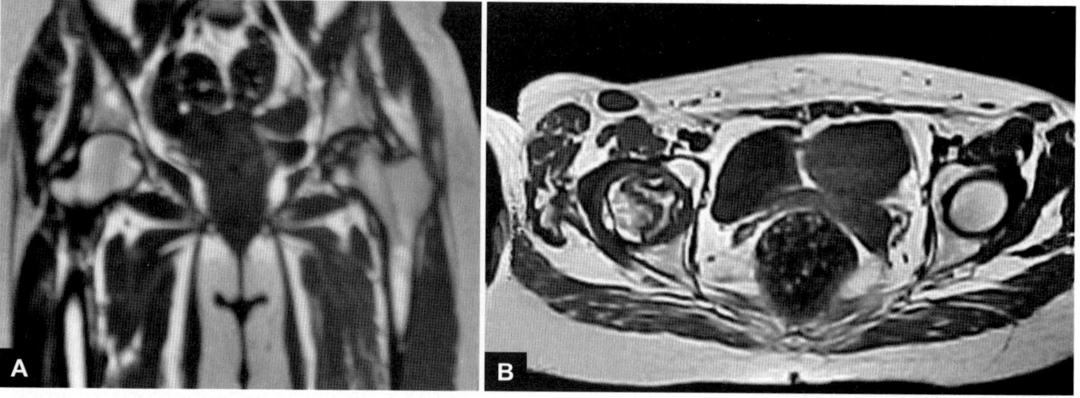

Figs 1.3A and B MRI scan of the same patient showing advanced changes in right hip

The best method for early osteonecrosis is radioisotope bone scan or magnetic resonance imaging. An MRI can detect the onset of osteonecrosis before the condition has had ample time to cause further damage to the affected bones. It is not until the bone condition has progressed to a serious stage that its effects can be viewed on X-ray, at which point it typically includes joint involvement and is too late (Figs 1.2 and 1.3).

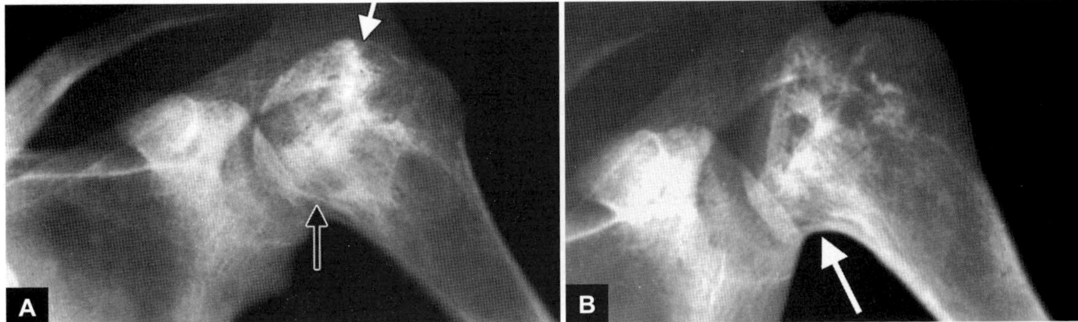

Figs 1.4A and B X-ray of shoulder of two patients showing multiple dense sclerotic spots fused to each other showing segmental involvement

Osteonecrosis is known to affect multiple locations in the axial and appendicular skeleton and is associated with diverse medical conditions and injury. Since the femoral head of the hip is the most common bone to be affected by osteonecrosis, symptoms often include limping and a great deal of pain in the groin. This topic of osteonecrosis of femoral head will be dealt in this monograph in detail, though other regions will also be discussed. Similar changes of osteonecrosis are noticed in humeral head (Figs 1.4A and B), vertebral end plates, distal femur, proximal tibia, anus, scaphoid, lunate, metatarsal heads, etc.

OSTEONECROSIS OF THE FEMORAL HEAD: AN INTRODUCTION

Osteonecrosis of the femoral head is presently recognized as a major musculoskeletal problem mostly affecting the young people. It is also known as *avascular necrosis* or *aseptic necrosis of bone* and is characterized by relentless progression in many cases despite treatment. Its significance lies in the fact that it mainly affects the young people in their productive years of life. The true prevalence of the disease is difficult to ascertain. In 5 to 18 percent of total patients undergoing total hip replacement in the US, the indication was reported to be advanced osteonecrosis of femoral head with secondary osteoarthritis[1,2] and approximately 45 percent of the primary total hip arthroplasties done in Taiwan.[3] Without treatment, more than 70 percent of femoral heads with osteonecrosis will collapse and require prosthetic replacement within three to four years of diagnosis.[3,4]

VASCULAR ANATOMY OF FEMORAL HEAD

The femoral head has a very precarious vascularity and is very prone to develop avascular necrosis following the injury and with known associated diseases. The hip joint capsule is a strong fibrous structure that encloses the femoral head and most of its neck. The capsule is attached anteriorly at the intertrochanteric line; posteriorly, however, the lateral third of the femoral neck is outside the capsule. That portion of the neck that is within the capsule has essentially no cambium layer in its fibrous covering to participate in the peripheral callus formation during the healing process. Therefore, healing of the femoral neck area is dependent on endosteal union alone. The blood supply to the femoral head and neck is complex. The femoral head derives its blood supply from the two largest tributaries of the profunda femoris; medial and lateral femoral circumflex arteries send branches that anastomose to form an extracapsular arterial ring, at the base of femoral neck. From this arterial ring, it sends ascending cervical arteries called as retinacular arteries which pierce the hip joint capsule and traverse along the neck of the femur deep to the synovial membrane. There are four major retinacular arteries, out of which the lateral retinacular artery is the most important blood supply to the femoral head and neck. The femoral head also receives blood supply from the artery of the ligament of head of femur, which branches from the obturator artery.

Many joint-preserving treatments, including hyperbaric oxygen, high-energy shock wave, electrical stimulation, core decompression, vascularized bone graft, and various osteotomies, have been developed in an effort to preserve the osteonecrotic femoral head in a precollapse stage.[5-12] Unfortunately, the success rates of all of these treatments vary widely, and there is no universally accepted treatment.[13]

Lately it has been observed that the incidence of osteonecrosis is steadily increasing (Figs 2.1A to D). The clinical entity affecting the femoral head is more important since it is commonly seen in young adults between the

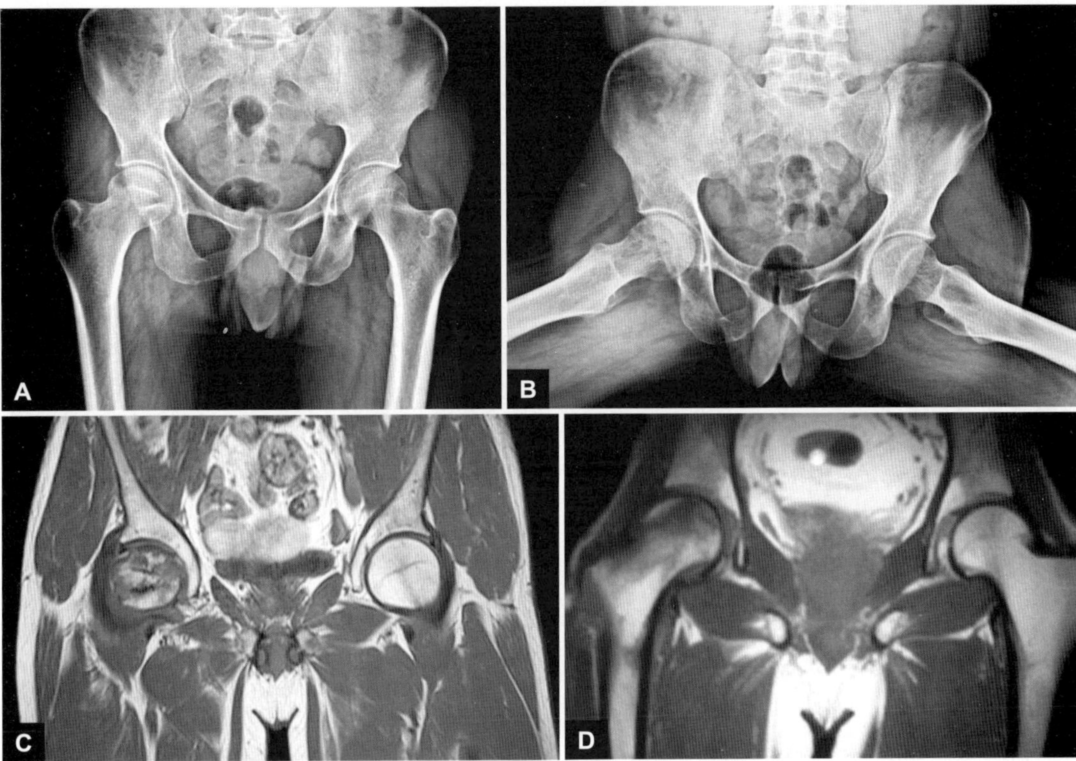

Figs 2.1A to D (A and B) Plain X-ray showing changes of osteonecrosis stage II/III with similar changes in MRI (C and D) In a young 35 years male alcoholic

ages of 20 to 40 years and is frequently bilateral (Figs 2.2A and B).[11,14-16] The disease most of the time results in severely disabling painful stiff hip in the early lifetime. The syndrome of segmental femoral head necrosis initially causes minimal pain and discomfort and is not noticed in many cases until deformity of the femoral head has already occurred and progressed to a great extent, and is likely to require arthroplasty (Figs 2.3A and B).[17]

HISTORICAL PERSPECTIVE (BULLOUGH 1997)[18]

It has been over a century since osteonecrosis was recognized as a clinical entity but unfortunately our knowledge about its pathophysiology and natural history is far from complete. The earliest documentation and probably one of the first reports of 'aseptic' necrosis of the femoral head was by James Russell, Professor of Clinical Surgery in Edinburgh in the year 1794. The gross appearance of bone necrosis was clearly described by James Paget in 1860. In 1888, Twynham published the first description of necrosis in a femoral head associated with Caisson's disease.[19] Another landmark paper was by Phemister in 1915, who described the microscopic findings in necrotic bone, comparing the changes in bone dying as result of infection (septic necrosis) with those resulting from a circulatory disturbance (aseptic necrosis).[20] Subsequently he reported the pathological and radiological changes seen in dead bone and the reparative process

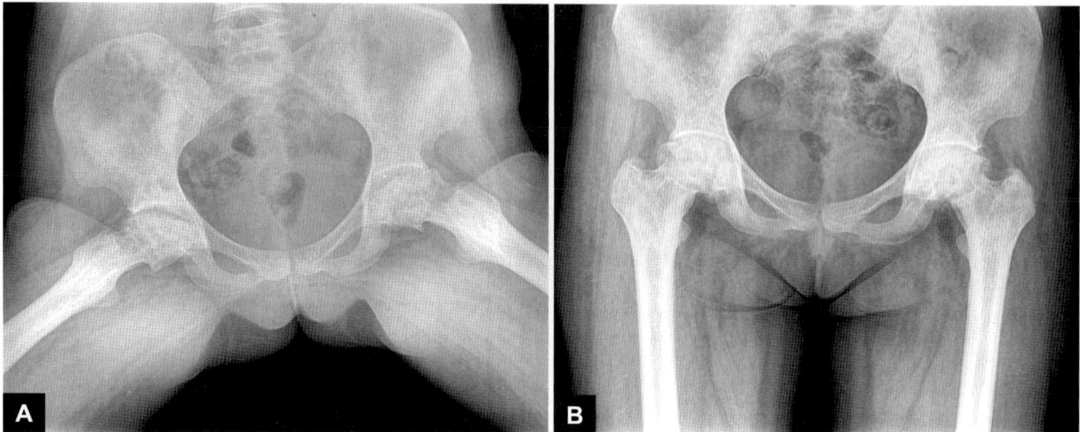

Figs 2.2A and B X-ray pelvis anteroposterior and Dunn's view showing bilateral advanced osteonecrosis of femoral head in 50 years female with sickle cell disease

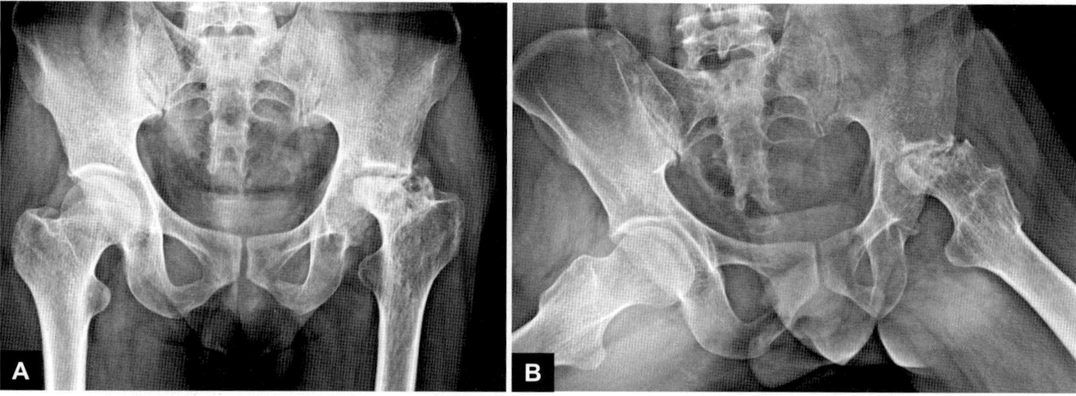

Figs 2.3A and B X-ray pelvis anteroposterior and Dunn's view showing advanced osteonecrosis of left femoral head with severe arthritic changes in 55 years alcoholic male

occurring around the dead bone following fracture, grafting and vascular occlusion.[21,22] He coined the term 'Creeping substitution' for this reparative process whereby the dead bone is finally removed after a layer of living bone has been deposited onto the pre-existing dead bone.[23] The earliest report of osteonecrosis with common associated conditions like alcoholism and use of steroids were published by Axhausen[24,25] and Pietrogrande and Mastromarino[26] respectively. Modell and Freeman[27] also confirmed the corticosteroid as a cause and reported a case of osteonecrosis in a patient with Cushing's disease. Increasing renal transplantation and postoperative steroid treatment provided Cruess et al.[28] with further evidence of association with steroid consumption. Catto published two articles describing in detail the destruction and reparative changes seen in osteonecrosis of the femoral head[29,30] following transcervical fracture neck femur.

In 1948, Chandler postulated that occlusion of the posterolateral retinacular artery leads to ischemic infarction and eventual collapse of the anterolateral area of the femoral head producing typical wedge shaped deformed femoral head on X-ray, which looks like the process of coronary artery disease. He coined the term *'Coronary disease of Hip'* which was widely accepted.[31,32]

Avascular necrosis of the femoral head is essentially a vascular disease and can be easily divided into two groups, traumatic and nontraumatic. In case of traumatic osteonecrosis of the femoral head (fracture neck femur, dislocation hip) it is attributed to disruption of extra-osseous circulation, reflecting the interruption of the blood supply of one or more major vessels to the femoral head. Osteonecrosis following fracture neck femur results from progressive ischemia rather than from acute infarction. In case of traumatic osteonecrosis one does not see any localized areas of subchondral infarction, as against nontraumatic osteonecrosis in which disruption of intraosseous circulation is most likely responsible for the disorder.[33] The ischemia is either due to occlusion of arteries or obstruction to venous drainage. Interruption of arterial supply or occlusion of venous drainage results in stasis and oxygen starvation. This results in bone cell death, which occurs because of disparity between the oxygen need of the bone cell and inability of the local circulation to meet the demand. Irrespective of the etiological condition it is well known that in the early phases of bone ischemia, the symptoms are minimal and X-rays are normal. Almost all the cases of bone necrosis pass through a preradiologic stage and even the earliest radiological changes indicate that the disease process had been in progress for some time. It is observed that in a high percentage of cases, eventually the other hip is involved regardless of the etiology. The lesion was observed to be bilateral in 50 percent of the patients of Merle De Aubingne et al.[14] in 72 percent patients of Boettcher and Bonfiglio[11] and 80 percent cases Ficat's.[16] This presents an opportunity to make the diagnosis on the opposite side prior to morphological failure of the femoral head. Most of the patients present with complaints of deep, throbbing pain in the groin and hip—initially intermittently, later more severe. Subsequently these patients complain of painful limited movements of the hip. A few patients may have radiating pain from the groin to the thigh and knee along with the medial aspect. In some patients the only complaint is discomfort and limp during weight-bearing. In later stages almost all patients develop painful stiff hips with grossly restricted movements, limiting squatting and sitting cross-legged. There are many problems and controversies in osteonecrosis. These exist in the areas of: etiopathology, method of diagnosis, and difference in the interpretation by imaging and surgical method of treatment.

NATURAL HISTORY OF OSTEONECROSIS

The natural history of symptomatic osteo-necrosis of the femoral head is generally one of relentless progression to collapse and incongruity of the joint, ultimately leading to requirement of total hip arthroplasty if the initial treatment consisted of nonoperative measures only. The study of the natural history of osteonecrosis is limited by a number of factors. These include selection of cases, diagnostic criteria and investigations used, inconsistencies in the manner in which the treatment modality is applied and the manner in which the results are reported. The above point is highlighted by two widely reported studies in the literature designed to address the efficacy of core decompression versus conservative treatment (Stulberg et al. 1991[34] and Koo et al. 1995[35]). The authors of these studies arrived at conflicting conclusions. Generally osteonecrosis of the femoral head in the adult is a progressive disease with most hips experiencing clinical and radiographic failure within two to three years after the onset of symptoms.[4-17] More recently, Aaron et al.[5] reported a study of 80 hips in 53 patients followed clinically and radiographically. Radiographic progression occurred regardless of Ficat stage with hips in Stage I showing more rapid progression than hips in Stage II or III. Overall clinical progression was seen in 69 percent and radiographic progression in 76 percent at a mean follow-up of 32 months.

Radiographic progression was also associated with progressive clinical failure.

Spontaneous Resolution of Osteonecrosis of the Femoral Head

The natural history of osteonecrosis of the femoral head, in general, is thought to be one of progressive disease if no intervention is undertaken. Untreated osteonecrosis of the femoral head is believed to carry a poor prognosis.[10,16] An emphasis has been placed on earlier intervention as it has been associated with an improved outcome.[36] With the advent of MRI, osteonecrosis of the femoral head has been found to be present in asymptomatic patients.[37-41] However, it is unknown whether surgical intervention is beneficial for patients with asymptomatic osteonecrosis of the femoral head. Spontaneous resolution of osteonecrosis of the femoral head can occur. The factors that appear to be related to resolution are:

1. Early, asymptomatic disease (Association Research Circulation Osseous Stage I)
2. Small lesion size (a modified index of necrotic extent of <25).

The phenomenon of spontaneous resolution may not be a rarity.[42] Of the 13 hips with asymptomatic disease that were identified in the prospective screening study of patients managed with organ transplantation, three (23%) showed evidence of spontaneous resolution.[42] Asymptomatic osteonecrosis of the femoral head is rarely diagnosed because screening MRI examinations are not routinely performed in clinical practice. Therefore, the identification of hips with asymptomatic osteonecrosis of the femoral head that undergoes spontaneous resolution is rare; however, the results of the present study suggest that the biologic phenomenon itself is not. All three patients had steroid-related osteonecrosis of the femoral head that had been diagnosed on the basis of MRI only after solid organ transplantation (including one kidney transplantation, one kidney-pancreas transplantation, and one lung transplantation).

Monitoring these patients closely for clinical signs and symptoms of disease progression and obtaining frequent serial magnetic resonance images are useful for identifying evidence of resolution. The reported prevalence of osteonecrosis of the femoral head in patients who have undergone a solid organ transplant has ranged from 3 to 41 percent.[43]

Asymptomatic Osteonecrosis

Nontraumatic osteonecrosis of the femoral head usually has an insidious onset in many patients which progresses to collapse of the femoral head and rapid destruction of the hip joint. Though many cases of osteonecrosis are diagnosed following the gradual onset of hip or groin pain, asymptomatic disease is sometimes diagnosed in the contralateral hip in a patient with symptomatically affected hip or detected during the process of screening of an at-risk population. Though the best treatment for asymptomatic osteonecrosis of the femoral head is not well-defined, the proper treatment should be addressed to the patient to avoid further progression which might be inevitable. Many authors believe that asymptomatic hips will eventually progress to collapse and the head may not be salvageable irrespective of the size of the lesion.

Hence, it is desirable to identify various factors which can guide to forestall the disease and avoid progression to collapse and avoid worse outcome of asymptomatic disease. There are a few criteria to determine the prevalence of the progression of asymptomatic lesions to symptomatic disease and collapse which might influence the prognosis of the disease. Various radiographic and demographic factors influence the progression of the disease, which include, size and location of the ischemic lesion, radiographic stage, and associated disease and risk factors. The treatment of asymptomatic osteonecrosis of the femoral head is a controversial issue. The natural history of asymptomatic osteonecrosis is important to identify the characteristics which will support operative or nonoperative treatment modalities. In the study by M Mont et al.[44,45] there was a prevalence of progression of disease to symptomatic disease in 59 percent and hence watchful waiting appears unlikely to be effective in the majority of patients. In the study by Hungerford and Jones on the natural history of asymptomatic osteonecrosis the success rate of surgical Core decompression was based on the size of the lesion, rather than symptoms.[46] Hernigou et al.[36] followed 40 patients with a small asymptomatic osteonecrosis lesion in one hip and symptomatic disease in the contralateral hip. They found progression of asymptomatic disease to symptomatic in 88 percent of the hips, with collapse occurring in 73 percent, at a mean of 92 months after diagnosis. Based on these findings, Hernigou recommended prophylactic joint-preserving surgical treatment of asymptomatic hips, irrespective of the size or location of the lesion. After the observation of M Mont,[44,45] they suggested that nonoperative treatment may be suitable for small and medially located lesions. Small lesions occupying <25 percent of the femoral head and those that spared involvement of the lateral two-thirds of the weight-bearing portion of the femoral head progressed to collapse in <10 percent of the hips, where it would be appropriate to treat these nonoperatively. However, given the high rate of progression of untreated lesions that do not meet these size and location criteria and the favorable success rate of head preserving surgeries, it is recommended that in patients with lesions involving the lateral two-thirds of the weight-bearing portion and lesions >25 percent of the femoral head should be subjected to early salvage surgery of the femoral head.

In a systematic review of the literature, it was found that asymptomatic osteonecrosis of the femoral head includes high risk of 84 percent progression of large lesions and substantial risk of progression in 25 percent cases of medium sized lesions. However, small and medially located lesions have < 10 percent risk of progression.

PRESENT STATUS: CONCLUSION

In a prospective, randomized trial in which the results of core decompression were compared with those of nonoperative treatment at a mean of 27 months, Stulberg et al.[34,47] reported a clinically successful result for only 2 of 23 patients who had been managed non-operatively. Steinberg et al. retrospectively reviewed the results of nonoperative treatment of 55 osteonecrosis hips and found radiographic progression in 92 percent (no numbers were given), with clinical progression in 84 percent, at a mean of 21 months.[48-54] Musso et al.[55] retrospectively reviewed the results for 50 osteonecrosis femoral heads that had been treated with modified weight-bearing, analgesics, and anti-inflammatory medications and found that 47 hips (94%) had progression of the disease, according to clinical or radiographic criteria, at a mean of 16 months.

Many reports in the literature regarding the natural history of nontraumatic osteonecrosis and the results of core decompression have documented marked differences in prognosis between hips that have had collapse and those that have not. However, the study performed by Bozic et al.[56] demonstrates the importance of distinguishing between patients who have cystic changes in the femoral head and those who have sclerotic changes only. Cystic changes in the femoral head as seen on plain radiographs were associated with more than a four-fold increase in the rate of overall failure after core decompression. This observation is consistent with the findings of Lennox et al.[57] who reported a combined rate of radiographic and clinical failure of 10 percent (2 of 20) in patients with Stage-IIA sclerotic disease compared with 7 of 11 patients with Stage-IIA cystic or osteoporotic disease. Thus, the available literature suggests relentless progression of disease in osteonecrosis and supports aggressive therapeutic intervention in all patients regardless of the clinical or radiographic features at presentation.

The long-term survival of hips in Ficat Stages I and II osteonecrosis after core decompression provides significant palliation and delays the need for further surgical treatment, sometimes for long periods. Total hip replacement is likely to improve with time, and therefore the delay in replacement in this group of young patients may also result in improvement in the results of arthroplasty. On the basis of our long-term results we would advocate the use of core decompression for precollapse stages of osteonecrosis. We also advise its use after minimal collapse in patients who fully understand the importance of delaying total hip replacement and who can be relied on to modify their activity level (Fairbank[58]). Given the relatively young mean age of our patients at the time of presentation, it is believed that preservation of the joint should be the goal of treatment of early-stage non-traumatic osteonecrosis. It is seen that patients who do not have cystic changes or collapse of the femoral head are most likely to benefit from core decompression. Furthermore, it is found that both a rapid onset of symptoms and the use of corticosteroids are independently associated with a poor outcome.

Data extracted from previously published studies suggest that asymptomatic osteonecrosis has a high prevalence of progression to symptomatic disease and femoral head collapse. While small, medially located lesions have a low rate of progression, the natural history of asymptomatic medium-sized, and especially large, osteonecrotic lesions, is progression in a substantial number of patients. For this reason, it may be beneficial to consider joint-preserving surgical treatment in asymptomatic patients with a medium-sized or large, and/or laterally located lesion.

REFERENCES

1. Mankin HJ. Nontraumatic necrosis of bone (osteonecrosis). N Eng J Med. 1992;326:1473-9.
2. Mont MA, Hungerford DS. Nontraumatic avascular necrosis of the femoral head. J Bone Joint Surg. 1995;77A:459-74.
3. Lai KA Shen WJ, Yang CY, Shao CJ, Shen WJ, Yang CY, Shai CJ, HSU JT, Lin RM. The use of alendronate to prevent early collapse of the femoral head in patients with nontraumatic osteonecrosis. J Bone Joint Surg Am. 2005;87:2155-9.
4. Steinberg ME. Recent advances in the management of osteonecrosis of the hip. Introduction. Semin Arthroplasty. 1998;9:181-3.
5. Aaron RK, Steinberg ME: Electrical stimulation of osteonecrosis of the femoral head. Semin Arthroplasty. 1991;2:214-21.
6. Alet J. Nontraumatic vascular necrosis of the femoral head: Past, present and future. Clin Orthop. 1992;277:12-21.
7. Arlet J, Ficat P. Forage-biopsie de la tete femorale dans l'osteonecrose primitive. Observations histo-pathologiques portant sur huit forgaes. Rev Rhumat. 1964;31:257-64.
8. Baksi DP. Treatment of post-traumatic avascular necrosis of the femoral head by multiple drilling and muscle- pedicle bone grafting. J Bone Joint Surg (Br). 1983;65B:268-73.
9. Baksi DP. Treatment of osteonecrosis of the femoral head by drilling and muscle-pedicle bone grafting. J Bone Joint Surg (Br). 1991;73B:241-5.
10. Beltran J, Knight CT, Zuelzer WA, et al. Core decompression for avascular necrosis of the femoral head: Correlation between long-term results and preoperative MR staging. Radiology. 1990;175:533-6.
11. Boettcher WG, Bonfigilo M, Smith K. Non-traumatic necrosis of the femoral head: II. Experiences in treatment. J Bone Joint Surg Am. 1970;52A:322-9.
12. Bradway JK, Morrey BF. The natural history of the silent hip in bilateral atraumatic osteonecrosis. J Arthroplasty. 1993;8:383-7.
13. Brinker MR, Rosenberg AG, Kull L, et al. Primary total hip arthroplasty using uncemented porous-coated femoral components in patients with osteonecrosis of the femoral head. J Arthroplasty. 1994;9:457-68.
14. Merle D' Aubingne R, Postal M. Mazabraud A, Massias P, Gueguen J. idiopathic necrosis of the femoral head in adults. J Bone Joint Surg Br. 1965;47B:612-33.
15. Ficat P, Arlet J, Hungerford DS (Eds). Ischaemia and Necrosis of Bone. Baltimore, MD, Williams & Wilkins, 1980.
16. Ficat RP. Idiopathic bone necrosis of the femoral head: Early diagnosis and treatment. J Bone Joint Surg Br. 1985;67B:3-9.

17. Cornell CN, Salvati EA, Pellicci. Long-term follow-up of total hip replacement in patients with osteonecrosis. Orthop Clin North Am. 1985;16:757-69.

18. Bullough PG. The morbid anatomy of subchondral osteonecrosis. In: Urbaniak JR, Jones JP (Eds); Osteonecrosis: Etiology, diagnosis, and treatment. Rosemont, IL: American Academy of Orthopaedic Surgeons; 1997.pp.69-72 (Monogram by AAOS 1997).

19. Twynham GE. A case of Caisson disease. Br Med J. 1888;1:190. Phemister DB; Necrotic bone and subsequent changes which it undergoes. JAMA. 1915;64:211-6.

20. Phemister DB. The recognition of dead bone based on pathological and X-ray studies. Ann Surg. 1920;72:466.

21. Phemister DB. Fractures of the Neck of the Femur, Dislocation of Hip, and Obscure Vascular Disturbances Producing Aseptic Necrosis of the Head of the Femur. Surg., Gynec., and Obstet. 1934;59:415-40.

22. Phemister DB. Changes in bones and joints resulting from interruption of the circulation. II.Nontraumatic lesions in adults with bone infarction, arthritis deformans. Arch Surg. 1940; 41:1455-82.

23. Phemister DB. Treatment of necrotic head of the femur in adults; J Bone Joint Surg Am. 1949; 31A, 55.

24. Axhausen G. Die Nekrose des In Osteonecrosis: Etiology, Diagnosis and Treatment. Urbaniak JR, Jones JP Jr (Eds); American Academy of Orthopaedic Surgeons, 1st edn, 1997; 69-72. proximalen Bruhstucks beim Schenkelhalsbruch und ihre Bedeeutung fur das Huftgelenk. Langenbeck Arch Klin Chir 1922;120:325-46.

25. Axhausen G. Uber anamische Inkarkte am Knowchensystem und ihre Bedeutung fur dies lehre von den primaren Epiphyseonekrosen. Arch Klin Chir. 1928;151:72.

26. Pietrogrande V, Mastromarino R. Osteopatda prolungata trattamento cortisonico. Ortop Traum Appar Mat. 1957;25:791-810.

27. Madell SH, Freeman LM. Avascular necrosis of the bone in Cushings Syndrome. Radiology 1964;83:1068-70.

28. Cruess RL, Blennerhassett J, MacDonald FR, et al. Aceptic necrosis following renal transplantation. J Bone Joint Surg. 1968;50A: 1577-90.

29. Catto M. A histological study of avascular necrosis of the femoral head after transcervical fracture. J Bone Joint Surg. 1965;47B:749-76.

30. Catto M. A histological appearances of late segmental collapse of the femoral head transcervical fracture. J Bone Joint Surg. 1965; 47B:777-91.

31. Chandler F. Aseptic necrosis of the head of the femur. Wis Med J. 1936;35:609.

32. Chandler FA. Coronary disease of the hip. Journal of International College of Surgeons. 1948;1:34-6.

33. Glimcher MJ, Kenzora JE. The biology of osteonecrosis of the human femoral head and its clinical implications: Part II. The pathological changes in the femoral head as an organ and in the hip joint. Clin Orthop. 1979;139:283-312.

34. Stulberg BN, Davis AW, Bauer TW, Levine M, Easley K. Osteonecrosis of the femoral head. A prospective randomized treatment protocol. Clin Orthop. 1991;268:140-51.

35. Koo KH, Kim R. quantifying the extent of osteonecrosis of the femoral head: A new method using MRI. J Bone Joint Surgery Br. 1995;77B:875-880-2593.

36. Hernigou A, Poignard A, Nogier, O Manicom. Fate of Very Small Asymptomatic Stage-I Osteonecrotic Lesions of the Hip: J Bone Joint Surgery Am. 2004;86:2589-93.

37. Lavernia CJ, Sierra RJ, Grieco FR. Osteonecrosis of the femoral head. J Am Acad Orthop Surg. 1999;7:250-61.

38. Fink B, Degenhardt S, Paselk C, Schneider T, Modder U, Ruther W. Early detection of avascular necrosis of the femoral head following renal transplantation. Arch Orthop Trauma Surg. 1997;116:151-6.

39. May DA, Disler DG. Screening for avascular necrosis of the hip with rapid MRI: preliminary experience. J Comput Assist Tomogr. 2000;24: 284-7.

40. Kopecky KK, Braunstein EM, Brandt KD, Filo RS, Leapman SB, Capello WN, Klatte EC. Apparent avascular necrosis of the hip: appearance and spontaneous resolution of MR findings in renal allograft recipients. Radiology. 1991;179:523-7.

41. Siddiqui AR, Kopecky KK, Wellman HN, Park HM, Braunstein EM, Brandt KD, Klatte EC, Capello WN, Leapman SB, Filo RS. Prospective study of magnetic resonance imaging and SPECT bone scans in renal allograft recipients:

evidence for a self-limited subclinical abnormality of the hip. J Nucl Med. 1993;34:381-6.

42. Marston SB, Gillingham K, Bailey RF, Cheng EY. Osteonecrosis of the femoral head after solid organ transplantation: a prospective study. J Bone Joint Surg Am. 2002;84:2145-51.

43. Edward Y Cheng, Issada Thongtrangan, Alan Laorr, Khaled J Saleh. Spontaneous of Osteonecrosis of the Femoral Head: J Bone Joint Surg Am. 2004;86:2594-9.

44. Mont MA, Hungerford DS. Non-traumatic avascular necrosis of the femoral head. J Bone Joint Surg. 1995;77A:459-74.

45. Mont MA, Carbone JJ, Fairbank AC. Core decompression versus nonoperative management for osteonecrosis of the hip. Clin Orthop. 1996;324:169-78.

46. Hungerford DS, Jones LC. Diagnosis of osteonecrosis of the femoral head. In Schoutens A, Arlet J, Gardeniers JWM, et al (Eds). Bone Circulation and Vascularisation in Normal and Pathological Conditions. New York, NY, Plenum Press. 1993.pp.265-75.

47. Stulberg BN, Singer R, Goldner J, Stulberg J. Uncemented total hip arthroplasty in osteonecrosis. A 2 to 10 year evaluation. Clin Orthop. 1997;334:116-23.

48. Steinberg ME, Brighton CT, Hayken GD, Tooze SE, Steinberg DR. Early results in the treatment of avascular necrosis of the femoral head with electrical stimulation. Orthop Clin North America. 1984;15:163-75.

49. Steinberg ME, Brighton CT, Steinberg DR, Tooze SE, Hayken GD. Treatment of avascular necrosis of the femoral head by a combination of bone grafting, decompression, and electrical stimulation. Clin Orthop. 1984;186:137-53.

50. Steinberg ME, Brighton CT, Hayken GD, Tooze SE, Steinberg DR. Electrical stimulation in the treatment of osteonecrosis of the femoral head—a 1-year follow-up. Orthop Clin North America. 1985;16:747-56.

51. Steinberg ME. Management of avascular necrosis of the femoral head—an overview. Instructional Course Lectures, American Academy of Orthopaedic Surgeons. Vol. 37, pp. 41-50. Park Ridge, Illinois, American Academy of Orthopaedic Surgeons, 1988.

52. Steinberg ME, Brighton CT, Corces A, Hayken GD, Steinberg DR, Strafford B, Tooze SE, Fallon M. Osteonecrosis of the femoral head. Results of core decompression and grafting with and without electrical stimulation. Clin Orthop. 1989;249:199-208.

53. Steinberg ME. Core decompression of the femoral head for avascular necrosis: indications and results. Canadian J Surg. 1995;38 (Supplement 1):S18-S24.

54. Steinberg ME, Hayken GD, Steinberg DR. A quantitative system for staging avascular necrosis. J Bone and Joint Surg Br. 1995;77-B(1):34-41.

55. Musso ES, Mitchell SN, Schink-Ascani M, Basset CAL. Results of conservative management of osteonecrosis of the femoral head. A retrospectivestudy. Clin Orthop. 1986;207:209-15.

56. Bozic KJ, Zurakowski D, Thornhill TS. Survivorship Analysis of Hips Treated with Core Decompression for Nontraumatic Osteonecrosis of the Femoral Head J Bone Joint Surg Am. 1999;81:200-9.

57. Lennox DW, Murrah RL, Ebert T, Carbone J. The efficacy and safety of core decompression of the hip as a treatment for osteonecrosis. Complicat. Orthop. 1993;47:39-42.

58. Fairbank AC, Bhatia D, Jinnah RH, Hungerfoed D. Long-term results of Core Decompression for ischaemic necrosis of the femoral head. J Bone and Joint Surg Br. 1995;77B(1):42-9.

3

MECHANISM OF DISEASE AND PATHOPHYSIOLOGY OF OSTEONECROSIS

ETIOPATHOLOGY

Pathogenesis refers to all the cellular events, reactions, and other pathological mechanisms occurring in the development and progression of the disease. The secret of pathophysiology lies in the vulnerable microcirculation of the femoral head. There are many theories of the pathogenesis of osteonecrosis of the femoral head. There are three main ways by which this circulation can get impaired:

1. Direct vascular interruption such as in trauma.
2. Intravascular occlusion of the blood vessels either by thrombotic occlusion such as in the case of hemoglobinopathies or by fat emboli such as in the case of alcohol or steroids.
3. Extravascular compression of the blood vessels such as in the case of intraosseous hypertension due to Cushing's syndrome.

Arterial occlusion seems to be the main contributing factor with two main mechanisms, thrombosis and emboli. The reduction of the blood supply leads to decrease in the delivery of oxygen to the osteocytes. Osteocyte necrosis occurs after two to three hours of ischemia, however osteocyte death is only observed histologically after 24 to 72 hours. Adipocyte necrosis and necrosis of the hematopoietic marrow occur before osteocyte necrosis. Variable areas of dead trabecular bone and bone marrow extending to the subchondral bone characterize osteonecrosis of the femoral head. The anterolateral segment of the femoral head is characteristically affected but no area is being spared. In adults the involved area does not revascularize and most radiographically evident lesions progresses until the femoral head collapses. The presumed mechanism of mechanical failure of femoral head is accumulated stress fractures of necrotic trabeculae that are not repaired[1-3] (Glimscher and Kenzora, 1979). The earliest sign of mechanical failure is the 'crescent sign'. In traumatic avascular necrosis, the mechanism is well understood and is because of extra-osseous disruption of vascular supply. In other instances the etiology is often proved on the basis of association with a particular risk factor. Exposure to corticosteroids and alcohol intake account for approximately 90 percent of all reported associated causes of avascular necrosis[4] (M Mont et al. 1995).

MECHANISM OF DISEASE

A number of different etiologies have been proposed for the causation of osteonecrosis. These include: the microembolization theory, the intraosseous hypertension theory, intravascular coagulation, and multifactorial causation of osteonecrosis.

Various theories for the pathogenesis of osteonecrosis are:

- Primary vascular abnormalities (occlusion of arterioles)
- Fat embolism
- Intravascular coagulation
- Accumulative cell stress theory
- Hypertrophy of fat cells
- Intramedullary hemorrhage.

It has been observed that the antero-superolateral segment of the femoral head undergoes necrosis first. This is obviously because of occlusion of posterolateral retinacular vessels or due to emboli from various sources finding their way through the microcirculation into the subchondral zone of the femoral head. This results into the weakening of the trabecular structure leading to multiple microfracture and finally collapse in the weight-bearing portion of the femoral head. This is the 'microembolization theory' for the pathogenesis of avascular necrosis of the femoral head[5-9] (Kenzora and Glimscher, Jones JP Jr 1965, 1992).

There is another concept for the formation of avascular necrosis of the femoral head: 'intraosseous hypertension theory'. According to this theory the femoral head bone functions as a closed compartment and the eventual infarction of weight-bearing bone is the end stage of the progressive compartment syndrome produced by increased intraosseous pressure.[10-14] The findings of increased bone marrow pressure at all stages and even in the early preradiologic stage supports this theory. It is presumed that there could be a combination of both the theories.[5,6] JP Jones proposed 'intravascular coagulation' as the missing link joining several unrelated risk factors that result in nontraumatic osteonecrosis.[15] It was proposed that the coagulopathy was not the cause of osteonecrosis but only an intermediary event initiated by an underlying etiologic factor.[16] The thrombotic threshold may be decreased in the various hypercoagulable patients with hereditary thrombophilia, hyperlipemia or antiphospholipid antibodies. Subsequent exposure to one or more additional risk factors facilitates thrombosis and bone infarction. 'Intravascular fat embolism' has been found to be one of the causative factors in the ischemic necrosis of the femoral head. Experimental studies, which were conducted by many workers, showed corticosteroid induced fat embolism causing avascular necrosis.[5,17-24] The experiments were conducted in rabbits and in all the specimens there was hyperlipidemia, fatty liver, systemic fat embolism, and fat embolism of the femoral head leading to focal osteocytic death of the cells of the femoral head.[8,18]

Fat Embolism

Osteonecrosis is associated with fat embolism which was demonstrated clinically and was confirmed experimentally.[7-25] In the subchondral region of the bone there is marked arteriolar and capillary distension which is essential to permit the passage of large fat globules and is limited by the confines of small haversian canal. Fat globules get deformed when compressed within the narrower channels. These are deformed in a cylindrical or oval shape which results in the advancement or penetration with terminal impaction of the fat globule. Intraosseous penetration is followed by focal intravascular coagulation, fibrin thrombus propagation, focal marrow necrosis, osteon anoxia and osteocytic death. End arteries in the bone are capable of blockage by very small emboli. Fat emboli may arise from a fatty liver, destabilization and coalescence of plasma lipoproteins and from disruption of fatty bone marrow or adipose tissue depots. Fat embolism also occurs in several clinical conditions which are associated with osteonecrosis, especially alcoholism, corticosteroid consumption, Cushing syndrome, hyperlipemia and so on. The alcohol-induced fatty liver is the most common source of continuous, low-grade and relatively asymptomatic showers of systemic fat emboli.

The pathophysiology of osteonecrosis because of fat embolism progresses in 5 stages:

1. ***Stage 0:*** Intraosseous fat embolism (resulting in the thrombotic process of focal intravascular coagulation).
2. ***Stage I:*** Focal osteonecrosis: (Mechanical from intraosseous vascular occlusion) (shows dead bone marrow and dead bone without repair).
3. ***Stage II:*** Chemical: Inflammatory (The repair process starts with recanalization of

the thrombosed vessel and revascularization, but without subchondral collapse or articular incongruity).

4. *Stage III:* Late segmental collapse (Collapse of the ischemic segment without any arthritic changes).

5. *Stage IV:* Stage of collapse and secondary arthritic changes.

List of associated conditions causing avascular necrosis in our series is shown in Table 3.1.

In our series we did not come across cases of osteonecrosis of the femoral head following Caisson's disease or Cushing syndrome.

The concepts of pathology and etiology must be separated since many diseases are associated with nontraumatic avascular necrosis of the femoral head and yet the clinical and radiological picture is similar.[8,18,26-31]

Pathogenesis

In spite of numerous studies, the pathogenesis of osteonecrosis of the femoral head is still unknown.[4,32] Proposed pathomechanisms include fat embolism[6-9] intravascular coagulation,[9] intraosseous hypertension[11-14] and fatty necrosis of osteocytes.[28] The significance of these mechanisms is highly controversial, as these findings cannot consistently be implicated in osteonecrosis[8] or verified in experimental models.[5,6] It is most likely that osteonecrosis results from multifactorial causes with each of the proposed mechanisms having a role.

There are multiple theories about pathogenesis. These include: thromboemboli in circulation from circulating fat, i.e. nitrogen bubbles, or abnormally shaped red blood cells (RBCs) seen in sickle cell disease, increased bone marrow pressure, i.e. obstruction of arteriolar and venous outflow, injury to wall of vessel by vasculitis, i.e. radiation damage, release of vasoactive factors in Gaucher's disease, altered lipid metabolism. Avascular necrosis is a multifactorial, heterogeneous group of disorders that lead to the final common pathology of mechanical failure of the femoral head. There are multiple etiologies

Table 3.1 List of diseases commonly associated with osteonecrosis of the femoral head

Sr. No.	Associated diseases (Causes)
1.	Sickle cell hemoglobinopathy
2.	Alcohol-induced
3.	Cortico steroid-induced
4.	Gaucher's disease
5.	Gout
6.	Systemic lupus erythematosis
7.	Following renal transplantation
8.	Idiopathic

for the disease, but the pathological condition is remarkably similar in all patients. The initial wedge-shaped usually anterolateral subchondral infarcted bone is covered with intact cartilage. A healing response may stabilize a small lesion. However in more than 90 percent of patients natural history demonstrates an ineffective healing response with resorption of bone predominantly and poor formation of new bone. The lack of repair at the center of the lesion and incomplete repair at the periphery leads to partial resorption of dead bone and replacement with fibrous and granulation tissue. Thickened trabeculae are formed by deposition of living bone directly on the dead bone. This produces radiographic appearance of alternating areas of osteosclerosis and cysts. Eventually, the unsupported cartilage collapses followed by increased destruction of the joint.

Any process, which evokes bone ischemia, is likely to result in increased bone marrow pressure, which would then; potentiate the ischemia.[12] By this mechanism such possible divergent etiologies as steroids, alcohol induced, fat embolism[5,8,31,33] as well as intraosseous lipocytes hypertrophy mechanism of Wang et al.[23] could produce similar effects of increased bone marrow pressure and decreased bone blood flow. It is said that ischemia provokes bone marrow edema and fibrosis, elevating bone marrow pressure, which further decreases the bone blood flow. This cycle of ischemia, edema and increased pressure culminates in bone cell death. The mechanical failure and continued weight-bearing results eventually in collapse of the femoral head and osteoarthritic changes. The natural history of osteonecrosis in most cases when there is no treatment attempt in modifying the disease process by medical, surgical or other means is collapse of the femoral head, destruction of articular cartilage and finally destructive and arthritic changes in the hip joint (Figs 3.1 to 3.5).

HISTOLOGY/BIOPSY

Histological study of biopsy from the femoral head showing trabecular bone with empty lacunae is the most definitive diagnostic finding of a avascular necrosis (Figs 3.6 to 3.14).

Findings at Core Biopsy

The characteristic clinical and radiographic features of osteonecrosis allow its recognition and initiation of treatment in most cases without histological diagnosis. However in early cases, noninvasive tests may not be conclusive and histopathology diagnosis may be appropriate.

The earliest change of osteonecrosis cannot be recognized by routine light microscopy but cytological changes have been detected by electron microscopy as early as 4 hours after experimental ischemia. At least 24 to 72 hours of anoxia may be required before autolysis can be recognized by light microscopy.[14]

The first recognizable signs of osteonecrosis are hemorrhage, loss of hemopoietic elements, loss of adipocyte nuclei and microvesicular fat, and necrosis of the bone marrow.

The histological picture of the next stage depends largely on geographic factors and thus both the age of the infarct and the extent of core biopsy will influence the histological appearance. If the infarct is not vascularized, then a central zone will remain acellular for

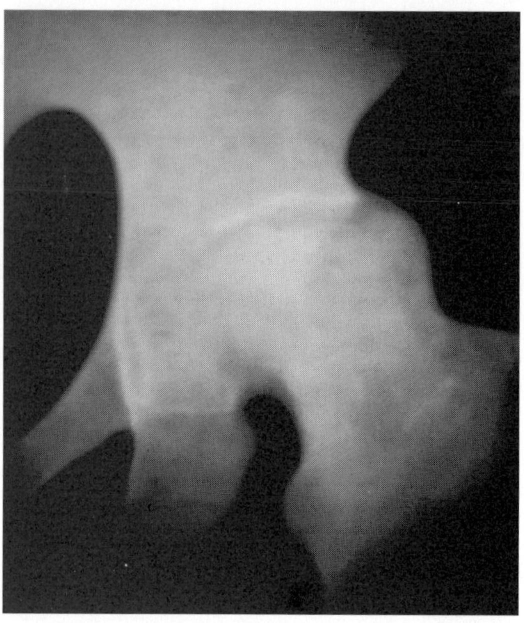

Fig. 3.1 X-ray showing advance osteonecrosis right femoral head in sickle patient

many years. Tissue at the interface between necrotic and viable bone reflects dynamic changes between repair and necrosis, the extent and rate of remodeling being influenced by many factors. These include local mechanical load, residual vascularity and metabolic factors. The subchondral portion of most osteonecrotic lesions retains the histological appearance of coagulative necrosis for months or even years. The absence of osteocyte nuclei has been used as evidence of necrosis, but this observation is of low sensitivity and specificity. Furthermore, osteocyte nuclei may persist in bone after an ischemic event.

The core biopsies that do not reach into the interface zone or the region of necrosis will show only histologically viable cancellous bone and will not be diagnostic. On the other hand the biopsies that reach the interface zone of established lesions will show deposition of new bone on the surface of necrotic trabeculae (creeping substitution). Dystrophic calcification of the fibrotic marrow may also be characteristic.

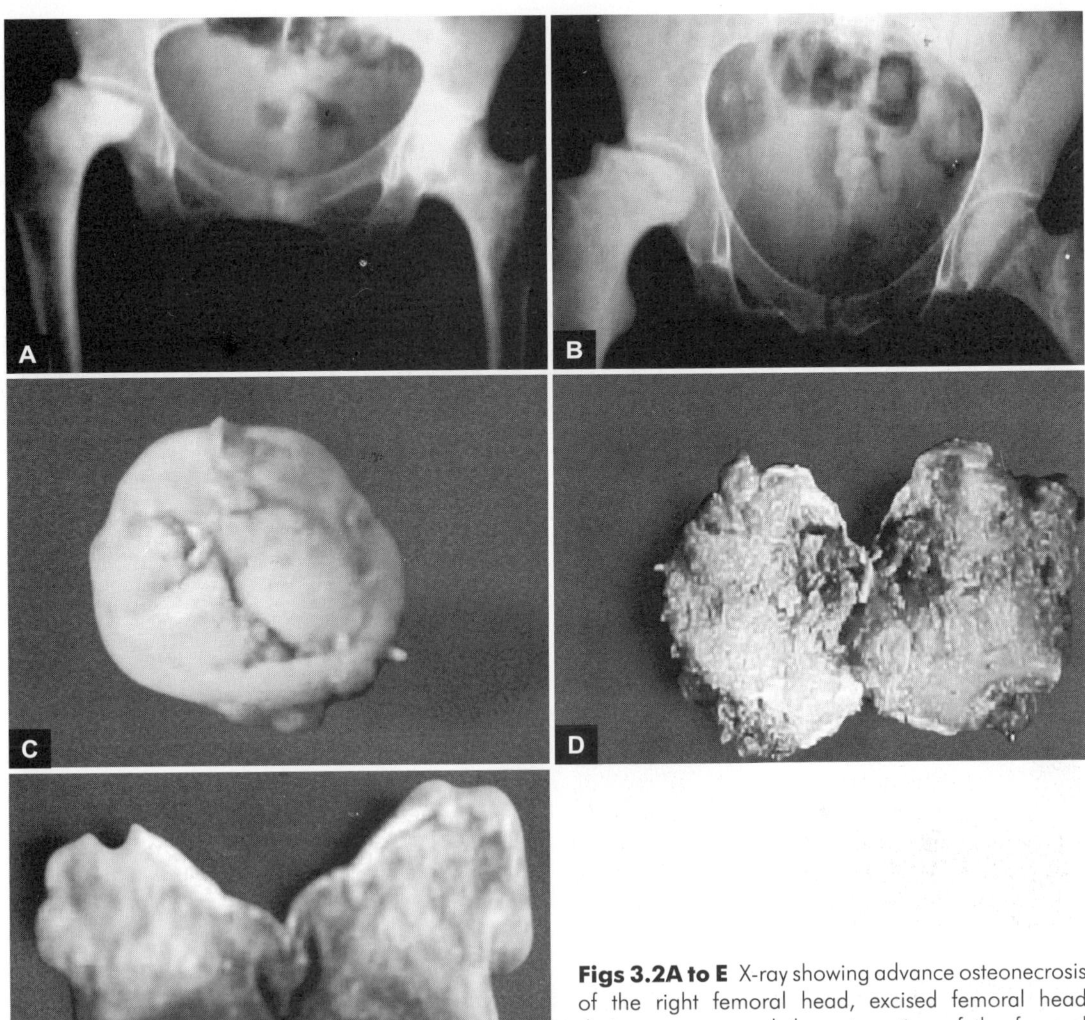

Figs 3.2A to E X-ray showing advance osteonecrosis of the right femoral head, excised femoral head during surgery, and the cut section of the femoral head which is sent for histopathology (*For color version of Figures 3.2C to E, see Plate 1*)

Histopathological Staging of Osteonecrosis

Four stages in the development of subchondral osteonecrosis have been defined morphologically, which correlates to radiographic appearances. The first stage is characterized predominantly by the presence of necrosis of both bone and bone marrow without any evidence of repair. In the second stage, reparative process is evident at the periphery of the necrotic region. The major feature of the third stage is segmental collapse of the articular surface. In the fourth stage features of secondary osteoarthritis develop. Morphological features of osteonecrosis are a composite of necrotizing and reparative processes, as observed in our biopsy study (Figs 3.6 to 3.14). Details of all stages including clinical features, macroscopic, microscopic and radiological

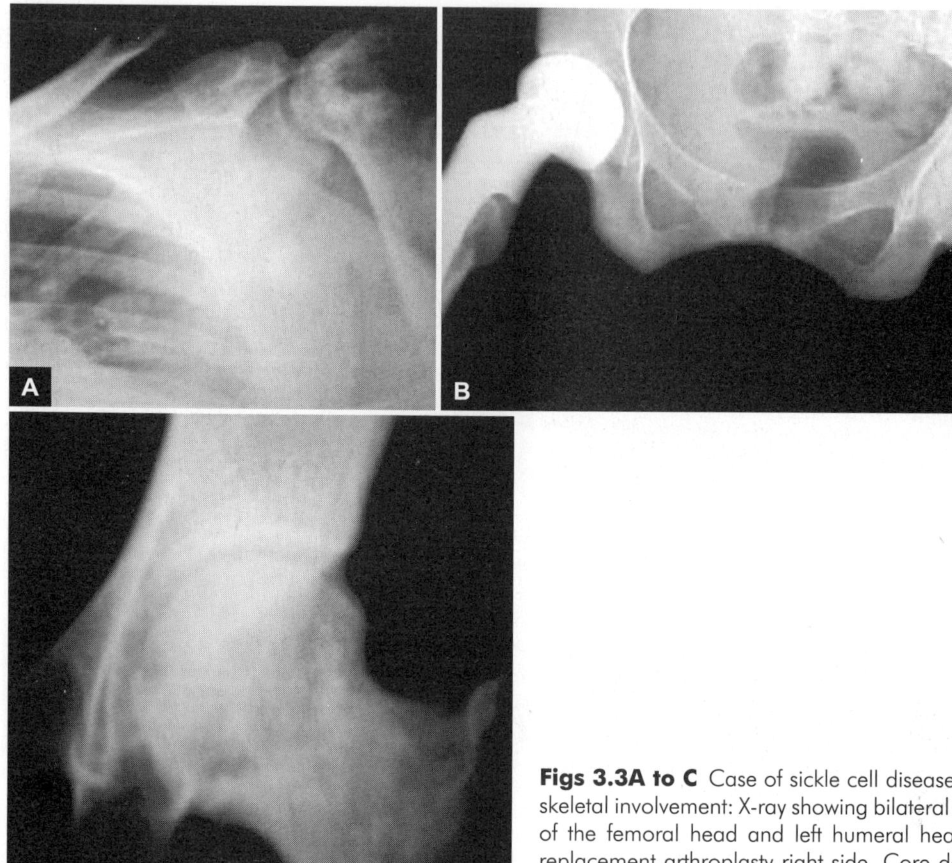

Figs 3.3A to C Case of sickle cell disease with multiple skeletal involvement: X-ray showing bilateral osteonecrosis of the femoral head and left humeral head, treated by replacement arthroplasty right side, Core decompression and free fibular graft left side and core decompression left humeral head

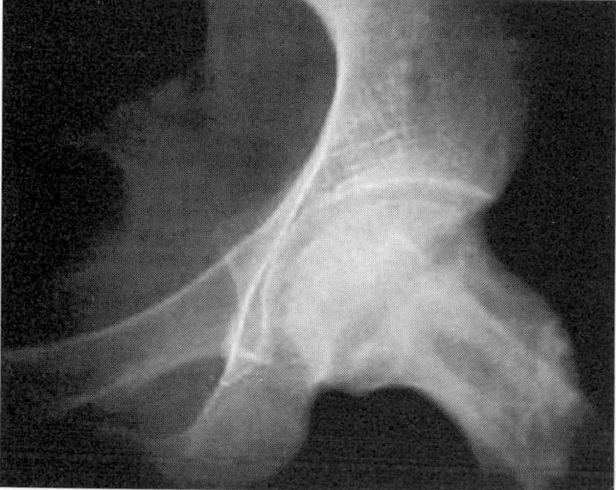

Fig. 3.4 X-ray showing osteonecrosis of the femoral head treated by core decompression and free fibular graft left side of the same patient, one year after surgery showing good vascularization

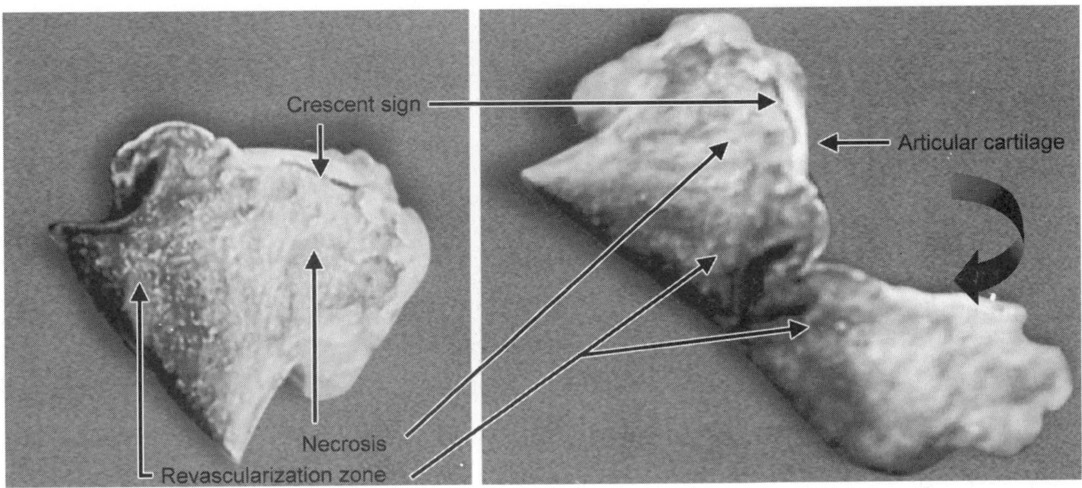

Fig. 3.5 Specimen of excised femoral head during replacement arthroplasty, showing gross appearance of the femoral head right hip *(For color version, see Plate 1)*

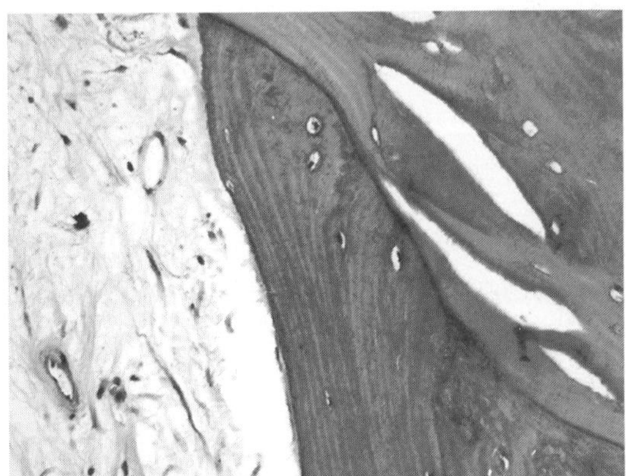

Fig. 3.6 Histopathology slide showing—Normal bone trabeculae with lacunae showing osteocytes *(For color version, see Plate 2)*

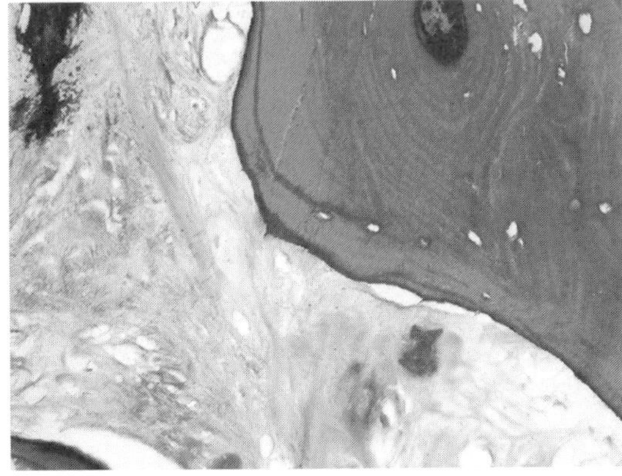

Fig. 3.7 Calcium deposit in necrotic marrow with nonviable trabeculae without osteophytes in lacunae *(For color version, see Plate 2)*

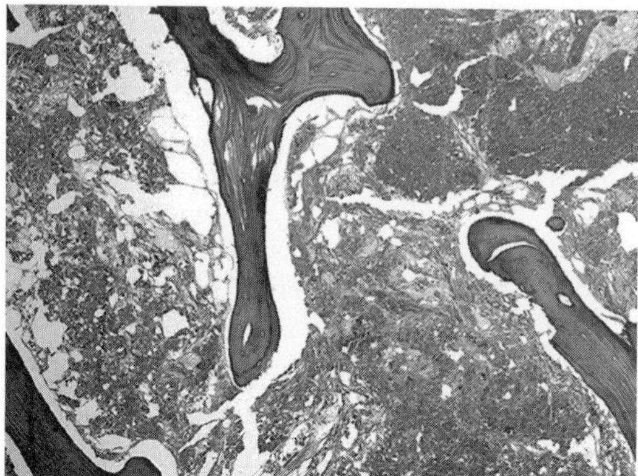

Fig. 3.8 Histopathology slide showing infarcted marrow (*For color version, see Plate 2*)

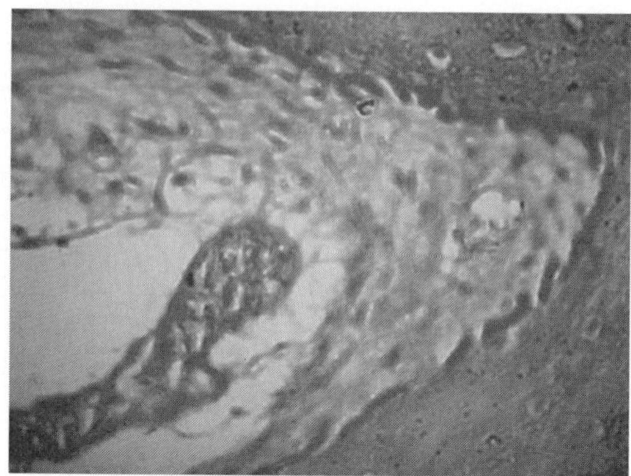

Fig. 3.11 Collagenized connective tissue at periphery (*For color version, see Plate 2*)

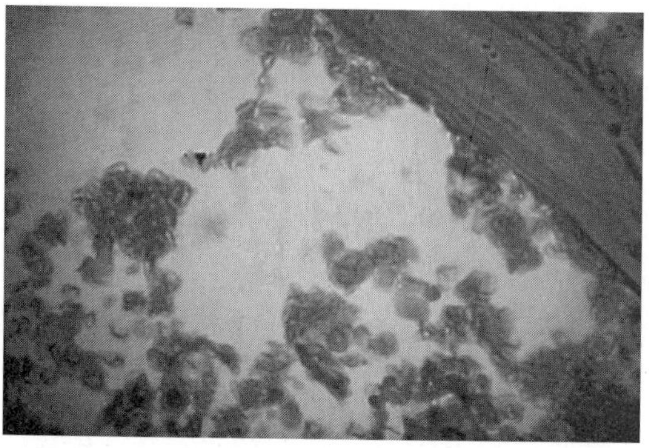

Fig. 3.9 Infarcted marrow with ghost cells in background (*For color version, see Plate 2*)

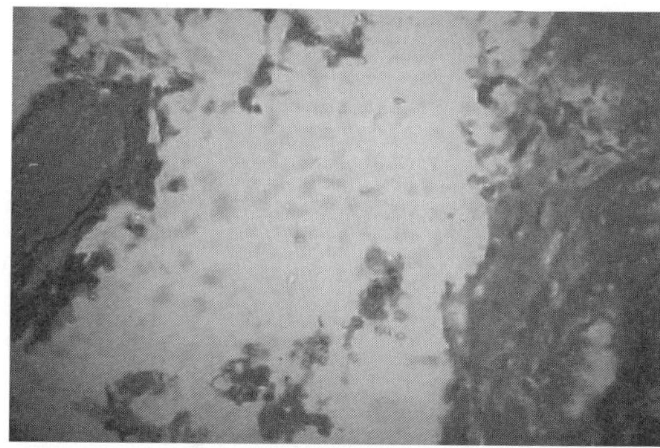

Fig. 3.12 Histopathology slide sickled RBCs with necrotic bone (*For color version, see Plate 3*)

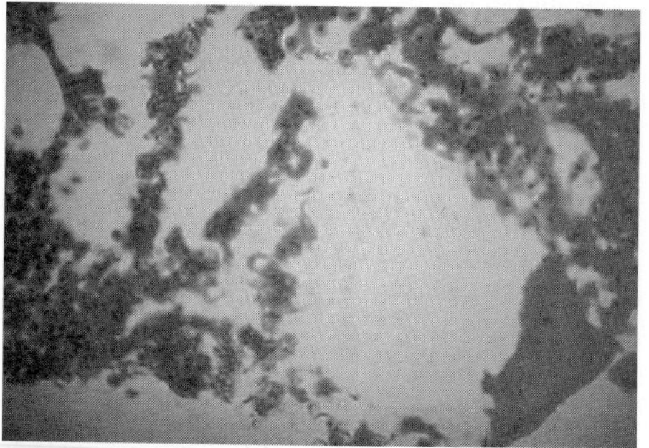

Fig. 3.10 Histopathology slide showing sickled RBCs with necrotic bone (*For color version, see Plate 2*)

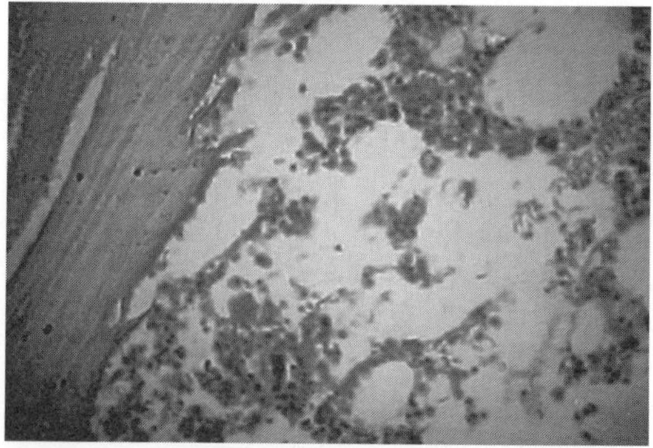

Fig. 3.13 Infarcted marrow with ghost cells in background (*For color version, see Plate 3*)

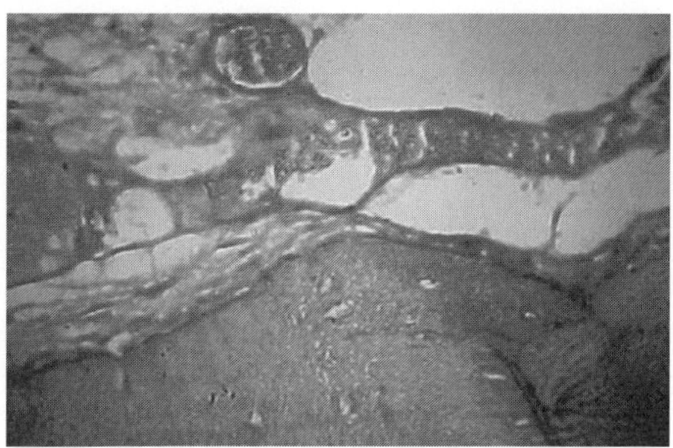

Fig. 3.14 Histopathology slide showing sickled RBC thrombus (*For color version, see Plate 3*)

appearance is described in the Table 3.2. Causes of osteonecrosis as shown in Table 3.3.

Morbid Anatomy and Histology

Four stages in the development of sub-chondral osteonecrosis have been defined morphologically. A number of studies have shown these to correlate with observed radiological changes.[10,11-17,34]

Stage I

Clinical features: Normal, No symptoms.

Macroscopic appearance: Wedge-shaped necrotic zone, marrow dull white, chalky, opaque in subarticular location. Necrotic zone surrounded by hyperemic bone.

Imaging: Normal.

Microscopic appearance

- Articular cartilage is viable. Bony end plate necrosis is seen corresponding to opaque yellow necrotic zone.
- The marrow elements are replaced by granular eosin material lodging cellular elements, cysts with lipid material.
- *In the bone:* osteocystic lacunae are empty or have a pale staining nucleus.
- At the margin of the infarct there is increased osteoclastic activity and inter-trabecular infiltration by proliferation of fibroblasts and capillaries.

Stage II

Clinical features: Occasional pain in the groin.

Macroscopic appearance: Overall shape of bone is preserved and articular surface is intact. Rim of bony sclerosis is seen at the periphery of the necrotic zone between the necrosis zone and unaffected marrow. Hyperemic zone is thicker than Stage I.

Imaging: Plain radiograph shows rim of sclerosis, increased uptake of radioactive Tc99m.

Microscopic appearance

- Advancing front of granulation tissue composed of lipid-laden macrophages, proliferating fibroblasts and capillaries seen at the periphery and extends into the central region of necrotic zone.
- Following closely behind this 'clean up' front is the second front composed of osteoblasts depositing a layer of new bone on pre-existing dead trabecular bone. Following this second front at a variable distance, a limited amount of both old dead and new living bone are removed by osteoclasts. The overall effect of these combined processes is to remove necrotic marrow, bone debris while maintaining the structural integrity of bone.

Stage III

Clinical features: Pain and limp with limited movements of the hip joint.

Macroscopic appearance: Alteration in the shape of the femoral head as a result of collapse of the necrotic region. Buckling or fragmentation of articular cartilage is seen. Fracture of trabecular bone associated with fracture of end-plate. The fracture of the trabecular bone could be because of the cumulative effect of micro-fractures within the necrotic zone induced by fatigue or weakness of trabeculae in the reparative front due to osteoclastic activity. There are focal concentration of stresses at the junction of thickened sclerotic trabeculae of reparative zone and necrotic trabeculae.

Table 3.2 Histopathological staging

Stages	Clinical features	Macroscopic appearance	Trabecular architecture on imaging	Microscopic examination
Stage I	Normal.	Wedge-shaped necrotic zone, marrow dull white, chalky, opaque in subarticular location. Necrotic zone surrounded by hyperemic bone.	Normal.	Articular cartilage viable. Bony end plate necrosis corresponding to opaque yellow necrotic zone. The marrow elements are replaced by granular eosin material lodging cellular elements, cysts with lipid material. In the bone—osteocystic lacunae are empty or have a pale staining nucleus. At the margin of the infarct there is increased osteoclastic activity and intertrabecular infiltration by proliferation fibroblasts and capillaries.
Stage II	Occasional pain in groin.	Overall shape of bone preserved and articular surface is intact. Rim of bony sclerosis is seen at the periphery of the necrotic zone between the necrosis zone and unaffected marrow. Hyperemic zone is thicker than Stage I.	X-ray showing rim of sclerosis. Increased uptake of radioactive Tc99m	Advancing front of granulation tissue composed of lipid-laden macrophages, proliferating fibroblasts and capillaries seen at the periphery and extending into the central region of necrotic zone. Following closely behind this 'clean-up' front is the second front composed of osteoblasts depositing a layer of new bone on pre-existing dead trabecular bone. Following this second front at a variable distance limited amount of both old dead and new living bone are removed by osteoclasts. The overall effect of these combined processes is to remove necrotic marrow, bone while maintaining the structural integrity of bone.

Contd...

Contd...

Stages	Clinical features	Macroscopic appearance	Trabecular architecture on imaging	Microscopic examination
Stage III	Pain and Limp with limited movements.	Alteration in the shape of the femoral head as a result of collapse of necrotic region. Buckling or fragmentation of articular cartilage. Fracture of trabecular bone associated with fracture of end plate. The fracture of trabecular bone could be because of cumulative effect of micro-fractures within the necrotic zone induced by fatigue. Weakness of trabeculae is the reparative front due to osteoclastic activity. Focal concentration of stress at the junction of thickened sclerotic trabeculae of reparative zone and necrotic trabeculae.	Apart from dense sclerosis of segmental involvement radiolucent zone is seen in the subchondral region called as "crescent sign".	Microscopically fractured trabeculae in the necrotic region appears as fragments of pulverized bony and cartilaginous detritus. The overlying cartilage may still appear viable. The fractures in the reparative zone will show abundance of fibrous tissue, cartilaginous tissue and reactive woven bone and have the appearance of ununited unstable fracture.
Stage IV	Symptoms of advanced degenerative changes gross restriction of movements with severe pain.	The initial events of necrosis, reparative process may not be very clear since most of the segment is collapsed. Articular cartilage is fragmented and disrupted. Usually there is a deep saddle shaped deformity following collapse of infarcted segmented with area of cartilaginous erosion and bony eburnation. Cut surface may show fragments of articular cartilage, dense fibrous connective tissue in the infarcted area surrounded by dense sclerotic bone.	X-ray shows collapsed femoral head with degenerative changes.	Microscopically few viable fragments of bone, necrotic bone within a layer of fibrous and cartilaginous tissue that includes granulation tissue and reactive woven bone are seen. The presence of bony and cartilaginous debris in the accompanying synovial and capsular tissue.

Table 3.3 Causes of osteonecrosis

Definite	Probable	
Major trauma fractures	Corticosteroids, high dosages	Blood clotting disorders
Dislocations	Alcohol	Pancreatitis
Caisson disease (deep sea divers)	Lipid disturbances	Kidney disease
Sickle cell disease	Connective tissue disease	Liver disease
Postirradiation	Postrenal transplant	Lupus
Chemotherapy		Smoking
Arterial disease		
Gaucher's disease		

Imaging: Apart from dense sclerosis of segmental involvement radiolucent zone is seen in the subchondral region called as crescent sign.

Microscopic appearance: Microscopically few viable fragments of bone, necrotic bone within a layer of fibrous and cartilaginous tissue that includes granulation tissue and reactive woven bone are seen. There is presence of bony and cartilaginous debris in the accompanying synovial and capsular tissue.

Stage IV

Clinical features: Symptoms of advanced degenerative changes, gross restriction of movements with severe pain.

Macroscopic appearance: The initial events of necrosis, reparative process may not be very clear since most of the segment is collapsed. Articular cartilage is fragmented and disrupted. Usually, there is deep saddle-shaped deformity following collapse of the infarcted segmented with area of cartilaginous erosion and bony eburnation. Cut surface may show fragments of articular cartilage, dense fibrous connective tissue in the infarcted area surrounded by dense sclerotic bone.

Imaging: X-ray shows collapsed femoral head with degenerative changes.

Microscopic appearance: Microscopically a few viable fragments of bone, necrotic bone within a layer of fibrous and cartilaginous tissue that includes granulation tissue and reactive woven bone are seen. The presence of bony and cartilaginous debris in the accompanying synovial and capsular tissue.

REFERENCES

1. Glimcher MJ, Kenzora JE. The biology of osteonecrosis of the human femoral head and its clinical implications: Part I. Tissue biology. Clin Orthop. 1979;138:284-309.
2. Glimcher MJ, Kenzora JE. The biology of osteonecrosis of the human femoral head and its clinical implications: Part II. The pathological changes in the femoral head as an organ and in the hip joint. Clin Orthop. 1979;139:283-312.
3. Glimcher MJ, Kenzora JE. The biology of osteonecrosis of the human femoral head and its clinical implications: Part III. Discussion of the etiology and genesis of the pathological sequelae; comments on treatment. Clin Orthop. 1979;140:273-312.
4. Mont MA, Hungerford DS. Non-traumatic avascular necrosis of the femoral head. J Bone Joint Surg. 1995;77A:459-74.
5. Kenzora JE, Steele RE, Yosipovitch ZH, et al. Experimental osteonecrosis of the femoral head in adult rabbits. Clin Orthop. 1978;130:8-46.
6. Kenzora JE, Glimcher MJ. Pathogenesis of idiopathic osteonecrosis: The ubiquitous crescent sign. Orthop Clin North Am. 1985;16:681-96.

7. Jones JP Jr, Engleman EP, Steinbach HL, et al. Fat embolization as a possible mechanism producing avascular necrosis. Arthrits Rheum. 1965;8:449.

8. Jones JP Jr, Jameson RM, Engleman EP. Alcoholism, Fat embolism, and avascular necrosis. J Bone Joint Surg Am. 1968;50A:1065.

9. Jones JP Jr. Intravascular coagulation and osteonecrosis. Clin Orthop. 1992;277:41-53.

10. Ficat RP. Idiopathic bone necrosis of the femoral head: Early diagnosis and treatment. J Bone Joint Surg Br. 1985;67B:3-9.

11. Zizic TM, Lewis C, Marcoux C, Hungerford DS, Stevens MB. Bone marrow pressure in Preclinical Ischemic Necrosis of Bone. Arthritis and Rheumatism. 1984;27(4):S66.

12. Hungerford DS, Lennox DW. The importance of increased intraosseous pressure in the development of osteonecrosis of the femoral head: Implications foor treatment. Orthop Clin North Am. 1985;16:4:635-54.

13. Bieber E, Hungerford DS. Diagnosis of Avascular Necrosis of the femoral head. Eastern Orthopaedic Association ransactions. 1985.p.25.

14. Hungerford DS, Jones LC. Diagnosis of osteonecrosis of the femoral head. In: Schoutens A, Arlet J, Gardeniers JWM, et al (Eds). Bone Circulation and Vascularisation in Normal and Pathological Conditions. New York, NY, Plenum Press; 1993.pp.265-75.

15. Jones JP Jr. Concepts of etiology and early pathogenesis of osteonecrosis. In: Schafer M (Ed). Instructional Course Lectures 43. Rosemont, IL, American Academy of Orthopaedic Surgeons; 1994.pp.499-512.

16. Jones JP Jr. Concepts of etiology and early pathogenesis of osteonecrosis. In: Schafer M (Ed). Instructional Course Lectures 43. Rosemont, IL, American Academy of Orthopaedic Surgeons; 1994.pp.500-12.

17. Roesingh GE, James J. Early phases of avascular necrosis of the femoral head in rabbits. J Bone Joint Surg Br. 1969;51B:165-76.

18. Fisher DE, Bickel WH. Corticosteroid induced avascular necrosis. A clinical study of seventy seven patients. J Bone Joint Surg Am. 1971;53A:859-73.

19. Fisher DE, Bickel WH, Holley KE, et al. Corticosteroid induced aseptic necrosis II. Experimental study. Clin Orthop. 1972;84:200-6.

20. Jaffe WL, Epstein M, Heyman N, Mankin HJ. The effect of Cortisone on femoral and Humeral head in Rabbits- An experimental study. Clin Orthop. 1972;82:221-8.

21. Cruess RL, Ross D, Crawshaw E. The etiology of steroid induced avascular necrosis of bone. A laboratory and clinical study. Clin Orthop. 1975;113:178-83.

22. Cruess RL. Osteonecrosis of bone: Currentconcepts as to etiology and pathogenesis. Clin Orthop. 1986;208:30-9.

23. Wang GJ, Sweet DE, Reger SI, et al. Fat cell changes as a mechanism of avascular necrosis of the femoral head in cortisone treated rabbits. J Bone Joint Surg Am. 1977;59A:729-35.

24. Kawai K, Tamaki A, Hirohata K. Steroid-induced accumulation of lipid in the osteocytes of the rabbit femoral head: A histochemical and electronmicroscopic study. J Bone Joint Surg Am. 1985;67A:755-63 .

25. Jones JP Jr, Sakovich L. Fat embolism of bone. A roentgenographic and histological investigations, with use of intra-arterial lipiodol, in rabbits. J Bone Joint Surg Am. 1966;68A:149-64.

26. Patterson RJ, Bickel WH, Dahlin DC. Idiopathic avascular necrosis of the head of the femur, a study of fifty-two cases. J Bone Joint Surg (Am). 1964;46A:612-33.

27. Merle d' Aubigne R, Postel M, Mazabraund A, Massias P, Gueguen J. Idiopathic necrosis of the femoral head. In adults. J Bone Joint Surg Br. 1965;47B:612-33.

28. Malka S. Surg Gynaec, Obst. 1966;123:1057.

29. Hunder GG, Warthington JW, Bickel NH. Avascular necrosis of the femoral head in a patient of Gout. JAMA. 1968;203(1):47-9.

30. Boettcher WG, Bonfigilo M, Smith K. Non-traumatic necrosis of the femoral head: II. Experiences in treatment. J Bone Joint Surg Am. 1970;52A:322-9.

31. Solomon L. Drug induced arthropathy and necrosis of femoral head. J Bone Joint Surg Br. 1973;55B:246-61.

32. Mont MA, Carbone JJ, Fairbank AC. Core decompression versus nonoperative management for osteonecrosis of the hip. Clin Orthop. 1996;324:169-78.

33. Jones JP Jr. Fat embolism and osteonecrosis. Orthop Clin North Am. 1985;16(4):595-633.

34. Bullough PG. The morbid anatomy of subchondral osteonecrosis. In Osteonecrosis: Etiology, Diagnosis and Treatment. Urbaniak JR, Jones JP Jr (Eds). American Academy of Orthopaedic Surgeons, 1st edn, 1997.

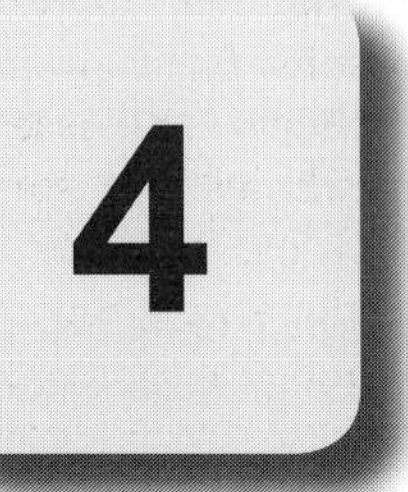

COAGULOPATHIES AND ASSOCIATED CONDITIONS CAUSING OSTEONECROSIS

Osteonecrosis is a multifactorial, heterogeneous group of disorders that lead to a common pathway of bone necrosis and mechanical failure of the femoral head. The ischemia is considered as a predominant mechanism of producing osteonecrosis. Various theories for the pathogenesis of osteonecrosis are:

1. Primary vascular abnormalities
2. Fat embolism
3. Intravascular coagulation
4. Accumulative stress theory
5. Hypertrophy of fat cells
6. Intramedullary hemorrhage.

INTRAVASCULAR COAGULATION

Intravascular coagulation of the intraosseous microcirculation consisting of capillaries and venous sinusoids progressing to generalized venous thrombosis, and less commonly retrograde arterial occlusion appears to be the genesis of osteonecrosis. Intravascular coagulation is only an intermediary event, which is triggered by some underlying risk factors.[1-4] The thrombotic threshold may be decreased in those hypercoagulable patients with hereditary thrombophilia and hyperlipidemia. Subsequent exposure to one or more additional risk factors should facilitate thrombosis and bone infarction. Decreased Protein C, Protein S or antithrombin III are some of the risk factors for osteonecrosis.

LIPID STORAGE DISORDERS

Lipid storage disorders like Gaucher's disease are associated with hyperviscocity, thrombocytopenia, and decreased factor IX and protein C.[4] Gaucher's cells are found in hepatic sinusoids, lungs and renal glomeruli. These large cells suddenly enter the circulation and cause fragmentation with intraosseous thrombosis and hemorrhage due to intravascular coagulation. Osteonecrosis may be caused by increased intraosseous from edema and hemorrhage.

SICKLE CELL HEMOGLOBINOPATHY

Osteonecrosis is commonly seen in an uncommon genetic disease, called Sickle cell disease (SCD) seen in certain communities in central India. The disease has multiple episodes of SC crisis, which produces marrow necrosis and intravascular coagulation. Bony changes occur mainly because of erythroid hyperplasia of the marrow and vascular insufficiency with infarction resulting from thrombosis.[5] There is increased blood viscocity, intraosseous stasis, capillary thrombosis and, finally infarction of the bone. There is erythrocyte sequestration with hypercoagulable state, increased platelet activation, increased thrombin generation, fibrin deposition and impaired fibrinolysis. Thrombosis results from activation of the coagulation system by a combination of fat and marrow embolism, thrombocytosis, hyper-fibrinogenemia and hyperviscocity and finally infarction of bone. The initial infarcts occur in the subchondral regions, where there is maximum sickling and where circulation through collaterals is very poor and limited. Such changes result in weakening of the trabecular structure leading to multiple micro-fractures and finally collapse in the weight-bearing portion of the femoral head and flattening.[5]

Hypercoagulability and Hyperlipedemia

Recent studies have revealed hereditary deficiencies of major natural anticoagulant mechanisms, i.e. Antithrombin III, Protein C, Protein S and resistance to activated Protein C that are associated with venous or arterial thrombosis which are labeled as primary prothrombotic states. Intravascular lipid[3,6] has been observed in histological studies of femoral heads from the patients of osteonecrosis with alcoholism and hypercortisonism. Intra-osseous arterial and venous thrombosis have been seen at the margins of osteonecrotic lesions.

Hyperlipemia and intravascular lipid may arise from fatty liver and may cause decreased intraosseous blood flow by hyperviscocity and lipid emboli resulting in osteonecrosis. Dis-ruption of fatty bone marrow or other adipose tissue is another source of fat emboli, especially seen in dysbaric phenomenon.[7] In alcoholism and hypercortisonism the lipid accumulates in subchondral osteocytes, which causes necrosis (Flow chart 4.1). Experimental studies, which were conducted by many workers, which also showed corticosteroid induced fat embolism causing avascular necrosis.[8-14] In alcoholics, there is a likelihood of the cumulative effect of alcohol consumption. The alcohol exposure threshold for associated osteonecrosis is about 150 liters of 100 percent ethanol. In alcoholics lipid emboli from fatty liver appear

to be the cause of osteonecrosis, whereas dysbaric osteonecrosis results from primary emboli or compressive effects on osseous vasculature from nitrogen bubbles. In systemic lupus erythematosis (SLE) osteonecrosis is probably because of coagulopathy. There are several risk factors in SLE—hyperlipemia, antiphospholipid antibodies, hypertension, hypercortisonism and co-existent infection.[15,16]

Osteonecrosis is characterized by necro-sis of the subchondral bone plate, associated with rapidly progressive arthropathy following collapse of the femoral head articular surface. Finally, there is joint destruction, which in initial stages may be associated with synovitis and cartilage destruction. There are areas of hypoxia in the femoral head with venous sta-sis, reduced blood flow and raised intraosseous pressure. Fibrin thrombi have been demon-strate in synovial and intraosseous venules of the femoral head. Hypercoagulability, relative hyperlipidemia and hypofibrinolysis are seen in osteonecrosis.

Thrombophilia and Hypofibrinolysis

In thrombophilia there is an increased ten-dency to develop thrombosis and in hypo-fibrinolysis there is reduced ability to dissolve the thrombi, both of which are pathogenic factors in the development of osteonecrosis. These conditions may predispose to thrombotic venous occlusion in bone, which leads to increased intramedullary pressure, anoxia, and ischemic bone death-which is characteristic of osteonecrosis (Fig. 4.1).

Thrombophilic disorders include: resis-tance to activated protein C, deficiency of protein C, and protein S. Hypofibrinolytic disorders include low stimulated plasminogen activator activity, high plasminogen activator inhibiter activity, and high lipoprotein. Intra-vascular coagulation of the intraosseous microcirculation progresses to thrombosis and arterial occlusion resulting in to osteonecrosis.

Flow chart 4.1 Mechanism of osteonecrosis

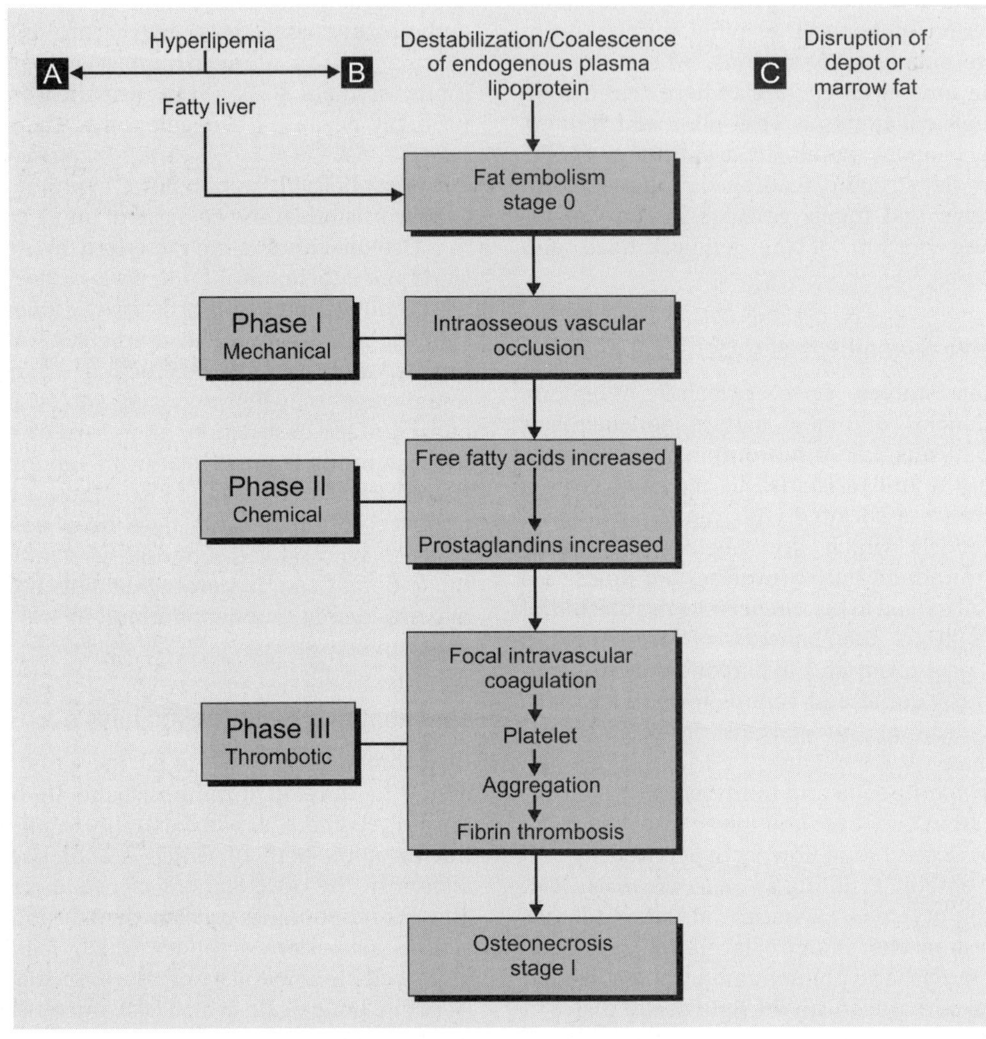

However, intravascular coagulation is only an intermediate event, which is triggered by some underlying etiologic risk factor. It is postulated that thrombophilia and hypofibrinolysis may lead to osteonecrosis via the same pathways.

◼ REFERENCES

1. Jones JP Jr. Intravascular coagulation and osteonecrosis. Clin Orthop. 1992;277:41-53.
2. Bick RL. Disseminated intravascular coagulation: objective laboratory diagnostic criteria and guidelines for management. Clin Lab Med. 1994;14:729-68.
3. Jones JP Jr. Concepts of etiology and early pathogenesis of osteonecrosis. In: Schafer M (Ed). Instructional Course Lectures 43. Rosemont, IL, American Academy of Orthopaedic Surgeons; 1994.pp.499-512.
4. Jones JP Jr. Osteonecrosis. In: Koopman WJ (Ed). Arthritis and allied conditions: A text book of Rheumatology, 13th edn. Baltimore, MD, Williams & Wilkins. 1977.pp.1923-42.

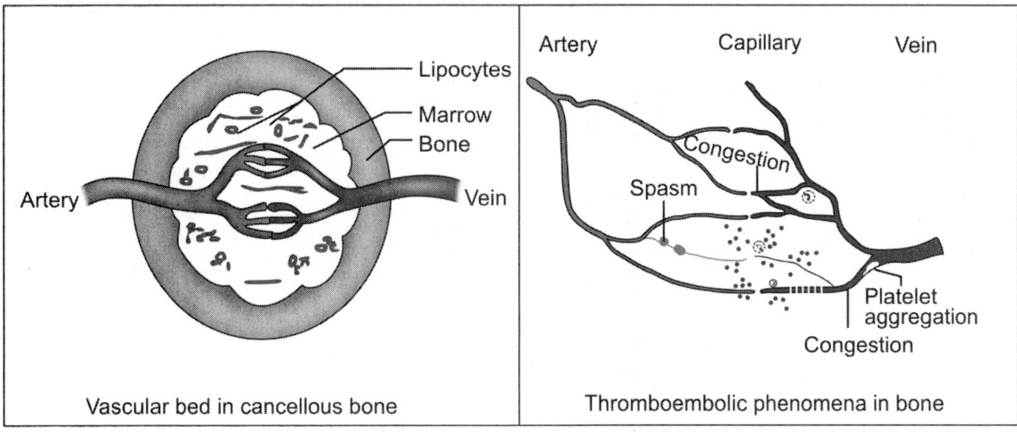

Fig. 4.1 Pathogenesis of osteonecrosis

5. Babhulkar Sudhir. Orthopaedic manifestations and bone changes in sickle cell haemoglobinopathy. Monogram by CBS Publishers; 1997.pp.15-23.

6. Jones JP Jr. Fat Embolism, intravascular coagulation, and osteonecrosis. Clin Orthop. 1993;292:294-308.

7. Jones JP Jr, Ramirez S, Doty SB. Pathophysiologic role of fat in dysbaric osteonecrosis. Clin Orthop. 1993;296:256-64.

8. Fisher DE, Bickel WH. Corticosteroid induced avascular necrosis. A clinical study of seventy-seven patients. J Bone Joint Surg Am. 1971;53A:859-73.

9. Fisher DE, Bickel WH, Holley KE, et al. Corticosteroid induced aseptic necrosis II. Experimental study. Clin Orthop. 1972;84:200-6.

10. Jaffe WL, Epstein M, Heyman N, Mankin HJ. The effect of Cortisone on femoral and Humeral head in Rabbits—an experimental study. Clin Orthop. 1972;82:221-8.

11. Cruess RL, Ross D, Crawshaw E. The etiology of steroid induced avascular necrosis of bone. A laboratory and clinical study. Clin Orthop. 1975;113:178-83.

12. Cruess RL. Osteonecrosis of bone: Current concepts as to etiology and pathogenesis. Clin Orthop. 1986;208:30-9.

13. Wang GJ, Sweet DE, Reger SI, et al. Fat cell changes as a mechanism of avascular necrosis of the femoral head in cortisone treated rabbits. J Bone Joint Surg Am. 1977;59A:729-35.

14. Kawai K, Tamaki A, Hirohata K. Steroid-induced accumulation of lipid in the osteocytes of the rabbit femoral head: a histochemical and electronmicroscopic study. J Bone Joint Surg Am. 1985;67A:755-63.

15. Ono K, Tohjima T, Komazawa T. Risk factors of avascular necrosis of the femoral head in patients with systemic lupus erythmatosus under high dose of corticosteroid therapy. Clin Orthop. 1992;277:89-97.

16. Shimamato Y, Suga K, Ohta A, et al. Risk factors for the development acute disseminated intravascualar coagulation with systemic lupus erythmatosus. Clin Rheumatol. 1995;14:176-9.

17. Jones JP Jr. Risk factors potentially activating intravascular coagulation and causing non-traumatic osteonecrosis. In: Osteonecrosis: Etiology, Diagnosis and Treatment. Urbaniak JR, Jones JP Jr (Eds); American Academy of Orthopaedic Surgeons, 1st edn. 1997. pp.89-96.

5

CLASSIFICATION: STAGING OF OSTEONECROSIS

Broadly two types of Osteonecrosis are recognised: Traumatic and Nontraumatic.

Traumatic Osteonecrosis

Osteonecrosis can occur in a bone with vulnerable vascular supply with or without associated risk factors. The incidence of traumatic osteonecrosis is known to vary with the location and severity of injury, type and timing of treatment and associated injuries.[1-3] Although the hip is the most common anatomic location for traumatic osteonecrosis after fracture neck femur or dislocation (Figs 5.1 and 5.2), other vulnerable sites include the scaphoid, talus and the proximal humerus.

Nontraumatic Osteonecrosis

This is usually a disease of the young people. In our series we had patients from the age of 4 onwards till the age of 60 years, and in children's it is not infrequently seen (Figs 5.3A and B). The average age of patients in a large series was found to be 38 years, with only 20 percent of patients being older than 50 years of age.[4] In another study, the mean age was reported to be 34 years. [5]

FACTORS ASSOCIATED WITH HIGH RISK

Nontraumatic osteonecrosis is usually associated with one or more risk factors. Approximately two-thirds of these are is related to alcohol abuse and corticosteroid intake.[4] The remaining one-third are associated with diverse conditions like decompression sickness, Sickle cell hemoglobinopathy, storage disorders like Gaucher's disease, pregnancy and coagulopathies. Other groups of patients prone to

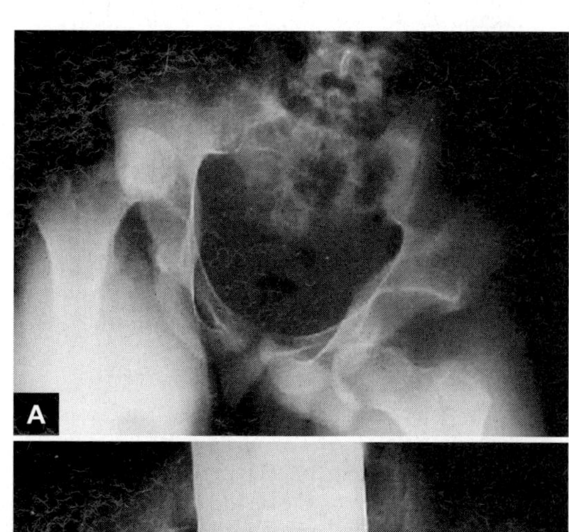

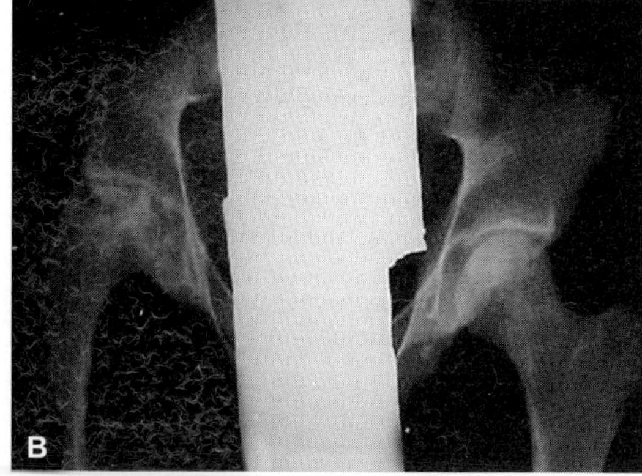

Figs 5.1A and B X-ray showing traumatic osteonecrosis after hip dislocation

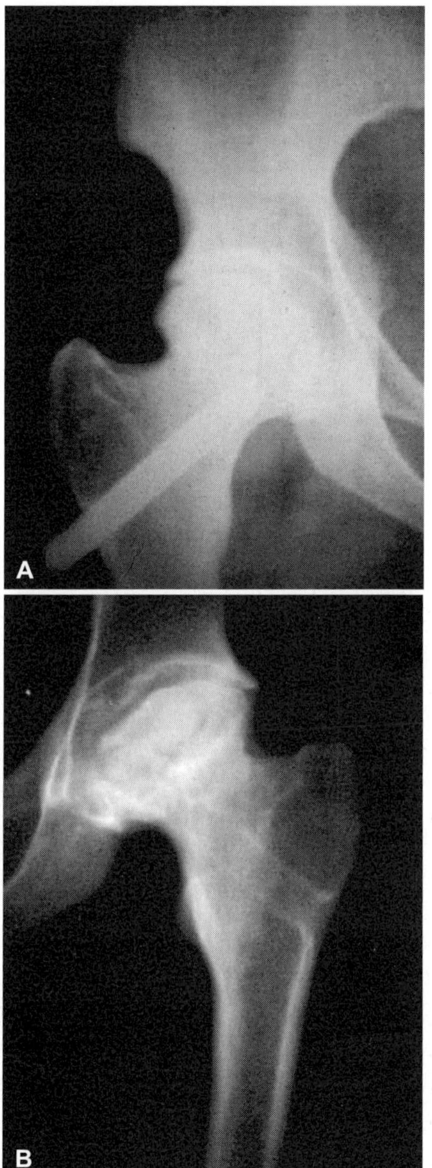

Figs 5.2A and B X-ray showing traumatic osteo-necrosis after fracture neck femur

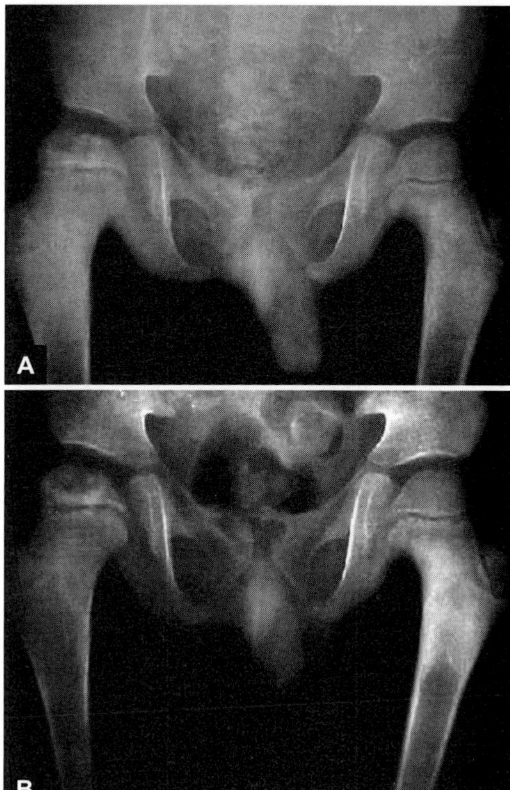

Figs 5.3A and B X-ray showing nontraumatic osteonecrosis in a 6-year-old child with Gaucher's disease

develop osteonecrosis include organ transplant recipients, and those with inflammatory bowel disease, and lupus erythematosus.[5]

Over the years a number of different systems of classification of osteonecrosis have been described. It is extremely difficult to compare the effectiveness of the different methods of treatment since there is no uniformity and effective method of classification and staging. Staging of the disease process is based on the natural progression of the untreated disease. In the majority of such systems, the progressive stages are identified in order to furnish guidelines for treatment designed to reverse or halt the progression of the disease. Various classification systems are discussed in detail.

Depending upon the presentation and radiographic appearance the osteonecrosis, has been classified by *Ficat and Arlet[6,7] in to:

Osseous Form (Classic Necrosis)

In this type, changes begin in the femoral head first and the hip joint is involved in later stages, after flattening and collapse of the head. Articular surface changes are seen only in advanced stages during the progress of osteonecrosis.

Osteochondral Form (Ischemic Coxopathy)

The joint space involvement begins with onset of disease in this form. The bone necrosis hides behind a mask of nonspecific bone changes and is interpreted as a secondary reaction to arthrosis. It looks similar to either early coxarthrosis or rheumatoid synovitis. The necrotic component is evident in some cases with terminal evolution towards sequestrum formation.

Depending upon the radiographic picture –osteonecrosis is also classified into:

A. Partial head type (Dissecans type): Non-progressive
B. Whole head affection (Perthes type): Advanced changes.

A. ***Affection of immature femoral head:***
   - Flattening
   - Epiphysio-metaphyseal overlap
   - Wide femoral neck
   - Upward progress of the lateral part of the femoral head
   - Medullary changes in infants

B. ***Affection of mature femoral head:***
   - Segmental involvement
   - Collapse of femoral head
   - Disruption of femoral head
   - Secondary arthritic changes

Various classifications proposed by different workers are described in detail:

- Neel Marcus et al.[8] (1973)—Florida system
- Steinberg et al.[9,10] (1984)—Philadelphia (Pennsylvania) system
- Ficat and Arlet[11] (1985)—French system
- ARCO Classification[12] (1991, 93)—Gardeniers

1. ***Marcus and Enneking's System[8]***

Stage	X-ray findings
I	Subtle mottled densities, scattered
II	Rim of increased density—peripheral infarct
III	Subtle flattening, radiolucent fracture line, subchondral bone
IV	Flattened femoral head, distinct step-off at the lateral margin
V	Increased asymmetry of the flattened dense femoral dome with narrowing of the acetabular cartilage
VI	Severe osteoarthritic changes, loss of evidence of initiating infarct

2. ***Steinberg's Classification[9,10]***

Stage	X-ray findings	MRI	CT
0	Normal roentgenogram, normal bone scan	+	+/-
I	Normal roentgenogram, abnormal bone scan	+	+/-
II	Sclerosis or cyst formation in the femoral head	+	+
III	Subchondral collapse (crescent sign) without flattening	+	+
IV	Flattening of head with joint narrowing or acetabular involvement	+	+
V	Flattening of head with joint narrowing and acetabular involvement	+	+
VI	Advanced degenerative changes in the hip joint	+	+

3. ***Japanese Investigation Committee's Classification***

Stage	X-ray findings
I	Pre-roentegenographic stage, only detectable by bone scintigraphy, MRI or core biopsy
II	Early stage, necrosis with or without less than 2 mm of collapse
III	Advanced stage, more than 2 mm of collapse
IV	Late stage, advanced stage associated with osteoarthritic changes

4. ***Ficat and Arlet Classification (1985)[11]***

Stage	Symptoms	Radiology (Bone Scan)	Pathological findings	Biopsy
0	None	None	-	-
I	None/ mild	Normal/cold spot-femoral head	Infarction of weight-bearing portion	Abundant dead marrow cells, osteoblasts and osteogenic cells
II	Mild	Density changes in femoral head/uptake positive	Spontaneous repair of infarcted area	New bone deposited between necrotic trabeculae
IIA		Sclerotic or cysts, Normal joint line, Normal head contour		
IIB		Osteoporosis/Sclerosis		
III	Mild to moderate	Loss of sphericity, flattening, collapse uptake +	Subchondral fracture, Collapse fragmentation of necrotic segment	Dead bone marrow and trabeculae around fracture
IV	Moderate to severe	Joint space narrowing, acetabular changes/ uptake +	Osteoarthritic changes	Degenerative changes in acetabulum

5. *Association Research Circulation Osseous Classification*

Finding	0	1	2	3	4
Finding	All present techniques normal or non-diagnostic	X-ray and CT are normal. At least One of the below is positive	No crescent sign: X-ray abnormal: Sclerosis, lysis, focal porosis	Crescent sign on the X-ray and/or flattening of articular surface of femoral head	Osteoarthritis joint space narrowing, acetabular changes, joint destruction
Finding	X-ray, CT, Scintigraph, MRI	Scintigraph, MRI, Quantitate on MRI	X-ray, CT, Scintigraph MRI, Quantitate MRI and X-ray	X-ray, CT only * Quantitate on X-ray	X-ray only
Finding	No	Medial	Central	Lateral	No
Finding	No	% Area Involvement Minimal A<15% Moderate B 15-30% Extensive C>30%	Quantitation Length of crescent A < 2 mm B 2-4 mm C > 4 mm	% Surface collapse dome depression A<15% B – 15-30% C> 30%	No

The Association Research Circulation Osseous (ARCO) has proposed a new international classification system including radiographs, computed tomography (CT), bone scans, and MRI. This classification system incorporates the Pennsylvania system based on lesion size and the Japanese system based on lesion location. Quantitation (% area involvement of femoral head, length of crescent sign, % surface collapse, and dome depression) and location of the lesion (medial, central or lateral) represent important prognostic factors. This ARCO classification has been proposed as the preferred system for the future; therefore, it will be used in this article.[12]

ARCO Osteonecrosis Classification—clinical, radiologic, and morphologic correlation (Histological) described below:

6. ***ARCO Classification (Histological)***

Findings	ARCO stage (Histological phase)				
	0(I)	I (II)	2 (III)	3 (IV)	4 (V)
Clinical	Normally no pain	Normally no pain	May have pain	Pain	Pain
Radiograph	Normal	Normal	Mottled and sclerotic rim	Crescent sign and/or flattening	Collapse
CT*	Normal	Normal	Mottled and sclerotic rim	Subchondral fracture	Collapse
Bone scan	Normal	Cold spot	Cold in hot spot	Cold in hotspot	Hot in hot spot
MRI*	Normal	Necrotic area and reactive interface	Necrotic area and reactive interface	Crescent sign	Collapse
Histology	Plasmostasis and marrow necrosis	Bone necrosis and inflammatory response	Reactive interface repair	Resorption and subchondral fracture	Flattening and cartilage destruction

The "General Assembly of ARCO" in Basel, Switzerland accepted the new classification in December 1991 as a "Proposal for an International Classification".

The Committee suggests strongly that the minimum requirements for reporting results on clinical and scientific work must include the following:

1. A clinical quantitation by means of any hip score rating, e.g. the Harris hip score
2. Staging according to this 'International Classification', in which the classification is meant to be minimum requirement.
3. Radiological and MRI quantitation to be reported separately from the clinical quantitation.
4. Therapeutic results on survival of the femoral head.

Histology should be done at every possible opportunity. It remains the 'Golden Standard'. although it is an invasive method, because it is also a curative procedure. A descriptive histological classification of the disease is not yet available and for the time being a "Simple Descriptive Histological Classification" was designed as a working scheme.

The silent hip: The difficulty in estimating the prevalence of osteonecrosis arises because the condition is asymptomatic in the early stages. The term 'Silent Hip' is applied to the asymptomatic hip in patients who present for the management of the contralateral painful hip. The reported incidence of bilaterality ranges from 6 to 72 percent.[13-15] Despite a high incidence of bilaterality only about 15 percent of patients report bilateral symptoms on initial presentation.[15]

■ REFERENCES

1. Herndon JH, Aufranc OE. Avascular necrosis of the femoral head in the adult. A review of its incidence in a variety of conditions. Clin Orthop. 1972;86:43-62.
2. Hougaard K, Thomsen PB. Traumatic posterior dislocation of the hip: prognostic factors influencing the incidence of avascular necrosis of the femoral head. Acta Orthop Traumat Surg. 1986;106:32-5.

3. Kruczynski J. Avascular necrosis of the proximal femur in developmental dislocation of the hip: Incidence, risk factors, sequlae and MR imaging for the diagnosis and prognosis. Acta Orthop Scand. 1996;268(suppl):1-48.

4. Mont MA, Hungerford DS. Non-traumatic avascular necrosis of the femoral head. J Bone Joint Surg Am. 1995;77A:459-74.

5. Jones JP Jr. Risk factors potentially activating intravascular coagulation and causing non-traumatic osteonecrosis. In: Osteonecrosis: Etiology, Diagnosis and Treatment. Urbaniak JR, Jones JP Jr (Eds); American Academy of Orthopaedic Surgeons, 1st edn; 1997.pp.89-96.

6. Ficat RP, Arlet J (Eds). Ischemie et Necrosis osseuses, Paris, France, Masson;1977.pp.224.

7. Ficat RP, Arlet J, Hungerford DS (Eds). Ischaemia and Necrosis of Bone. Baltimore, MD, Williams & Wilkins;1980.pp.53-74.

8. Marcus ND, Enneking WF, Massam RA. The silent hip in idiopathic aseptic necrosis: treatment by bone grafting. J Bone Joint Surg (Am). 1973;55A:1351-66.

9. Steinberg ME, Hayken GD, Steinberg DR. A new method for evaluation and staging of avascular necrosis of the femoral head in Arlet J, Ficat RP, & Hungerford DS (Eds): Bone Circulation. Baltimore, MD, Williams & Wilkins;1984.pp. 398-403.

10. Steinberg ME, Hayken GD, Steinberg DR. A quantitative system for staging avascular necrosis. J Bone Joint Surg Br. 1995;77B:34-41.

11. Ficat RP. Idiopathic bone necrosis of the femoral head: Early diagnosis and treatment. J Bone Joint Surg Br. 1985;67B:3-9.

12. Gardeniers JWM. ARCO international classification of osteonecrosis. ARCO News. 1993; 5:79-82.

13. Bradway JK, Morrey BF. The natural history of the silent hip in bilateral atraumatic osteonecrosis. J Arthroplasty. 1993;8:383-7.

14. Hungerford DS, Jones LC. Diagnosis of osteonecrosis of the femoral head. In: Schoutens A, Arlet J, Gardeniers JWM, et al (Eds): Bone Circulation and Vascularisation in Normal and Pathological Conditions. New York, NY, Plenum Press; 1993.pp.265-75.

15. Kozinn SC, Wilson PD Jr. Adult hip diseae and total hip replacement. Clin Symp. 1997;39: 1-32.

6

EARLY DIAGNOSIS

In the earliest stage of the disease, X-rays appear normal and the diagnosis is made using isotope bone scan or MRI.[1-5] Once it is seen on X-ray, it is not actually the dead bone that can be seen but the healing response of the living bone to the area of the dead necrotic bone. The advanced stages of osteonecrosis begin when the dead bone starts to fail mechanically through a process of microfractures of the bone. Eventually, this will result in further damage to the femoral head and other side of the joint, requiring major joint reconstruction.[6-10]

The natural history of osteonecrosis of the femoral head before the development of the crescent sign or before the collapse of the femoral head has never been well defined.[11,12] The possibility of progression to collapse is thought to be increased after the development of an abnormality that can be seen on plain radiograph and such a possibility and the course of collapse may be highly variable and unknown. Hence, early diagnosis is important prior to the appearance of radiological changes.[1,13] Early diagnosis leads to a better outcome. A high index of suspicion is essential. Pain deep in the groin is the most common symptom and signs can be unremarkable. However, pain signs could be like pain with flexion and internal rotation, antalgic gate, decreased range of movement and clicking in the hip at later stages when the fragment is collapsed. Complaints of groin or hip pain in a patient with a known predisposing cause for avascular necrosis should arouse a suspicion and must be thoroughly investigated. All these patients have positive clinical signs highly suggestive of osteonecrosis of the femoral head. Loss of internal rotation of the hip and positive axis deviation test is one such finding, which is highly suspicious of osteonecrosis. Whenever there is sectoral involvement of the femoral head, axis deviation test is positive.[4,5] Normally, if the hip is flexed more than 90 degree with flexed knee, the knee and patella faces towards the opposite shoulder, whereas if it faces the same axilla or shoulder, it should be considered as positive axis deviation test. Whenever the test is positive in the patients with loss of internal rotation, they should be investigated by X-rays, bone scan and MRI to confirm the diagnosis.[1-10,14-22]

Presently MRI, and isotope bone scans (rarely CT scan) have replaced the invasive procedure of functional bone investigations. Similarly, in a patient of osteonecrosis of the femoral head, the opposite hip is regarded as high-risk and close watch is kept on such a patient for at least a year or two. MRI and bone scanning are of great value if the X-rays are negative in patients with a high index of suspicion for osteonecrosis of the femoral head. All the investigations are unnecessary if the X-rays are positive (Figs 6.1 and 6.2). Although X-ray examination is of limited value in making early diagnosis, it has considerable value in staging.[1,3,23-26] Once any deformity appears in the subchondral plate or early collapse of the femoral head is evident radiologically, the prognosis is poor. Bone scan studies are done in 'high-risk patients' when hip symptomatology

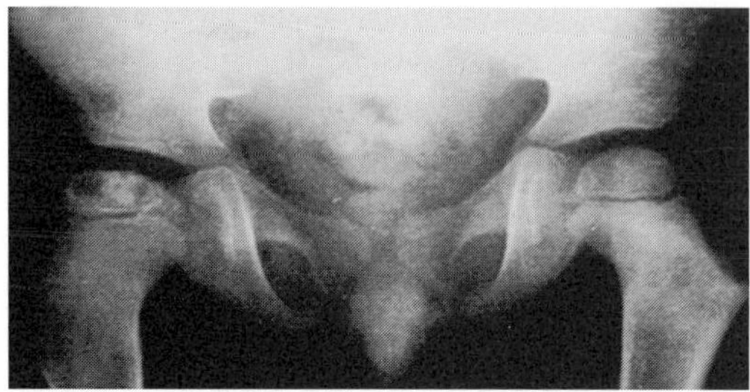

Fig. 6.1 X-ray of young child of 5 years with changes of osteonecrosis similar to Perthe's disease in a case of sickle cell disease

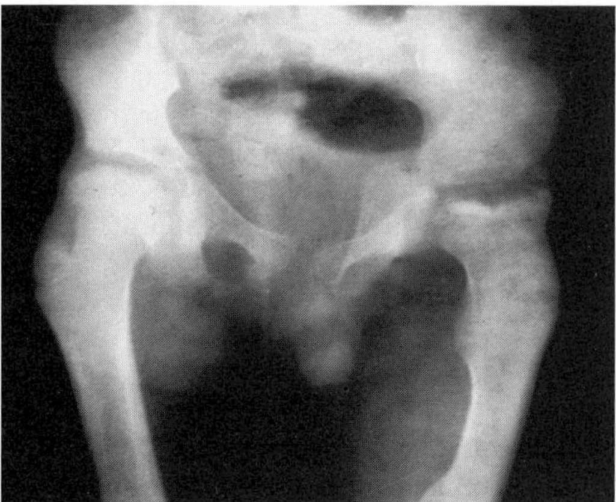

Fig. 6.2 X-ray of another young child of 4 years with changes of osteonecrosis similar to Perthe's disease in a case of sickle cell disease

is associated with conditions commonly seen in association with osteonecrosis like, sickle cell disease, corticosteroid consumption, alcohol abuse, lupus erythmatosus, hepato-renal disorders and so on, routinely and subsequently at regular intervals. If suspicion is very high even with negative bone scan, core decompression and biopsy used to be a routined procedure but with the availability of MRI, we now closely observe these patients and avoid invasive procedure.[27] Commonly, the patients present after radiographic changes are seen and at times with advanced osteoarthritic changes. If the deformity occurs because of involvement of the subchondral bone or even early collapse of supportive cancellous bone,

which is evident radiologically, the prognosis is very poor.

The success of the treatment of osteonecrosis is related to the stage at which the treatment is initiated. Description of the methods used to make an accurate diagnosis early in the disease process are (diagnostic modalities currently available):[1-10,28]

- Radiography
- Scintigraphy
- Functional bone investigations (FBI)
- Magnetic resonance imaging (MRI)
- Computed tomography (CT)
- Histopathology.

History and Clinical Examination

- Pain
- Painful range of movements, especially on forced internal rotation
- Positive axis deviation test
- History of associated risk factor
- High index of suspicion.

The contralateral hip in a patient of unilateral osteonecrosis must be carefully evaluated since the bilateral prevalence is reported to be 50 to 80 percent.[12,28,29]

Investigations

- Radiographic evaluation
- Diagnostic criteria.

The diagnosis of osteonecrosis should be considered as established if any of the following are found:[29,30]

- Pathognomonic radiographic changes (collapse of the femoral head, anterolateral sequestration, crescent sign[30,31]).
- A double line on T2-weighted MRI.
- Increased uptake surrounding a photo-penic area of bone scan (cold in hot).
- Positive finding on bone biopsy showing empty lacunae involving multiple adjacent trabeculae.

In the more advanced stages of the disease and/or when more of the joint is damaged, it is less likely that the natural joint can be preserved. Fortunately, joint replacement procedures today are highly successful, even in the relatively young patients affected by osteonecrosis. It is always the physician's desire to preserve the normal joint whenever possible. Unfortunately many patients do not visit the orthopedic surgeon until their joint is at an advanced stage of the disease.

REFERENCES

1. Ficat RP. Idiopathic bone necrosis of the femoral head: Early diagnosis and treatment. J Bone Joint Surg Br. 1985;67B:3-9.
2. Arlet J. Nontraumatic avascular necrosis of the femoral head: Past, present and future. Clin Orthop. 1992;277:12-21.
3. Marcus ND, Enneking WF, Massam RA. The silent hip in idiopathic aseptic necrosis: treatment by bone grafting. J Bone Joint Surg (Am). 1973;55-A:1351-66.
4. Babhulkar SS. Osteonecrosis of the femoral head (in young individuals) Indian Journal of Orthopaedics. 2003;37(2):77-86.
5. Babhulkar SS. Osteonecrosis of the femoral head: Treatment by Core decompression and vascular pedicle grafting, Indian Journal of Orthopaedics. 2009;43(1):27-35.
6. Glimcher MJ, Kenzora JE. The biology of osteonecrosis of the human femoral head and its clinical implications: Part I. Tissue biology. Clin Orthop. 1979;138:284-309.
7. Glimcher MJ, Kenzora JE. The biology of osteonecrosis of the human femoral head and its clinical implications: Part II. The pathological changes in the femoral head as an organ and in the hip joint. Clin Orthop. 1979;139:283-312.
8. Glimcher MJ, Kenzora JE. The biology of osteonecrosis of the human femoral head and its clinical implications: Part III. Discussion of the etiology and genesis of the pathological sequelae; comments on treatment. Clin Orthop. 1979;140:273-312.
9. Hungerford DS, Jones LC. Diagnosis of osteonecrosis of the femoral head. In Schoutens A, Arlet J , Gardeniers JWM, et al (Eds): Bone Circulation and Vascularisation in Normal and Pathological Conditions. New York, NY, Plenum Press. 1993.pp.265-75.
10. Boettcher WG, Bonfigilo M, Smith K. Non-traumatic necrosis of the femoral head: II. Experiences in treatment. J Bone Joint Surg Am. 1970;52A:322-9.
11. Ohzono K, Saito M, Takaoka K, Ono K, Saito S, Nishina T, Kadowaki T. Natural history of atraumatic avascular necrosis of the femoral head. J Bone Joint Surg Br. 1991;73:68-72.
12. Bradway JK, Morrey BF. The natural history of the silent hip in bilateral atraumatic osteonecrosis. J Arthroplasty. 1993;8:383-7.
13. Ficat P, Arlet J, Hungerford DS (Eds). Ischaemia and Necrosis of Bone. Baltimore, MD, Williams and Wilkins, 1980.
14. May DA, Disler DG. Screening for avascular necrosis of the hip with rapid MRI: preliminary experience. J Comput Assist Tomogr. 2000; 24:284-7.
15. Kramer J, Hofmann S, Imhof H. The non-traumatic femur head necrosis in the adult: II. Radiologic diagnosis and staging. Radiologe. 1994;34:11-20.
16. Lang P, Genant HK, Jergesen HE, et al. Imaging of the hip joint: Computed tomography versus magnetic resonance imaging. Clin Orthop. 1992;274:135-53.
17. Mitchell DG, Steinberg ME, Dalinka MK, et al. Magnetic resonance imaging of the ischaemic hip: Alterations within the osteonecrotic, viable, and reactive zone. Clin Orthop. 1989;244: 60-77.
18. Mitchell MD, Kundel HL, Steinberg ME, Kressel HY, Alavi A, Axel L. Avascular necrosis of the hip: comparison of MR, CT, and scintigraphy. AJR. Am J Roentgenol. 1986;147:67-71.
19. Mitchell DG, Rao VM, Dalinka MK, Spritzer CE, Alavi A, Steinberg ME,Fallon M, Kressel HY. Femoral head avascular necrosis: correlation of MRI, radiographic staging, radionuclide imaging, and clinical findings. Radiology. 1987; 162:709-15.
20. Coleman BG, Kressel HY, Dalinka MK, Scheibler ML, Burk DL, Cohen EK. Radiographically negative avascular necrosis: detection with MR imaging. Radiology. 1988;168:525-8.
21. Mitchell DG, Steinberg ME, Dalinka MK, et al. Magnetic resonance imaging of the ischaemic hip: Alterations within the osteonecrotic, viable, and reactive zone. Clin Orthop. 1989;244:60-77.
22. Koo KH, Kim R. Quantifying the extent of osteonecrosis of the femoral head: A new method using MRI, J Bone Joint Surg Br. 1995;77B:875-80.
23. Steinberg ME, Hayken GD, Steinberg DR. A new method for evaluation and staging of avascular necrosis of the femoral head in Arlet J, Ficat RP, and Hungerford DS (Eds): Bone Circulation.

Baltimore, MD, Williams and Wilkins; 1984.pp. 398-403.

24. Steinberg ME, Hayken GD, Steinberg DR. A quantitative system for staging avascular necrosis. J Bone Joint Surg Br. 1995;77B:34-41.

25. Ficat RP. Idiopathic bone necrosis of the femoral head: Early diagnosis and treatment. J Bone Joint Surg Br. 1985;67B:3-9.

26. Steinberg ME, Brighton CT, Steinberg DR, Tooze SE, Hayken GD. Treatment of avascular necrosis of the femoral head by a combination of bone grafting, decompression, and electrical stimulation. Clin. Orthop. 1984;186:137-53.

27. Takatori Y, Kokubo T, Ninomiya S, Nakamura S, Morimoto S, Kusaba I. Avascular necrosis of the femoral head. Natural history and magnetic resonance imaging. J Bone and Joint Surg Br. 1993;75B(2):217-21.

28. Hungerford DS, Jones LC. Diagnosis of osteonecrosis of the femoral head. In Schoutens A, Arlet J, Gardeniers JWM, et al. (Eds): Bone Circulation and Vascularisation in Normal and Pathological Conditions. New York, NY, Plenum Press; 1993.pp.265-75.

29. Kozinn SC, Wilson PD Jr. Adult hip disease and total hip replacement. Clin Symp. 1997;39:1-32.

30. Gardeniers JWM. ARCO international classification of osteonecrosis. ARCO News. 1993; 5:79-82.

31. Norman A, Bullough P. The radiolucent crescent line: An early diagnostic sign of avascular necrosis of the femoral head. Bull Hosp Joint Dis. 1963;24:99-104.

7

IMAGING MODALITIES

Osteonecrosis is a disease characterized by ischemic death of bony and marrow tissues. Different imaging modalities provide different information on the mineralized and non-mineralized component of the bone. Early diagnosis and proper staging of the disease are important for planning the treatment and improving clinical outcome.[1-19] The advent of magnetic resonance imaging (MRI) has dramatically improved the diagnosis of osteonecrosis.[20-28]

RADIOGRAPHY

The standard technique should include anteroposterior (AP) view of the pelvis and frog leg lateral (Dunn's) views of both hips. The plain radiographs are of limited use in the early stages but plain radiography findings are characteristic in stages 3 and 4 and at this stage any additional imaging modality is not required for final diagnosis.[29,30] Plain radiography is unable to detect changes during the ischemic stage and changes become apparent only after the process of repair has started. Another limitation of plain radiographic findings is poor inter- and intraobserver correlation.[31,32] Despite this plain radiographs remain the first imaging step as they can help in differentiating osteonecrosis from a number of other causes of painful hip joint and are also useful for staging of the disease. Both ARCO's classification and Steinberg staging for osteonecrosis of the femoral head are used for clinical assessment and planning the treatment.[1,2,7,8,13]

Osteonecrosis of the femoral head generally affects anterolateral segment, which is placed superiorly in the femoral head. Cancellous bone placed posteriorly is also projected in this area in anteroposterior (AP) view. It is, therefore, difficult to diagnose osteonecrosis of the femoral head on AP view, when changes are minimal. We routinely perform Dunn's view in addition to the AP view whenever osteonecrosis of the femoral head is suspected. However, tangential radiographs would delineate the entire femoral head nicely for more accurate assessment of the size of the necrotic segment. In early stages (preradiological), plain radiograph will not reveal any findings and diagnosis can only be done by functional bone investigation. Bone scan or MRI, if one suspects osteonecrosis of femoral head especially in high-risk patients (Figs 7.1 and 7.2).[3,4,33-39] The earliest changes on X-ray are diffuse or spotty osteoporosis, sclerosis or mixed picture (Figs 7.3 and 7.4).

At times a mixture of osteoporosis, sclerosis and cystic changes is seen. Subsequently, a small infarct occurs as a rim of increased repair process. Then the femoral head appears subtly flattened and at this stage 'crescent sign' is seen (Figs 7.5 to 7.7). Later there is fissuring and collapse of the necrotic segment changing the contour of the femoral head with a definite step at the margins of the infarcted zones. Finally the femoral head collapses and secondary osteoarthritic changes are seen, initially in the femoral head and subsequently even on the acetabular side (Fig. 7.8).

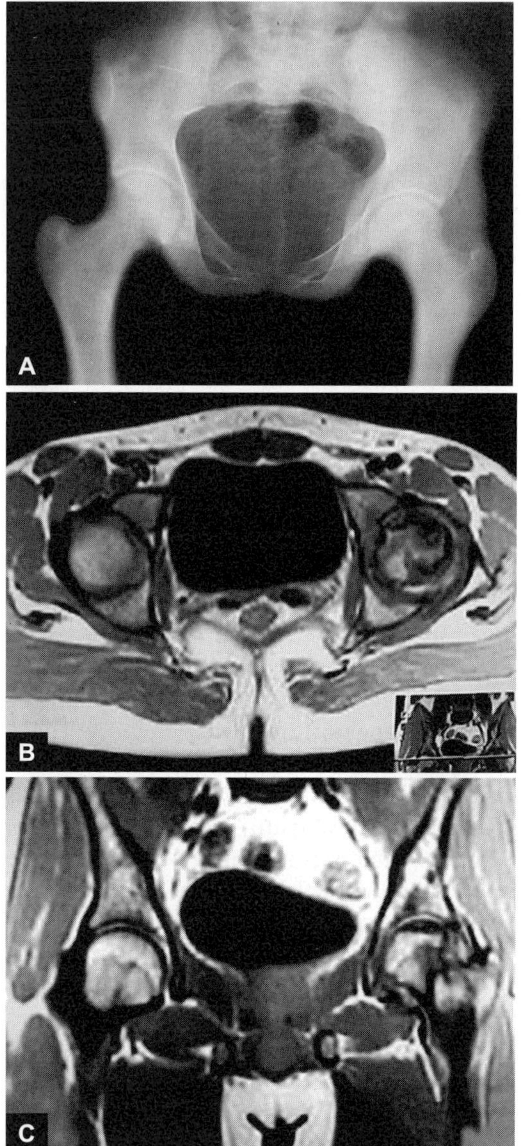

Figs 7.1A to C (A) X-ray of young girl of 20 years with all clinical signs of osteonecrosis left femoral head, not showing any evidence of necrosis. Stage I of osteonecrosis; (B and C) MRI showing early changes of sectoral involvement in left femoral head

Noninvasive Technique

Noninvasive techniques like isotope bone scan, CT scan and MRI are useful mainly for

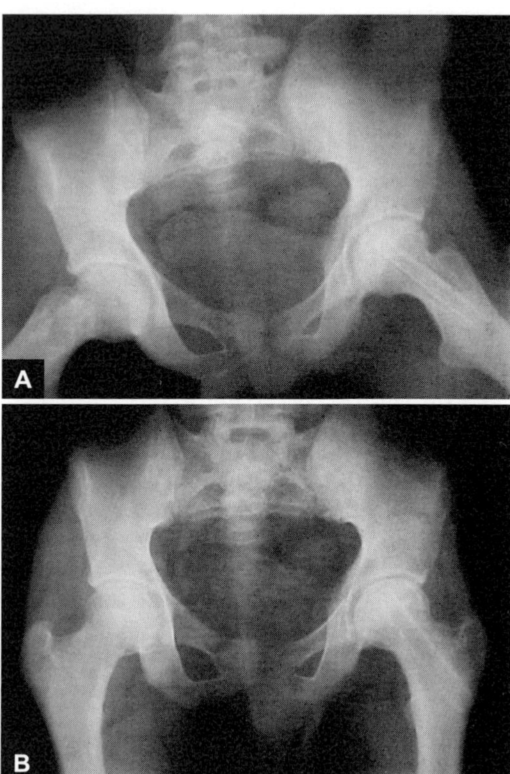

Figs 7.2A and B (A) X-ray pelvis of the same patient; (B) After core decompression and free fibular grafting

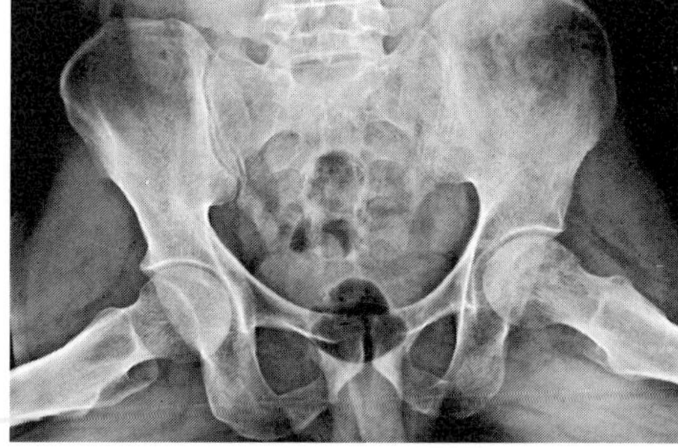

Fig. 7.3 Plain radiogram of PBH in abduction and external rotation shows subchondral sclerosis in the right femoral head, the head contour is maintained, the joint space is normal and the acetabular margin appears normal—stage II osteonecrosis

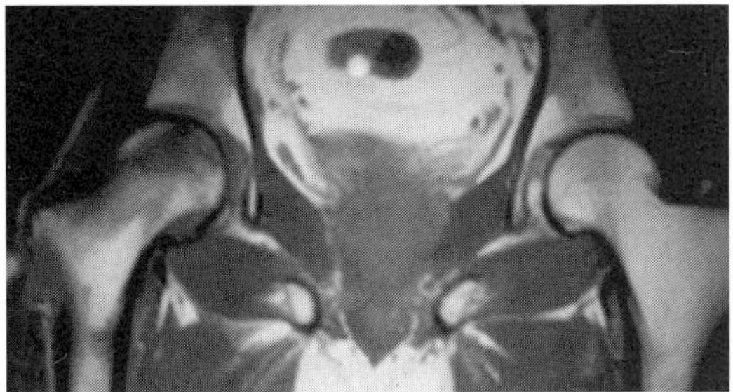

Fig. 7.4 MRI of same patient of Figure 7.3—coronal T1W-MR image shows geographic subarticular lesion showing fatty marrow signal, and outlined with hypointense margin, with preserved head contour and joint space stage II osteonecrosis

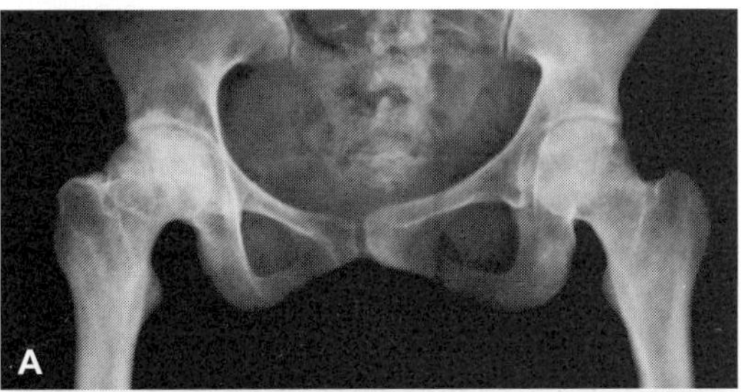

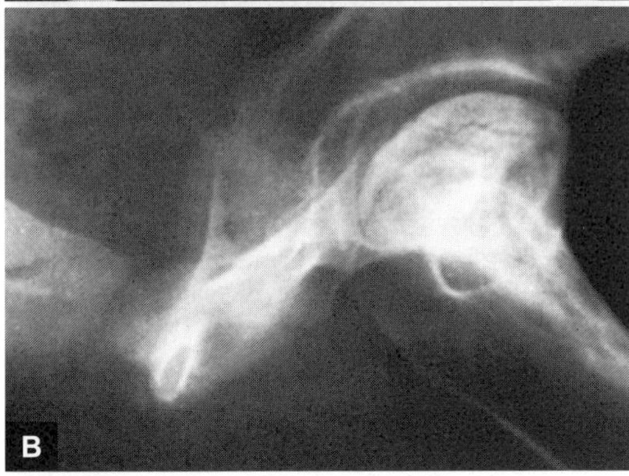

Figs 7.5A and B (A) Plain radiogram of pelvis with both hips shows sclerosis in right femoral head with subtle flattening of contour and subchondral crescentic lucency. Joint space is preserved—stage III osteonecrosis; (B) Showing classical crescent sign-subchondral fracture. Left femoral head appears to be normal

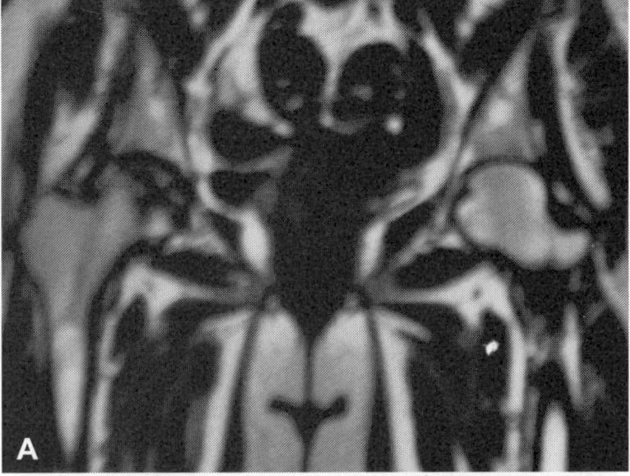

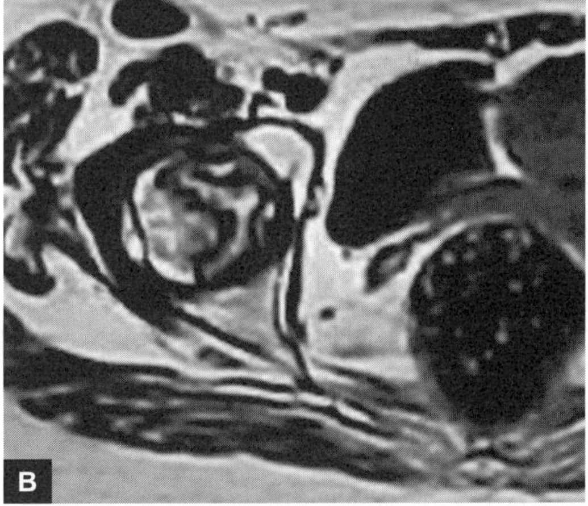

Figs 7.6A and B (A) MRI-T1W coronal image on left and axial image on right image of same patient (Fig. 7.5); (B) Subchondral hypointense signal, and subtle flattening of head contour, stage III osteonecrosis right side

screening high-risk patients and achieving early diagnosis.[39-44] These investigations offer a unique opportunity (before radiological changes are evident) to diagnose osteonecrosis of the femoral head in its early form.

Bone Scintigraphy: Bone Scanning

The standard technique should include three-phase scintigraphy and anterior and posterior planar scans. Bone scintigraphy can visualize the regional blood flow, but is not able to measure the efficiency of the vascular supply or repair mechanism. The early changes of osteonecrosis may be evident as early as 24 hours, which shows reduced vascularity on flow phase and photopenic area in the femoral head

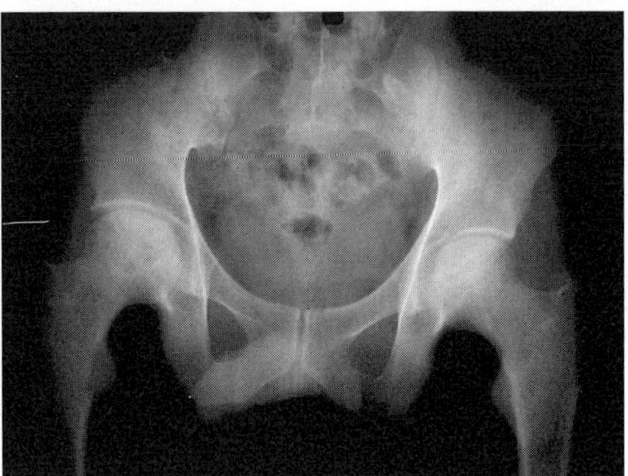

Fig. 7.7 X-ray of pelvis with both hips shows sclerosis in the right femoral head with crescent shaped lucency. The acetabulum appears normal and the joint space is preserved, appears to be a stage III osteonecrosis. The left femoral head also shows increased density without subchondral crescentic lucency—stage II osteonecrosis

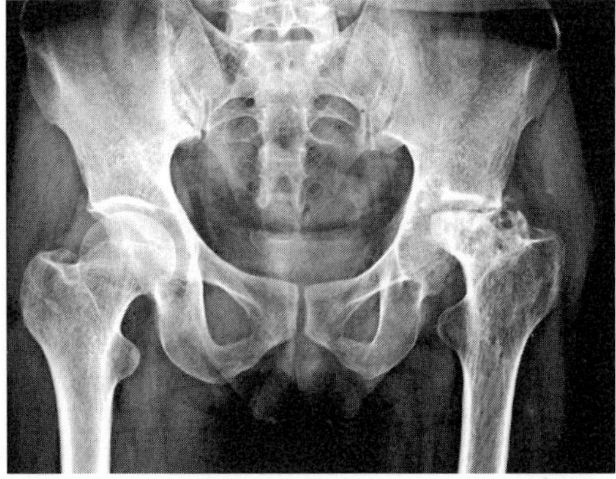

Fig. 7.8 Plain X-ray of pelvis with both hips shows collapse of left femoral head with subarticular sclerosis on either side of the joint. The joint space is reduced with signs of osteoarthritis—stage IV osteonecrosis. The opposite femoral head appears normal

on delayed images. After few days and weeks photopenic area in the femoral head may be surrounded by a rim of increased tracer uptake (Figs 7.9 and 7.10). In late stages the femoral head is distorted in shape and is reduced in size and shows increased tracer concentration due to bone remodeling. The interruption of blood

supply, detected as cold spot, is a nonspecific pattern and can be found in several other bone marrow processes.[30] The repair process with revascularization, detected as a hot spot is the most common finding but is nonspecific. Only a combination of cold in hot spot represents a diagnostic pattern for osteonecrosis.[30,39,40] Thus, bone scan is highly sensitive for detection of early osteonecrotic changes but the specificity is low to allow a definitive diagnosis of osteonecrosis.

Conway JJ et al. and Calver R et al. has proposed a four-stage approach to scintigraphic pattern in primary aseptic necrosis of femoral head: the first stage or early stage usually is demonstrated by absent activity in a portion or all of the femoral head and is associated with normal radiographs (Figs 7.9 and 7.10). This is usually found within 5 weeks' of onset of symptoms. The second stage or early vascularization usually occurs within 4 months where early radiographic changes may be seen. On bone scan one may see a lateral column of revascularization, considered to be the result of posterolateral position of superior capsular artery (Figs 7.11 and 7.12). The third stage, or base filling occurs at about 10 months after onset and is generally represented by diffuse zones of increased activity (Figs 7.13 and 7.14). The fourth stage, is last stage and represents a return to normal activity with no zones of increased activity to be seen in the epiphysis and is noticed after 18 to 24 months following onset of symptoms.

Bone scintigraphy in osteonecrosis is indicated for patients with risk of multifocal lesions when MRI is not available or for patients at high-risk for osteonecrosis who have persistent pain despite negative MRI.[39] Technetium 99 methylene-di-phosphate bone scanning is a useful technique. In general, the reactivity of bone around the infarcted segment shows an increased uptake of isotopes on the delayed image. This represents an accumulation of the radionuclide in the area of increased bone turnover at the junction of dead and reactive bone. Although increased uptake alone can be seen in reflex sympathetic dystrophy, transient osteoporosis, infarction,

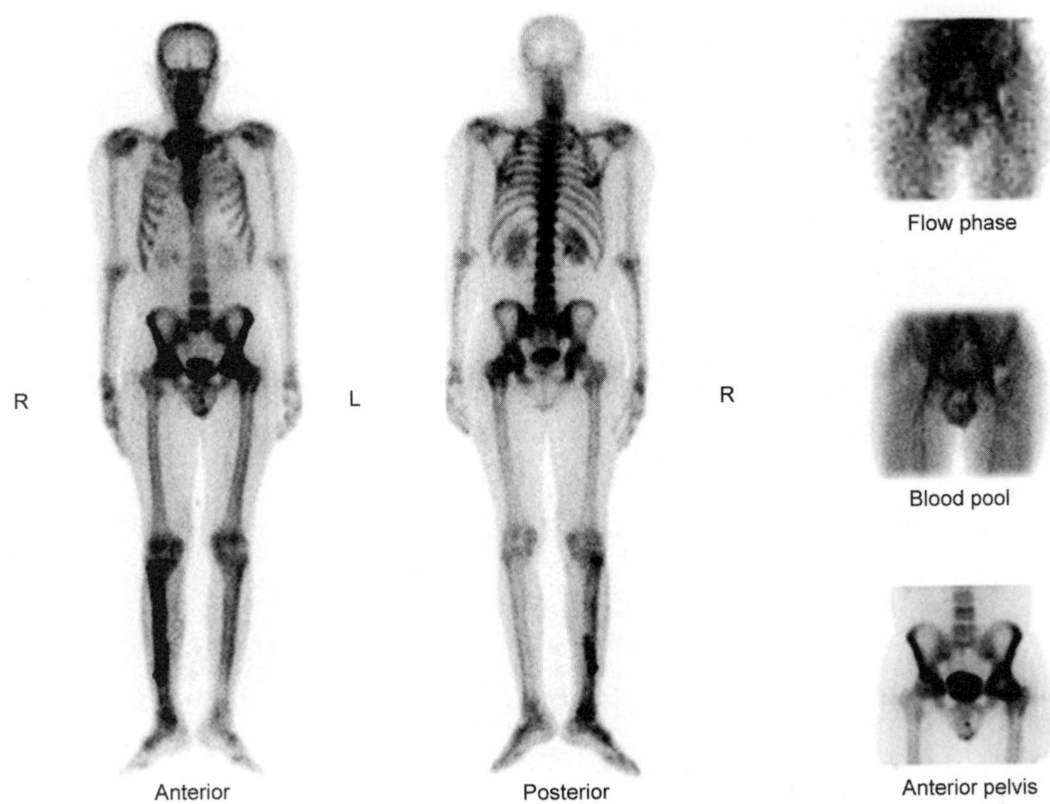

Fig. 7.9 Radioisotope bone scan showing normal flow phase. Blood pool not showing any abnormal soft tissue uptake. Anterior pelvis shows increased tracer uptake in obliquely linear fashion involving the neck of left femur with photopenic (Cold) area involving superomedial aspect of femoral head with a hot rim of activity suggesting early case of stage I osteonecrosis of the femoral head

tumors, etc. a photopenic area surrounded by an area of increase activity are most consistent with a diagnosis of osteonecrosis (Figs 7.13 and 7.14). Since bone scan is a low cost investigation in osteonecrosis, its use is recommended in patients who has a negative radiograph for osteonecrosis, no risk factors and unilateral symptoms. If the bone scan is negative patient should be observed and followed, and MRI may be advised in case of strong clinical suspicion.

MAGNETIC RESONANCE IMAGING

Magnetic resonance imaging (MRI) is the most accurate imaging modality for the diagnosis of osteonecrosis of femoral head, especially in the early stages when there are only bone marrow changes. Conventional MRI studies may be false negative in evaluating the earliest lesions in which the cellular integrity of the necrotic fatty marrow is intact or when the lesion is very small and under the resolution of MRI. An accuracy of more than 90 percent is reported with routine MRI techniques.[15,21,22,30,39] The preferred equipment and imaging technique should include at least 0.5 tesla units, 3 mm slice thickness, body coil with coronal sections of both hips, and T1 and T2 weighted images.[39,40] An additional fat suppression sequence will increase the accuracy of MRI.[39]

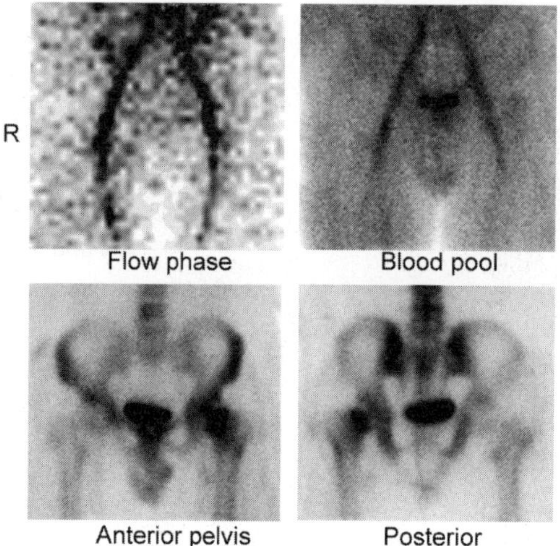

Fig. 7.10 Radioisotope bone scans showing normal flow phase. Blood pool not showing any abnormal soft tissue uptake. Anterior pelvis shows increased tracer uptake in obliquely linear fashion involving the neck of left femur with photopenic (Cold) area involving superomedial aspect of femoral head with a hot rim of activity suggesting osteonecrosis stage I/ II of the femoral head

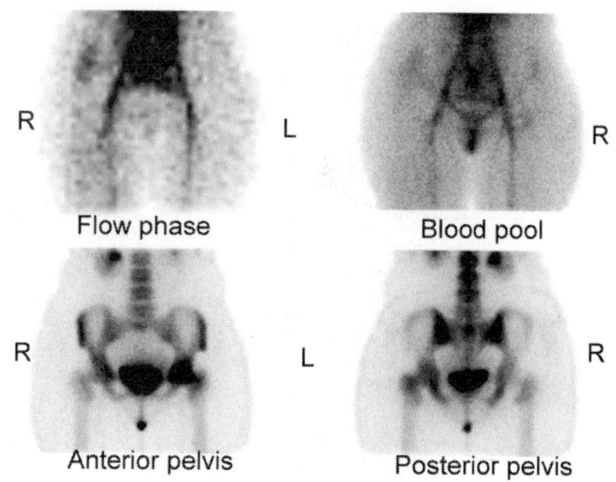

Fig. 7.11 Radioisotope bone scans showing normal flow phase—perfusion. Blood pool not showing any abnormal soft tissue uptake. Delayed static images of anterior pelvis shows a photopenic (Cold) area involving left femoral head with a hot rim of activity suggestive of stage II osteonecrosis of femoral head

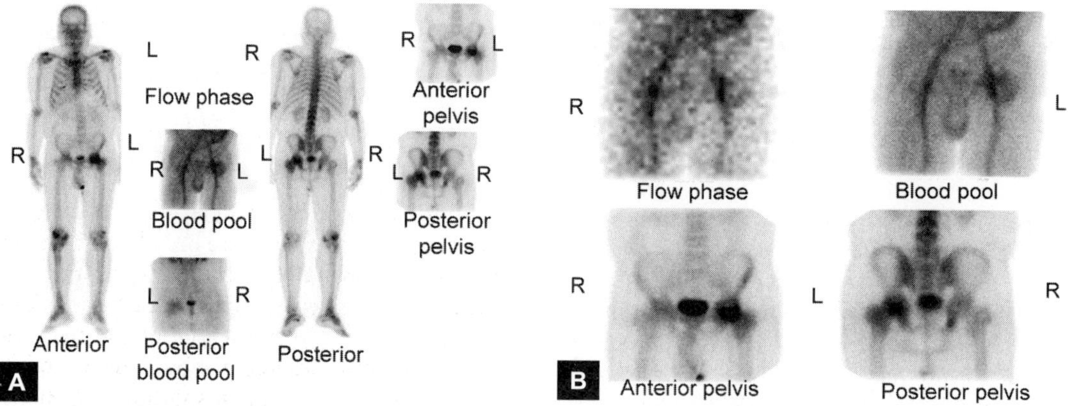

Figs 7.12A and B The perfusion phase reveals no focal hyperemia. The blood pool phase reveals significant soft tissue uptake and increased early bone uptake by left femoral head. The delayed static image of anterior and posterior pelvis shows a photopenic (Cold) area involving the superomedial aspect of left femoral head with a hot rim of activity suggestive of stage II osteonecrosis of left femoral head

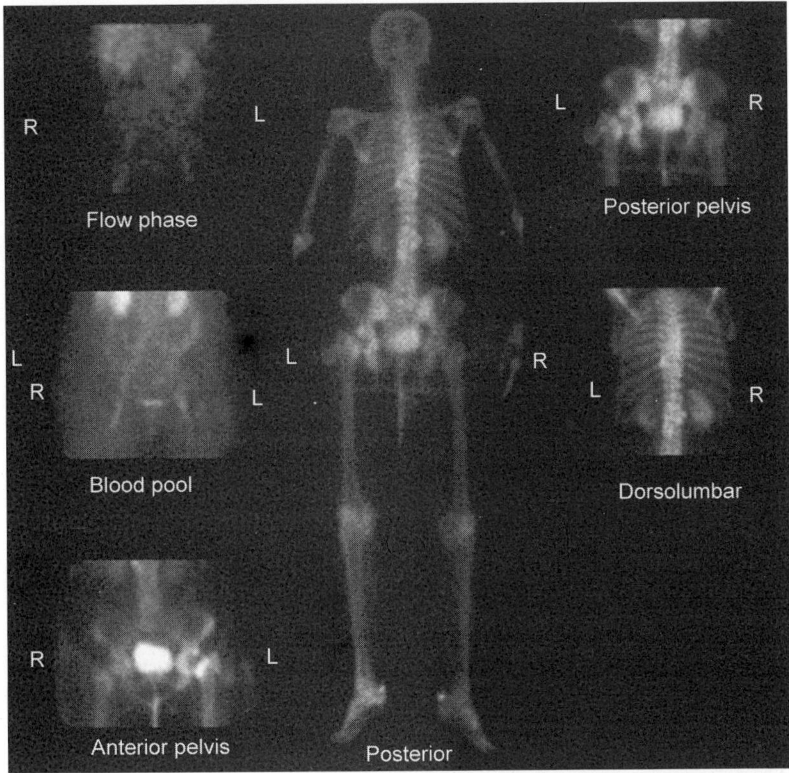

Fig. 7.13 Radioisotope bone scan showing normal flow phase. Blood pool not showing any abnormal soft tissue uptake. Anterior pelvis shows increased tracer uptake in obliquely linear fashion involving the neck of left femur with photopenic (Cold) area involving superomedial aspect of femoral head with a hot rim of activity suggesting early case of stage I osteonecrosis of the femoral head *(For color version, see Plate 4)*

Stage I Osteonecrosis

The earliest finding in osteonecrosis is a single density line (a low-intensity signal) on T1 generated image that presumably represents the separation of normal and ischemic bone. Double line on T2 generated image a signal including line represents hypervascular granulation tissue. MRI is used to outline the area of involvement. It can show the revascularization front and can provide objective evidence of changes in the tissues in response to treatment. It also allows sequential evaluation of a symptomatic lesion, which is not seen on plain radiograph. Rarely histopathological examination has revealed changes of osteonecrosis in patients who had negative MRI. [40]

Characteristic MRI signal alterations in the anterosuperior portion of the femoral head surrounded by a band of low-signal intensity on T1- and T2-weighted images represent the diagnostic criteria of osteonecrosis on MRI. The occurrence of a double-line sign on the T2-weighted image represents a pathognomonic osteonecrosis sign, but its absence does not eliminate the diagnosis of osteonecrosis (Figs 7.15 and 7.16). [39-41] An additional MRI finding in osteonecrosis is a joint effusion, which can be graded on T2-weighted images. [38-41]

The limitation of MRI in osteonecrosis is indicated by the lack of clear prognostic criteria

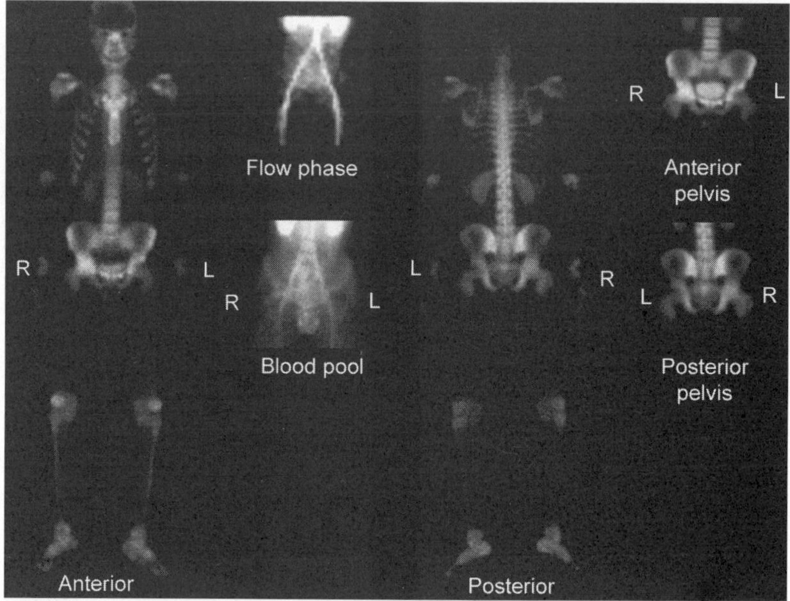

Fig. 7.14 The delayed anterior pelvis shows abnormal diffusely increased tracer uptake by the entire right femoral head suggestive of delayed or revascularization phase of osteonecrosis—stage III of right femoral head (*For color version, see Plate 5*)

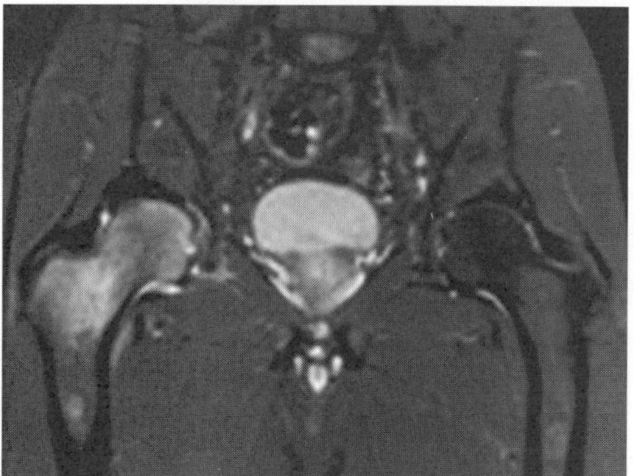

Fig. 7.15 MR-coronal stir image showing—diffuse marrow edema in the right femoral head and neck

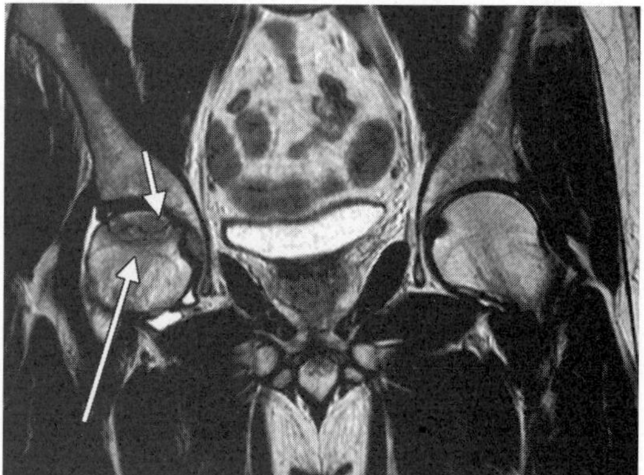

Fig. 7.16 MRI-double line sign of osteonecrosis. Coronal T2W image shows a geographic lesion in the subarticular aspect of right femoral head, lined by an inner thin T2 hypointense (longer arrow) and outer T2 hyperintense (short arrow) margin

for the signal alterations.[40-42] Furthermore, MRI is less sensitive than radiography and, especially CT in detecting subchondral fractures or early femoral flattening.[30,39,43]

MRI is more sensitive and accurate than plain radiography (Figs 7.17 to 7.19). The extent as measured on an AP radiograph is not the same as in a mid coronal MRI and that in lateral radiograph does not correspond

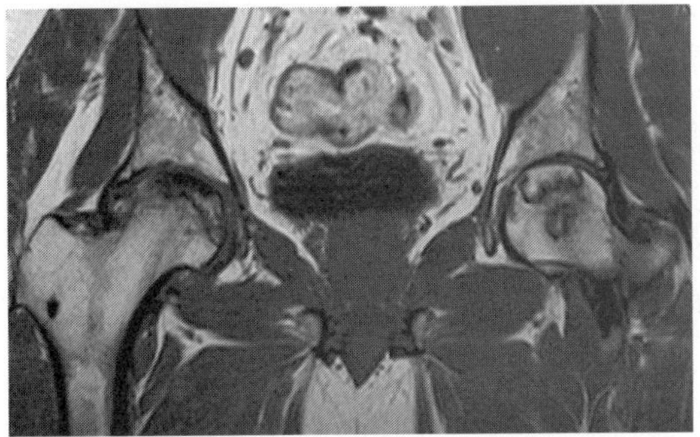

Fig. 7.17 MR-T1 weighted image—subarticular geographic lesion in left femoral head, outlined by hypointense margins, and showing central fat signal. Head contour is maintained. No subchondral fracture is seen. The acetabular margin appear normal, stage II osteonecrosis. Right femoral head shows a similar lesion, but with subchondral T1 hypointense signal s/o sclerosis, and with flattening of head contour. The acetabular rim however, appears uninvolved—osteonecrosis stage III

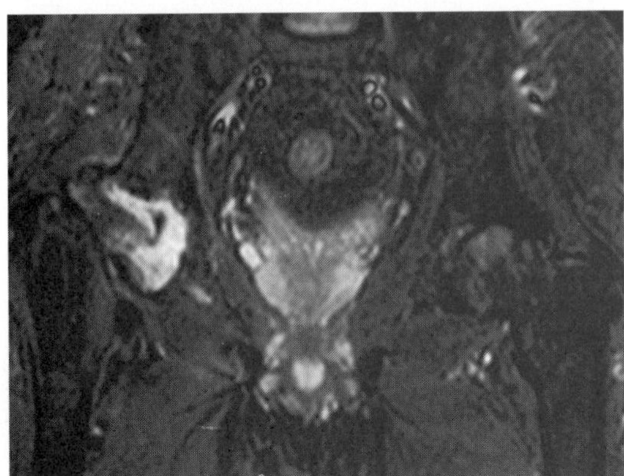

Fig. 7.18 MR-coronal stir image. A small geographic area of marrow edema is seen in the left femoral head in subarticular region—possibly stage I osteonecrosis. Complete collapse of right femoral head with reduced joint space—erosive changes in acetabular rim—suggestive of stage IV osteonecrosis. Synovial effusion is also seen on right

to a midsagittal MRI. The extent of necrotic portion at the initial MRI scan predicts the risk of collapse of femoral head. Quantifying the extent of osteonecrosis of femoral head can be

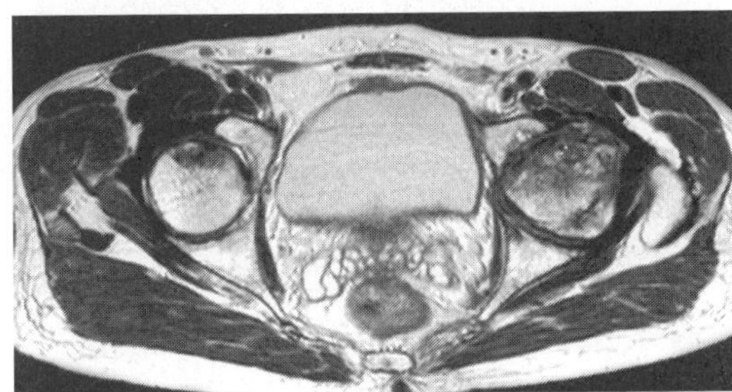

Fig. 7.19 MRI-axial T2W image of the same patient shows the osteoarthritic changes, in the form of reduced joint space, subarticular sclerosis which appear hypointense, on either side of the joint, with formation of subchondral T2 hyperintense small cysts, in the anterior acetabulum, osteonecrosis—stage II right side, stage IV on left side

a major predictor of future collapse which can be clinically useful in the management of early stage osteonecrosis of the femoral head and can be a major predictor of future collapse which can be clinically useful in the management of early stage osteonecrosis femoral head.[44]

The midcoronal: (A) and midsagittal (B) sections which showed the largest diameter of femoral head were used for the measurement.

$A/180 \times B/180 \times 100 =$ Index of necrotic segment

Small necrosis 33

Medium necrosis 34–66

Large necrosis 67–100.

Computed Tomography

Computed tomography (CT) is particularly useful in detecting subtle collapse of the femoral head when conventional radiographs appear normal (Table 7.1).[39] Additional multiplanar two-dimensional reconstruction in the coronal and sagittal planes are helpful for ARCO's staging and surgical planning. The complex architecture of the trabeculae in the femoral head allows early recognition of the patchy repair process on CT.[20] This so-called 'asterisk sign' represents an early but nonspecific osteonecrosis pattern.[20,30]

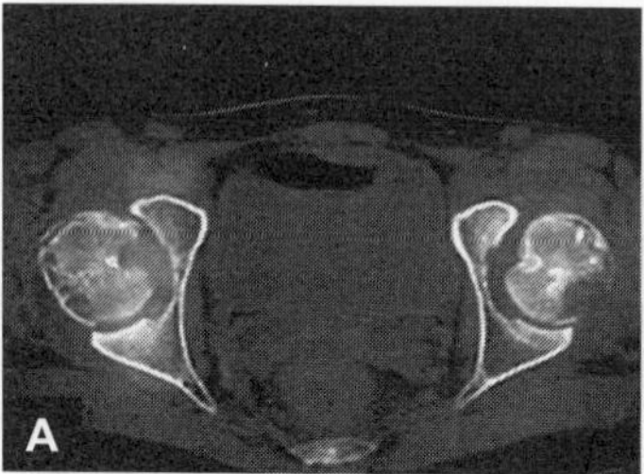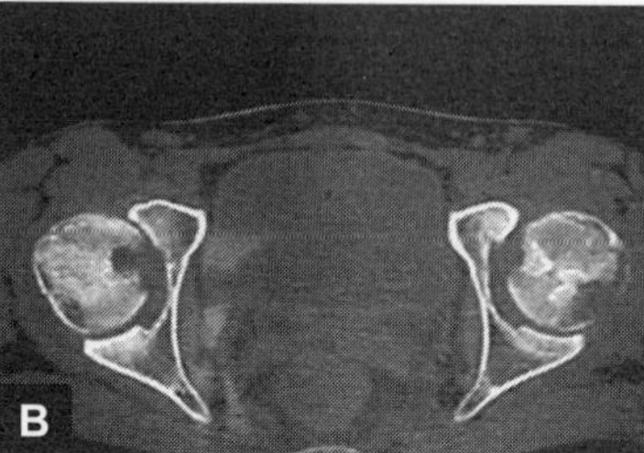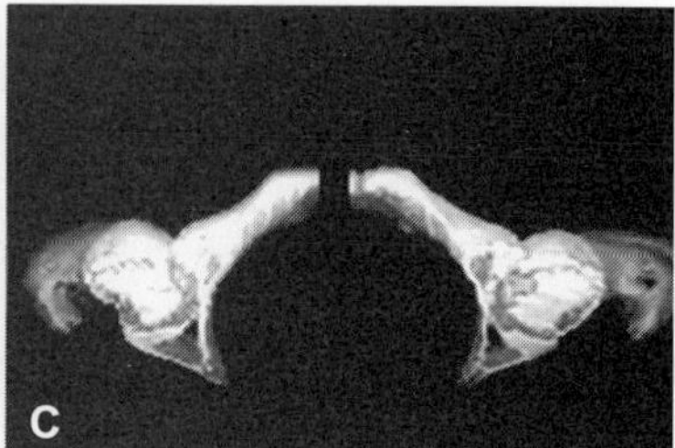

Figs 7.20A to C CT scan pelvis showing changes of osteonecrosis with subchondral cystic changes and subchondral fracture

The main advantage of CT compared to other imaging modalities is the accurate detection of subchondral fracture or early femoral collapse (Figs 7.20A to C). It is expensive and exposes the patient to considerable amounts of radiation and it is usually unnecessary for establishing the diagnosis of osteonecrosis.

Additional Imaging Studies

Digital subtraction angiography: With the use of this technique Wheeless et al.[45] have demonstrated vessel abnormalities in 31 percent of control hips compared to 94 percent of osteonecrosis hips. The vessel abnormalities were significantly higher in subgroups with an additional risk factor. Their results may indicate that there is a population that is at risk for osteonecrosis as a result of anomalies of the macrovascular circulation to the femoral head.

Imaging Correlated Histomorphology of Osteonecrosis

The typical histomorphologic lesion of osteonecrosis is described as subchondral area of multiple necrotic bony trabeculae, surrounded by marrow tissue in different stages of necrosis and demarcated from the underlying living bone and marrow by zones of fibrovascular marrow regeneration, active bone formation and remodeling.[6,15,33] These microscopic criteria are generally regarded as the 'gold-standard' for the diagnosis of

Table 7.1 MAGID Revised radiographic staging. Magid D, Fishman EK, Scott WW, et al. 1985 (Based on CT Multiplanar Reconstruction Criteria)

Plain film staging	CT multiplanar reconstruction	
0 (Normal)	Stage	Definition or explanation
	0	No change
I (Preradiographic)	I	May be defined by further research into density measurement, trabecular assessment and other factors
II	IIa	Subtle, early sclerosis and osteoporosis, Trabecular coarsening (Arrested asterisk sign) Distinct to definite foci of sclerosis, osteoporosis
	IIb	Early subchondral rim or crescent sign
III	IIIa	Contour at risk. Advanced subchondral undermining large cysts
	IIIb	Early alteration in contour or subchondral fracture
IV	IV	Marked collapse of femoral head significant acetabular involvement

osteonecrosis.[46] In clinical practice, particularly for early diagnosis in the precollapse stage, one has to rely on various noninvasive imaging modalities.[1]

The classic staging of femoral head osteonecrosis, described by Ficat,[1] was based on standard radiographs, a positive functional bone exploration and bone biopsy findings. This clinical staging had poor correlation with the histopathological staging described by Arlet and Ficat[6,7] as early type I and II with marrow changes alone were not detectable on plain radiographs and only the late type IV correlated with the plain radiographic finding of bone repair. This classification therefore, had limited clinical relevance and prognostic value.

The new ARCO classification is based on newer imaging techniques and is expected to correlate with histomorphologic findings.[13,14,17-20]

■ DETERMINATION: LESION SIZE IN OSTEONECROSIS OF THE FEMORAL HEAD

A number of studies have confirmed that the size of the necrotic lesion is an important factor in predicting the outcome of and determining the treatment for hips with osteonecrosis.[1-17] The Ficat and Arlet staging system that is currently often used for treatment decisions is based on the radiographic stage and clinical symptoms, without consideration of the extent of necrosis.[7]

To date, however, nonquantitative systems of staging are still in frequent use, and there is no general agreement to the best method for determining the extent of involvement. An ideal evaluation method that would be most useful to clinicians would need to meet several conditions. It should be simple and easy to use with regard to performing measurements. It should include the measurement of necrotic extent in the coronal as well as the sagittal plane because the measurement in one plane alone is not accurate for predicting further collapse of the femoral head. It should be reproducible within and between observers and should successfully predict the progression of early stage osteonecrosis. It should be based on MRI rather than radiography because MRI is more accurate in the evaluation of the extent of osteonecrosis and can provide a three dimensional assessment of the extent of the lesion.[21-24] Many authors have expressed concern that volumetric measurements are technically too demanding for general use and have thus accepted the use of a simpler but perhaps less accurate method. In 1974, Kerboul et al.[47] developed a simple and easy-to-use method of combined necrotic angle measurement. They measured the arc of the femoral surface involved by necrosis on both an anteroposterior and a lateral radiograph of the femoral head and then calculated the sum of the two angles.

In 1984, Steinberg et al.[8] developed staging systems for osteonecrosis on the basis of plain radiographic findings.[8] The major contribution of their classification was the addition of quantitation of femoral head involvement. The extent of head involvement with osteonecrosis was quantified by angular measurements of the arc of involvement from standard radiographs. In 1995, Steinberg et al. proposed a comprehensive quantitative system.[48] Hips affected with osteonecrosis were grouped into seven stages (0 to VI) and three grades (mild, moderate, and severe) for stages I to V. The merit of their method was the maximized utility of routine anteroposterior and lateral radiographs in the staging and grading of hips of stage II through V, and they have now incorporated MRI into their system. However, the method was too complicated to be used by clinicians and the reproducibility of the method was not acceptable.

Steinberg et al. studied and examined anteroposterior and lateral radiographs of 42 hips with established osteonecrosis. These hips were graded as being at stages II, III, or IV according to the University of Pennsylvania system of classification and staging.[8,48] They relied primarily on MRI for the evaluation of lesions in hips that appeared normal on radiographs but abnormal on bone scan or MRI (Stage I).

The extent of involvement for each hip was determined separately with the use of three techniques of evaluation: quantitative digital image analysis;[13,14,23] the necrotic angle of Kerboul et al;[47] and the "index of necrotic extent" of Koo and Kim,[44] as modified by Cherian et al.[49] It should be noted that the technique of Koo and Kim and the modification described by Cherian et al were used originally to evaluate magnetic resonance images; however, they were easily adapted for the evaluation of anteroposterior and lateral radiographs in the present study. Only hips with lesions that were clearly outlined on anteroposterior and lateral radiographs were selected. These radiographs were then traced onto tracing paper, showing the outline of the entire femoral head and neck as well as the necrotic segment. Two examiners agreed on the limits of the necrosis before tracing. By using this technique rather than working from the original radiographs themselves, the possibility of interobserver differences in estimating lesion size was reduced. Angular and volumetric measurements were made directly from these tracings.

In 1991, Ohzono et al.[50,51] introduced the concept of radiographic location of the lesion to correlate with prognosis. The findings on anteroposterior radiographs were used to classify the lesions into three categories. Type-A lesions occupied the medial one-third or less of the weightbearing portion of the femoral head and rarely progressed. Type-B lesions occupied the medial two-thirds or less of the weightbearing portion and had a prognosis of intermediate severity. Type-C lesions occupied more than the medial two-thirds of the weight-bearing portion and had the worst prognosis. In 1994, Sugano et al.[52,53] used coronal MRI scans instead of anteroposterior radiographs. This system was based on coronal-plane images and described the location of the lesion. However, measurement in the coronal plane alone was not accurate to quantify the necrosis.

In 1993, Lafforgue et al.[54] measured three quantitative parameters on contiguous MRI sections, corresponding to the 2 cm-wide medial portion of the femoral head: the angle filled by the osteonecrosis, the percentage of weightbearing femoral cortex involved with osteonecrosis, and the percentage of the femoral head surface involved with osteonecrosis. The values were strikingly lower in the group with good clinical or radiographic outcomes compared with those with poor outcomes and appeared to be accurate for use in the prediction of the outcome of osteonecrosis. However, this method was rather complicated for clinical application.

In 1995, Koo and Kim[44] estimated the extent of osteonecrosis as determined from a combination of coronal and sagittal MRI scans. The arc of the necrotic portion in the midcoronal image (A) and that in the midsagittal image (B) were used to quantify the extent of necrosis by the formula: $(A/180) \times (B/180) \times 100$. There was a strong correlation between this index and the risk of collapse, and the index was a major predictor of future collapse. However, to obtain the index, a conversion table or a calculator was necessary.

Volumetric Measurement

The volume of the necrotic lesion was determined with the use of a simple computerized program. The process involved outlining the entire femoral head as well as the necrotic segment on the both the anteroposterior and lateral radiographic projections, determining the percentage of necrosis in each of these views separately, and then multiplying these two values (Fig. 7.21). This was done with the use of a Graphire System. This method derives a reasonable approximation of the percent of the femoral head that is necrotic. These measurements have been previously compared with measurements that were obtained from three-dimensional magnetic resonance images.[55-60]

Combined Necrotic Angle of Kerboul et al.

In 1974, Kerboul et al.[47] using an anteroposterior radiograph and a lateral radiograph

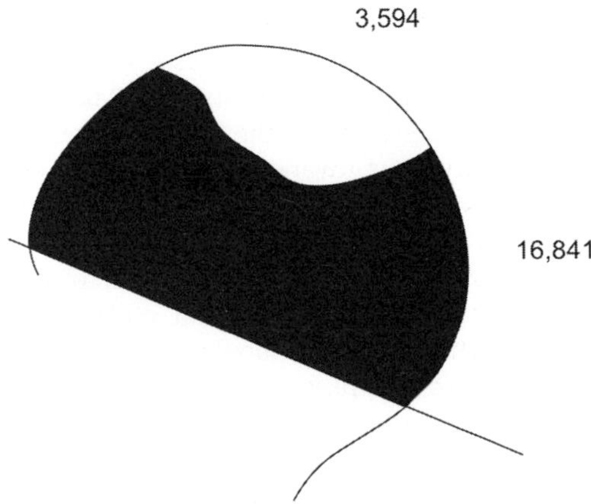

Fig. 7.21 Computer-generated tracing of an antero-posterior radiograph of a femoral head with an area of necrosis, shown in white. Similar measurements are made from the lateral radiograph. Both measurements are then used to determine the percent volume of the head that is necrotic, as described in the text

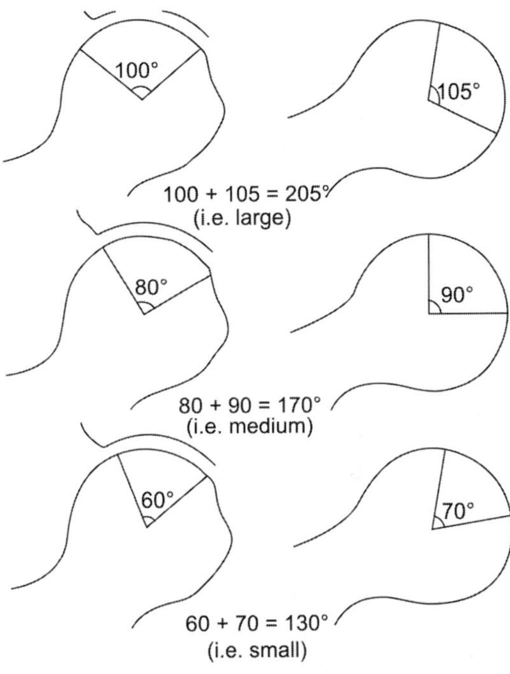

Fig. 7.22 Method of measuring lesion size as described by Kerboul et al. 1974. Diagram shows how the extent of the necrosis was recorded

of the same hip, measured the angle that resulted from drawing a line from the center of the femoral head to the two margins of the necrotic segment. They then calculated the sum of the two measurements. This method of calculation has been referred to by some as the "Combined necrotic angle"[47] (Figs 7.22 and 7.23). Kerboul et al. considered the extent of the necrosis to be large when the sum of these angles was ≥200°; small, when ≤160°; and medium, when between 159° and 199° or (small when 160° or less). They reported that when the combined angle is more than 200° the clinical outcome is poorer than when the combined angle is smaller.

When the sum was ≥ 200°, the clinical outcome was worse than when the sum was <200°.

In the study, midcoronal and midsagittal MRI scans were used instead of anteroposterior and lateral radiographs, and the combined angles predicted the subsequent risk of collapse more successfully. In the current study, the combined necrotic angle for ten of fifteen hips with Ficat stages IIA and IIB could not be measured with the use of the conventional

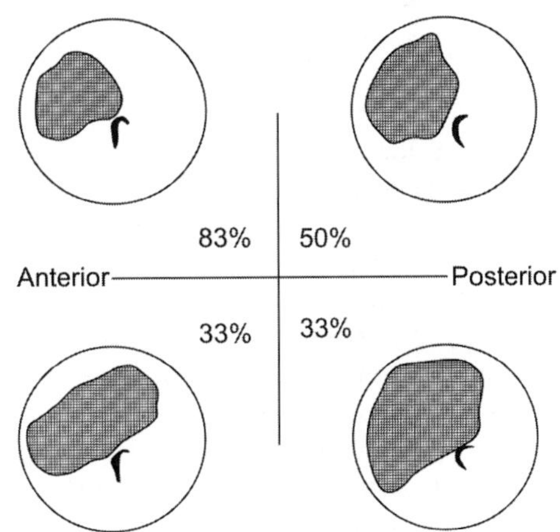

Fig. 7.23 Method of measuring lesion size as described by Kerboul et al. 1974. Diagram showing the influence of size and situation of the necrosis on the result of osteotomy

Kerboul method because the necrotic margin was not evident in the subchondral area on the radiographs. In the remaining five hips, the combined necrotic angle differed by 1° to 58° (mean, 26°) between the measurements made from the radiographs and those made from the magnetic resonance images.

Index of Necrotic Extent (Koo and Kim)

In 1995, Koo and Kim[44] used a modification of the Kerboul angular measurements in which the two angular measurements were calculated on midsagittal and midcoronal magnetic resonance images rather than on anteroposterior and lateral plain radiographs. The weightbearing surface of the femoral head was described as occupying a 180° angle; therefore, by dividing these angular measurements initially by 180 and then multiplying the coronal value by the sagittal value and then by 100, they derived a "percent" of the articular surface involved. On the basis of these values, they classified hips as having small (33%), medium (34–66%), and large (>66%) areas of necrosis and referred to this method of calculation as the "index of necrotic extent" or "index of necrosis."

The "Modified Index of Necrotic Extent," Described by Cherian et al. in 2003[49]

It is believed by some authors to be a more accurate indication of lesion size. Cherian et al. measured the lesion at its greatest diameter in both the coronal and sagittal planes rather than at the midcoronal and midsagittal planes. They compared both of these indices as well as a simple visual estimate of lesion size by evaluating 39 hips with stage I or stage II osteonecrosis. Hips evaluated by visual estimate were grouped by lesion size: small lesions consisted of lesions with <15 percent of head involvement; medium lesions, 15 to 30 percent; and large lesions, >30 percent. When only angular measurements were used, hips were grouped into only two categories: those with lesions encompassing <40 percent of the entire head and those with lesions encompassing ≥40 percent of the entire head.

Very little collapse was seen in the former group, whereas significant collapse was encountered in the group with larger lesions ($p < 0.05$). The authors concluded that these three methods of measurement were reproducible and reliable for quantitative evaluation of the extent of osteonecrosis and that they were clinically useful for the identification of hips at greatest risk of subchondral collapse. In the present study, by calculating this index on plain radiographs rather than on serial magnetic resonance images, the lesion was in fact measured at its maximum size. Thus, these measurements corresponded more closely to the modified index than to the original index that was described by Koo and Kim.[55-60]

With the use of the modified necrotic index, the distribution of lesions into small, medium, and large categories was much more even than when Kerboul angles were used. There was also a much closer correlation in lesion size between volumetric measurements and the necrotic index than with the Kerboul angle. Simply redefining the limits of measurements for small, medium, and large lesions might appear to improve the correlation with this technique, but it does not overcome the inherent problems of this method.

These factors have been considered primarily in reference to the femoral head prior to collapse. Once collapse has occurred, the extent of collapse and the amount of surface involved should be determined. If the joint is affected, one must evaluate the degree of joint-line narrowing and the extent of acetabular involvement, if present. It is essential to employ an effective and accurate method for determining the extent of involvement of both the femoral head and the acetabulum. This evaluation must be done not as an isolated series of measurements but as a part of a comprehensive system for staging osteonecrosis. In this way it will be possible to establish a prognosis, determine the most effective method of treatment, follow progression or remission, and compare the effectiveness of various methods of management.

CONCLUSION

The combined necrotic angle of the current study can be calculated in a simple, easy-to-use, and reproducible manner. It is based on biplanar MRI scans and provides a three-dimensional assessment of the extent of the necrosis. The categorization of femoral head osteonecrosis according to the combined necrotic angle measurement from midcoronal and midsagittal magnetic resonance imaging scans may accurately predict the risk of subsequent collapse of the femoral head. We believe that studies of the effectiveness of any surgical treatment to prevent collapse should be limited to the hips in the moderate and high-risk groups because surgical intervention in the low-risk group may be hard to justify. Further studies concerning the reliability of this method are required.

Quantitative volumetric measurements appear to be the most reliable method to measure the true size of a three-dimensional osteonecrotic lesion of the femoral head. Volumetric measurement is more accurate than angular measurement and can be performed easily with modern technology. Angular measurements, although somewhat simpler to conduct than volumetric measurements, may provide only a rough estimate of lesion size, partly due to the considerable differences in outline or location of the necrotic segments. Nevertheless, determination of lesion size must be part of a comprehensive system of staging of this disease, which includes the evaluation of other parameters, such as the extent and degree of articular surface involvement and the status of the hip joint and the acetabulum.

IMAGING STUDIES IN BRIEF

Radiography

Plain radiographic findings are unremarkable in the early stages of the disease. In mild-to-moderate disease, radiographs demonstrate sclerosis and changes in bone density. In advanced disease, bone deformities, such as flattening, subchondral radiolucent lines (crescent sign), and collapse of the femoral head, are evident.

Magnetic Resonance Imaging

- MRI is the most sensitive study and is the imaging procedure of choice, with an overall sensitivity of more than 90 percent. The specificity of MRI is also very high. The use of gadolinium is particularly useful in early detection.
- MRI findings include decreased signal intensity in the subchondral region on both T1- and T2-weighted images, suggesting edema (water signal) in early disease. This relatively nonspecific finding is often localized in the medial aspect of the femoral head. This abnormality is observed in 96 percent of cases.
- The next stage is characterized by a reparative process (reactive zone) and shows low-signal intensity on T1-weighted scans and high signal intensity on T2-weighted scans. This finding is diagnostic for osteonecrosis.
- Advanced osteonecrosis is characterized by deformity of the articular surface and by calcification, which are easily detected by radiography and CT scan.

Radionuclide Bone Scan

- In early osteonecrosis, osteoblastic activity and blood flow are increased; thus, the sensitivity of radionuclide bone scan is better than that of plain films at this stage .
- The central area of decreased uptake is surrounded by an area of increased uptake. This phenomenon is known as the doughnut sign and indicates the reactive zone surrounding the necrotic area.[61]
- Limitations of bone scan include the following:
  - In early osteonecrosis, bone scan is less sensitive than MRI.
  - Findings are nonspecific.

– Results are difficult to interpret if disease is bilateral. In unilateral disease, the healthy side can be used for comparison.

CT Scan

- CT scan shows sclerosis in the central part of the femoral head as an asterisk sign.
- Changes in the anterior part of the femoral head are easily observed.
- CT scan is a good modality to assess the extent of the disease and calcification, but it is not as sensitive as MRI.

■ REFERENCES

1. Ficat P, Arlet J, Hungerford DS (Eds). Ischaemia and Necrosis of Bone. Baltimore, MD, Williams and Wilkins, 1980.
2. Marcus ND, Enneking WF, Massam RA. The silent hip in idiopathic aseptic necrosis: treatment by bone grafting. J Bone Joint Surg (Am). 1973;55A:1351-66.
3. Hungerford DS. Bone marrow pressure, venography and core decompression in ischemic necrosis of femoral head-Hip Society meeting, Proceedings. 1979.pp.218-37.
4. Hungerford DS, Dennis W Lennox. The importance of increased intraosseous pressure in development of avascular necrosis of femoral head; Implication of treatment; Orthopaedic clinics of North America. 1985:16;635-68.
5. Hungerford DS, Jones LC. Diagnosis of osteonecrosis of the femoral head. In: Schoutens A, Arlet J, Gardeniers JWM, et al (Eds). Bone Circulation and Vascularisation in Normal and Pathological Conditions. New York, NY, Plenum Press. 1993.p.265.
6. Arlet J. Nontraumatic avascular necrosis of the femoral head: Past, present and future. Clin Orthop 1992;277:12-21.
7. Ficat RP. Idiopathic bone necrosis of the femoral head: Early diagnosis and treatment. J Bone Joint Surg Br 1985;67B:3-9.
8. Steinberg ME, Hayken GD, Steinberg DR. A new method for evaluation and staging of avascular necrosis of the femoral head. In: Arlet J, Ficat RP, Hungerford DS (Eds). Bone Circulation. Baltimore, MD, Williams and Wilkins. 1984.pp. 398-403.
9. Steinberg ME, Brighton CT, Hayken GD, Tooze SE, Steinberg DR. Early results in the treatment of avascular necrosis of the femoral head with electrical stimulation. Orthop. Clin. North America. 1984;15:163-75.
10. Steinberg ME, Brighton CT, Steinberg DR, Tooze SE, Hayken GD. Treatment of avascular necrosis of the femoral head by a combination of bone grafting, decompression, and electrical stimulation. Clin. Orthop. 1984;186:137-53.
11. Stulberg BN, Levine M, Bauer TW, et al. Multimodality approach to osteonecrosis of the femoral head. Clin Orthop. 1989;240:181-93.
12. Stulberg BN, Davis AW, Bauer TW, Levine M, Easley K. Osteonecrosis of the femoral head. A prospective randomized treatment protocol. Clin. Orthop. 1991;268:140-51.
13. Gardeniers JWM. ARCO committee on terminology and staging (report from the Nijmegen meeting). ARCO Newsletter. 1991;3: 153-9.
14. Steinberg ME, Hayken GD, Steinberg DR. A quantitative system for staging avascular necrosis. J Bone Joint Surg Br. 1995;77B:34-41.
15. Mont MA, Hungerford DS. Non-traumatic avascular necrosis of the femoral head. J Bone Joint Surg Am. 1995;77A:459-74.
16. Steinberg ME, Bands RE, Parry S, et al. Does lesion size affect the outcome in avascular necrosis? Clin Orthop. 1999;367:262-71.
17. Babhulkar SS. Osteonecrosis of the femoral head (in young individuals). Indian Journal of Orthopaedics. 2003;37(2):77-86.
18. Gardeniers JWM. ARCO international classification of osteonecrosis. ARCO News. 1993;5: 79-82.
19. Gardeniers JWM. ARCO Committee on Terminology and Staging. The ARCO perspective for reaching one uniform staging system of osteonecrosis. In: Schoutens A, Arlet J, Gardeniers JWM, Hughes SPF (Eds). Bone circulation and vascularization in normal and pathological conditions. New York: Plenum Press. 1993.pp.375-80.
20. Dihlmann W. CT analysis of the upper end of the femur: The asterisk sign and ischaemic bone necrosis of the femoral head. Skeletal Radiol. 1982;8:251-8.
21. Mitchell MD, Kundel HL, Steinberg ME, et al. Avascular necrosis of the hip: comparison of MR, CT, and scintigraphy. AJR. Am J Roentgenol. 1986;147:67-71.

22. Mitchell DG, Rao VM, Dalinka MK, et al. Femoral head avascular necrosis: correlation of MR imaging, radiographic staging, radionuclide imaging, and clinical findings. Radiology. 1987;162:709-15.

23. Coleman BG, Kressel HY, Dalinka MK, et al. Radiographically negative avascular necrosis: detection with MR imaging. Radiology. 1988;168:525-8.

24. Mitchell DG, Steinberg ME, Dalinka MK, et al. Magnetic resonance imaging of the ischaemic hip: Alterations within the osteonecrotic, viable, and reactive zone. Clin Orthop. 1989;244:60-77.

25. Norman A, Bullough P. The radiolucent crescent line: An early diagnostic sign of avascular necrosis of the femoral head. Bull Hosp Joint Dis. 1963;24:99-104.

26. Markisz JA, Knowles RJ, Altchek DW, et al. Segmental patterns of avascular necrosis of the femoral heads: early detection with MR imaging. Radiology. 1987;162:717-20.

27. Bassett LW, Gold RH, Reicher M, Bennett LR, Tooke SM. Magnetic resonance imaging in the early diagnosis of ischemic necrosis of the femoral head. Preliminary results. Clin Orthop. 1987;214:237-48.

28. Hauzeur JP, Pasteels JL, Schoutens A, et al. The diagnostic value of magnetic resonance imagingin non-traumatic osteonecrosis of the femoral head. J Bone Joint Surg Am. 1989; 71:641-9.

29. Herndon JH, Aufranc OE. Avascular necrosis of the femoral heead in the adult. A review of its incidence in a variety of conditions. Clin Orthop. 1972;86:43-62.

30. Resnick D, Niwayama G. Osteonecrosis: Diagnostic techniques, specific situations, and complications. In: Resnick D (Ed). Diagnosis of Bone and joint Disorders, 3rd edn. Phildelphia, PA, WB Saunders. 1995;5:3495-3558.

31. Kay RM, Lieberman JR, Dorey FJ, et al. Inter- and Intra-observer variation in staging patients with proven avascular necrosis of the hip. Clin Orthop. 1994;307:124-9.

32. Smith SW, Meyer RA, Connor PM, et al. Interobserver reliability and interobserver reproducibility of the modified Ficat classi-fication system of osteonecrosis of the femoral head. J Bone Joint Surg Am. 1996;78A:1702-6.

33. Glimcher MJ, Kenzora JE. The biology of osteonecrosis of the human femoral head and its clinical implications: Part I. Tissue biology. Clin Orthop. 1979;138:284-309.

34. Glimcher MJ, Kenzora JE. The biology of osteonecrosis of the human femoral head and its clinical implications: Part II. The pathological changes in the femoral head as an organ and in the hip joint. Clin Orthop. 1979;139:283-312.

35. Glimcher MJ, Kenzora JE. The biology of osteonecrosis of the human femoral head and its clinical implications: Part III. Discussion of the etiology and genesis of the pathological sequelae; comments on treatment. Clin Orthop. 1979;140:273-312.

36. Jones JP Jr, Engleman EP, Steinbach HL, et al. Fat embolization as a possible mechanism producing avascular necrosis. Arthrits Rheum. 1965;8:449.

37. Jones JP Jr, Jameson RM, Engleman EP. Alcoholism, Fat embolism, and avascular necrosis. J Bone Joint Surg Am. 1968;50A:1065.

38. Jones JP Jr. Intravascular coagulation and osteonecrosis. Clin Orthop. 1992;277:41-5.

39. Kramer J, Hofmann S, Imhof H. The non-traumatic femur head necrosis in the adult: II. Radiologic diagnosis and staging. Radiology. 1994;34:11-20.

40. Beltran J, Herman LJ, Burk JM, et al. Femoral head avascular necrosis: MR imaging with clinical-pathologic and radionuclide correla-tion. Radiology. 1988;166:215-20.

41. Beltran J, Knight CT, Zuelzer WA, et al. Core decompression for avascular necrosis of the femoral head: Correlation between long-term results and preoperative MR staging. Radiology. 1990;175:533-6.

42. Shimizu K, Moriya H, Akita T, et al. Prediction of collapse with magnetic resonance imaging of avascular necrosis of the femoral head. J Bone Joint Surg Am. 1994;76A:215-23.

43. Lang P, Genant HK, Jergesen HE, et al. Imaging of the hip joint: Computed tomography versus magnetic resonance imaging. Clin Orthop. 1992;274:135-53.

44. Koo KH, Kim R. Quantifying the extent of osteonecrosis of the femoral head: A new method using MRI. J Bone Joint Surg B. 1995; 77-B:875-80.

45. Wheeless CR, Lins RE, Knelson MH, Urbaniak JR. Digital substraction angiography in patients with osteonecrosis of the femoral head. In: Urbaniak JR, Jones JP (Eds). Osteonecrosis-Etiology, Diagnosis and treatment. American Academy of Orthopaedic Surgeons, 1st edn. 1997.pp.241-245.

46. Kenzora JE, Glimcher MJ. Pathogenesis of idiopathic osteonecrosis: The ubiquitous crescent sign. Orthop Clin North Am. 1985; 16:681-96.

47. Kerboul M, Thomine J, Postel M, et al. The conservative surgical treatment of idiopathic aseptic necrosis of the femoral head. J Bone Joint Surg Br. 1974;56B:291-6.

48. Steinberg ME, Hayken GD, Steinberg DR. A quantitative system for staging avascular necrosis. J Bone Joint Surg Br. 1995;77B:34-41.

49. Cherian SF, Laorr A, Saleh KJ, et al. Quantifying the extent of femoral head involvement in osteonecrosis. J Bone Joint Surg Am. 2003;85A: 309-15.

50. Ohzono K, Saito M, Takaoka K, et al. Natural history of atraumatic avascular necrosis of the femoral head. J Bone Joint Surg Br. 1991;73: 68-72.

51. Ohzono K, Saito M, Sugano N, et al. The fate of nontraumatic avascular necrosis of the femoral head: A radiologic classification to formulate prognosis. Clin Orthop. 1992;277:73-8.

52. Sugano, N, Takaoka K, Ohzono K, et al. Prognostication of nontraumatic avascular necrosis of the femoral head. Significance of location and size of the necrotic lesion. Clin. Orthop. 1994;303:155-64.

53. Sugano N, Ohzono K, Masuhara K, Takaoka K, Ono K. Prognostication of osteonecrosis of the femoral head in patients with systemic lupus erythematosus by magnetic resonance imaging. Clin Orthop. 1994;305:190-9.

54. Lafforgue P, Dahan E, Chagnaud C, et al. Early-stage avascular necrosis of the femoral head: MR imaging for prognosis in 31 cases with at least 2 years of follow-up. Radiology. 1993; 187:199-204.

55. Yong-Chan Ha, Woon Hwa Jung, Jang-Rak Kim, et al. Prediction of collapse in femoral head osteonecrosis: a modified kerboul method with use of magnetic resonance images. J Bone Joint Surg Am. 2006;88:35-40.

56. Kim YM, Ahn JH, Kang HS, Kim HJ. Estimation of the extent of osteonecrosis of the femoral head using MRI. J Bone Joint Surg Br. 1998;80B: 954-8.

57. Kopecky KK, Braunstein EM, Brandt KD, et al. Apparent avascular necrosis of the hip: appearance and spontaneous resolution of MR findings in renal allograft recipients. Radiology. 1991;179:523-7.

58. Seiler JG 3rd, Christie MJ, Homra L. Correlation of the findings of magnetic resonance imaging with those of bone biopsy in patients who have stage-I or II ischemic necrosis of the femoral head. J Bone Joint Surg Am. 1989;71:28-32.

59. Theodorou DJ, Konstantinos NM, Beris AE, Theodorou SJ, Soucacos PN. Multimodal imaging quantitation of the lesion size in osteonecrosis of the femoral head. Clin Orthop. 2001;386:54-63.

60. Hernigou P, Lambotte JC. Volumetric analysis of osteonecrosis of the femur: Anatomical correlation using MRI. J Bone Joint Surg Br. 2001;83:672-5.

61. Gottshalk A, Hoffer PB, Potchen EJ, Berger HJ. Book on Diagnostic Nuclear Medicine, Chapter on Radionuclide Studies in Avascular Necrosis: Published by Williams & Wilkins, 2nd edn. 1979.pp.1042-4.

8

BONE MARROW EDEMA SYNDROME AND OSTEONECROSIS

Bone marrow edema syndrome (BMES) of the femoral head is a rare disorder and its relationship with osteonecrosis is controversial. The bone marrow edema pattern of signal intensity changes on MR images, decreased on T1 weighted and increased on T2 weighted is a nonspecific finding encountered with several entities, including transient osteoporosis, transient bone marrow edema syndrome, osteonecrosis, trauma, infection and infiltrative neoplasm. Transient osteoporosis is an unusual but distinct syndrome characterized by self-limiting pain and radiographically evident osteopenia, and can be distinguished from other causes of bone marrow edema pattern, particularly osteonecrosis, on the basis of clinical findings and the development of radiographically evident focal osteopenia within eight weeks after the onset of pain. This is an important distinction, since all patients with transient osteoporosis recover completely, without any intervention.[1] The condition of BMES is characterized by disabling pain in the hip without any previous trauma with clinical signs of osteonecrosis without any radiographic evidence of osteopenia limited to the hip region and by a typical signal pattern on MRI. BMES of the femoral head, transient osteoporosis of the hip and osteonecrosis may not be completely distinct and separate entities, but may be related to common cause which remains unclear, but expresses different pathological effects. The condition may remain asymptomatic and may heal spontaneously; hence this disorder is underdiagnosed as compared to other causes of osteonecrosis. Wison et al.[2] reported ten patients with debilitating hip or knee pain with bone scan showing increased uptake in the involved joint with MR images showing decreased signal intensity of the bone marrow with normal conventional radiographs. These authors called this as "The transient bone marrow edema syndrome". These signal changes were quite different from focal lesions typical of osteonecrosis.[3,4] Although BMES is a rare disorder as compared to osteonecrosis, both conditions are associated with known risk factors and associated diseases causing osteonecrosis in the middle aged men and pregnant women in third trimester. Curtis and Kincaid[5] first described transient demineralization of the hip in pregnancy in 1959.

PATHOGENESIS

Intravascular coagulation of intraosseous microcirculation progressing to generalized venous thrombosis, and at times to retrograde arterial occlusion is probably the cause for osteoncrosis and BMES. The exact cause is unknown, but the abnormalities of vascular factors, altered lipid metabolism, and decreased fibrinolysis, which may result in multiple small thrombotic episode and may occur within the marrow, causing coagulopathy. A possible hypothesis is that the ischemia time and the deficiency in blood flow relative to normal perfusion are insufficient to cause significant irreversible osteocytic necrosis, though little fatty marrow may undergo necrosis and this necrotic damage is limited. Ischemic hypoxia temporarily injures the bone cells, which remains marginally viable and eventually recovers. The trabeculae donot lose their osteocyte. In BMES, there might be rapid plasmin activation by a fibrinolytic system. Fibrinolysis begins on the arterial side and normally progresses through microcirculation to the venous system. In BMES there is complete fibrinolysis of the extraosseous and intraosseous thrombi within a few minutes to two hours after the acute ischemic insult, which results into adequate reflow through pre-existing extraosseous and intraosseous circulation.

There is increased intraosseous pressure in BMES, which is likely to be the cause of severe pain. Reperfusion of partially necrotic terminal arterioles, capillaries and sinusoids reults in hemorrhage and edema. Depletion of the clotting factor during intravascular coagulation further aggravates the interstitial hemorrhage and produces secondary edema. A minimum of two hours of complete ischemia and total anoxia is required to cause irreversible osteocytic necrosis. The lack of reflow in osteonecrotic lesion is in contrast to the increased blood flow with reactive hyperemia and hypervascularity that occurs in BMES lesions following reperfusion. There is a relationship between ischemia time and intraosseous blood flow. There is a variable zone of borderline necrosis between the threshold of classic reversible BMES and classic irreversible osteonecrosis. In this transitional zone, there may be incomplete fibrinolysis with residual thrombosis and multiple islands of ischemic hypoxia. These microinfarctions probably do not progress or coalesce, because relatively normal marrow is interspersed between these multifocal lesions, which may spontaneously heal by a process of fibrovascular proliferation and osteoclastic resorption. In BMES, MRI reveals joint effusion, which is associated with increased intraosseous pressure.

It is possible to differentiate BMES and osteonecrosis of the head of the femur from plain X-rays, bone scan and MRI. Bone scan picture of osteonecrosis may be similar, although the increased uptake is usually more limited to the femoral head and less intense. Occasionally uptake of isotope over the anterosuperior portion of the femoral head is decreased forming a photopenic area or cold spot, which is almost pathognomic of osteonecrosis and is never seen in BMES. Classically it is recognized as focal subchondral signal intensity changes. Appearance of bone marrow on MRI[6] reveals low signal intensity on T1W and high signal intensity from the femoral head to the intertrochanteric region on T2W images. This diffuse, as opposed to focal, homogenous lesion, which corresponds to the area of increased activity on the bone scan. The lesions which are circumscribed by a rim of low signal intensity on T1 weighted image or double line sign on T2 weighted image, consisting of concentric low and high signal intensity bands, represent the interface between osteonecrotic and viable bone. It is noted that low intensity signals in osteonecrosis of the femoral head may take several forms, including homogeneous regions of decreased signal intensity, inhomogeneous areas of low intensity, bands of low intensity, or rings of low intensity around central regions of high signal intensity.[7] On plain radiography, there are no changes around the hip region, unlike in osteonecrosis where the appearance is of mottled radiolucent area surrounded by an area of sclerosis. There is segmental involvement in the anterosuperior subchondral area of the head of the femur in osteonecrosis.[5] MRI shows a mottled low-signal lesion in T1W images in osteonecrosis and a high-signal lesion in the bone marrow suggesting marrow edema on T2W images.[3,6] There are several recent reports of patients with hip pain, focal loss of radiodensity, positive bone scans and the appearance of bone marrow edema on MRI, without the specific MRI signs of osteonecrosis. This syndrome is called as transient marrow edema syndrome and as transient osteoporosis.[6,8,9] All the authors regard it as a condition which regresses spontaneously after 6 to 12 months and needs no surgical intervention.[8] However, a few authors consider it as an early phase of osteonecrosis, which without surgical treatment, may progress to the full-form of osteonecrosis with collapse of the femoral head.[8,9] Turner et al.[10] reported five patients who were initially seen with pain in the hip and bone marrow edema pattern on MRI, which subsequently showed focal changes of osteonecrosis which was proved by histopathology. It appears that osteonecrosis occasionally manifests a bone marrow edema pattern on MR images, and there is slight controversy as to whether BMES represents a very early, reversible stage of osteonecrosis.[3] The relationship between BMES, osteonecrosis and the incidence of progression from BMES to osteonecrosis is still not very clear.[9-32]

Several treatment options have been reported. Conservatively nonsteroidal antinflammatory drugs and limited weight-bearing may be advocated.[4,19,20] Various surgical options have been recommended for rapid and complete reduction of symptoms and intractable pain by core decompression with a return to normal MRI signal patterns, based on the theory that pain in the BMES and osteonecrosis is caused by elevated intramedullary pressure.[9] Core decompression enabled the faster recovery than in the conservatively treated group of the patients.[9]

■ REFERENCES

1. Hayes CW, Conway WF, Daniel WW. MR imaging of bone marrow edema pattern: transient osteoporosis, transient bone marrow edema syndrome, or osteonecrosis. Radiographics. 1993;13:1001-11.
2. Wilson AJ, Murphy WA, Hardy DC, Totty WG. Transient osteoporosis: Transient bone marrow edema: Radiology. 1988;167(3):757-60.
3. Guerra JJ, Steinberg ME. Distinguishing transient osteoporosis from avascular necrosis of the hip. J Bone Joint Surg Am. 1995;7A:616-24.
4. McCarthy EF. The pathology of transient regional osteoporosis. Iowa Orthop J. 1998;18:35-42.
5. Curtis PH, Kincaid WE. Transitory demineralization of the hip in pregnancy—a report of three cases. J Bone Joint Surg Am. 1959;41A:1327-33.
6. Bloem JL. Transient osteoporosis of the hip: MR imaging. Radiology. 1988;167:753-5.
7. Robinson HJ Jr, Hartleben PD, Lund G, et al. Evaluation of magnetic resonance imaging in the diagnosis of osteonecrosis of the femoral head, J Bone Joint Surg Am. 1989; 71A:650-63.
8. Takatori Y, Kokubo T, Ninomiya S, Nakamura T, OkutsuI, Kamogawa M. Transient osteoporosis of the hip: Magnetic resonance imaging. Clin Orthop. 1991;271:190-4.
9. Hofmann S, Engel A, Neuhold A, et al. Bone marrow oedema syndrome and transient osteoporosis of the hip. J Bone Joint Surg Br. 1993;75B:210-3.
10. Turner DA, Templeton AC, Seizer PM, et al. Femoral Capital osteonecrosis: MR finding of diffuse marrow abnormalities without focal lesions. Radiology. 1989;171:135-40.
11. Diwanji SR, Cho YJ, Xin ZF, Yoon TR. Conservative treatment for transient osteoporosis of the hip in middle-aged women. Singapore Med J. 2008;49(1):e17-21.
12. Ma FY, Falkenberg M. Transient osteoporosis of the hip: An atypical case. Clin Orthop. 2006; 445:245-9.
13. Shifrin LZ, Reis ND, Zinman H, Besser MI. Idiopathic transient osteoporosis of the hip. J Bone Joint Surg Br. 1987;69B(5):769-73.
14. Wood ML, Larson CM, Dahners LE. Late presentation of a displaced subcapital fracture of the hip in transient osteoporosis of pregnancy. J Orthop Trauma. 2003;17(8):582-4.
15. Balakrishnan A, Schemitsch EH, Pearce D, McKee MD. Distinguishing transient osteoporosis of the hip from avascular necrosis. Can J Surg. 2003;46(3):187-92.
16. Cahir JG, Toms AP. Regional migratory osteoporosis. Eur J Radiol. 2008;67:2-10.
17. Bramlett KW, Killian JT, Nasca RJ, Daniel WW. Transient osteoporosis. Clin Orthop. 1987;222:197-202.
18. Karagkevrekis CB, Ainscow DAP. Transient osteoporosis of the hip associated with osteogenesis imperfecta. J Bone Joint Surg Br. 1998;80B:54-5.
19. Varenna M, Zucchi F, Binelli L, Failoni S, Gallazzi M, Sinigaglia L. Intravenous pamidronate in the treatment of transient osteoporosis of the hip. Bone. 2002;31(1):96-101.
20. Kibbi L, Touma Z, Khoury N, Arayssi T. Oral bisphosphonates in treatment of transient osteoporosis. Clin Rheumatol. 2008;27:529-32.
21. Samdani A, Lachmann E, Nagler W. Transient osteoporosis of the hip during pregnancy: a

case report. Am J Phy Med Rehabil. 1998;77(2): 153-6.

22. Gupta P, Sharma S, Gupta S, Singh D, Agarwal A, Chauhan V. Transient osteoporosis of hip—a case report. Indian J Orthop. 2005;39(4):257-9.

23. Curtis PH, Kincaid WE. Transitory demineralization of the hip in pregnancy: a report of three cases. J Bone Joint Surg Am. 1959:41A; 1327-33.

24. Bezer M, Gokkus K, Kocaoglu B, Erol B, Guven O. Transient osteoporosis of the hip in pregnancy: a report of three cases. Acta Orthop Traumatol Turc. 2004;38(3):229-32.

25. Ergun T, Lakadamyali H. The relationship between MRI findings and duration of symptoms in transient osteoporosis of the hip. Acta Orthop Turc. 2008;42(1):10-1.

26. Uematsu N, Nakayama Y, Shirai Y, et al. Transient osteoporosis of the hip during pregnancy. J Nippon Med Sch. 2000;67(6):459-63.

27. Koo KH, Ahn IO, Song HR, Kim SY, Jones JP. Increased perfusion of the femoral head in transient bone marrow edema syndrome. Clin Orthop. 2002;402:171-5.

28. Bloem JL. Transient osteoporosis of the hip: MR imaging. Radiology. 1988;167:753-5.

29. Guerra JJ, Steinberg ME. Distinguishing transient osteoporosis from avascular necrosis of the hip. J Bone Joint Surg Am. 1995;77A: 616-24.

30. Hayes CW, Conway WF, Daniel WW. MR imaging of bone marrow edema pattern: transientosteoporosis, transient bone marrow edema syndrome, or osteonecrosis. Radiographics. 1993;13:1001-11.

31. Martinez MW, Thomas MR. 54-year-old man with hip pain. Mayo Clin Proc. 2005;80(6): 803-6.

32. McCarthy EF. The pathology of transient regional osteoporosis. Iowa Orthop J. 1998;18: 35-42.

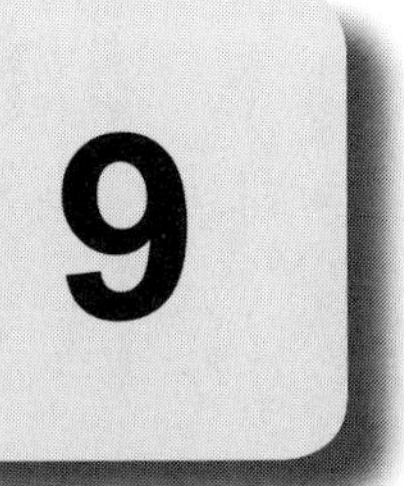

PREGNANCY AND OSTEONECROSIS

Pfeiffer[1] was the first to report in 1957 the relatively rare association of osteonecrosis of the femoral head with pregnancy, but a detailed description was reported by Curtis and Kincaid[2] in 1959. A variety of mechanisms has been implicated in the causation of osteonecrosis, which includes mechanical vascular interruption, thrombosis and embolism, injury to the vessel walls and vascular occlusion. Osteonecrosis of the femoral head can occur in association with pregnancy in the absence of other known risk factors for the disease. These women are healthy with no other history of known risk factors for osteonecrosis or trauma. The demography of pregnant women with osteonecrosis and women with idiopathic osteonecrosis is different and distinguishes from each other. The nonpregnant women with idiopathic osteonecrosis are generally older than pregnant women with the average age of 30 to 32 years, and they are generally heavier and obese. They have equal prevalence of affection right and left hip, with 50 percent involvement of bilateral hips; pregnant women with osteonecrosis have bilateral incidence of 31 percent with high prevalence of left side involvement, seen in primigravid women with small body frames.[3,4]

The pregnant patient presents with constant pain around the hip, at times intermittent, extending to the groin and lateral thigh. The diagnosis of osteonecrosis in the evaluation of hip pain during pregnancy is often delayed. The pain in the hip or groin in pregnant women may be because of two similar conditions occurring during pregnancy and the condition might be misdiagnosed.[3]

1. Ttransient osteoporosis of hip with pregnancy
2. Osteonecrosis of the femoral head with pregnancy.

Transient osteoporosis of the hip with pregnancy most frequently occurs in the third trimester and is characterized by acute onset of pain in the groin.[2] Ranges of movements are painful and are restricted at the extremes with abnormal gait, since the weightbearing exacerbates the symptoms.[5,6] Laboratory tests are usually normal. The initial X-rays may appear normal since the osteopenia follows symptoms by four to eight weeks, and the remineralization continues for 6 to 8 weeks after the resolution of symptoms.[7-10] The disease is usually self-limiting, and protected weight-bearing, pain control, and prevention of pathological fractures are sufficient treatment until resolution occurs, typically within eight weeks postpartum.[11] The etiology of transient osteoporosis of the hip of pregnancy is unknown. Suggested causes, although not proved, includes increased maternal demand of calcium: changes in the blood flow; and viral, neurologic, arthritic, inflammatory factors or a variant of reflex sympathetic dystrophy. The patient usually presents with acute symptoms of pain with limited mobility. Radiograph reveals generalized osteopenia, and bone scan shows diffuse high signal uptake. Whereas MRI shows consistent features which includes diffuse bone marrow edema pattern signal.

Prolonged reactive hyperemia on reflow and persistent hypervascularity, causes transient demineralization of the bone marrow edema which is seen radiographically as osteopenia. Usually within three to six months, the marrow hypervascularity subsides, the osteoid mineralization, and the radiolucent and osteopenic lesion spontaneously heals with extensive new bone formation. This syndrome of transient osteoporosis of the hip is characterized by pain of varying severity in one or both hips or thighs and develops during the last trimester of pregnancy. Roentgenograms show a spotty demineralization with sharply localized margins, involving one or both femoral heads, a small part of the femoral neck, and the acetabulum. The pain subsides and the roentgengraphic appearance returns to normal within several months after delivery.

In contrast osteonecrosis in association with pregnancy may be progressive, and the final outcome may include the collapse of the femoral head, articular surface and development of degenerative joint disease. A number of factors are likely to contribute to the development of osteonecrosis in pregnant women. Amongst potential factors, theories of venous congestion and hypercoagulability are prominent. Pregnancy is well known to produce a hypercoagulable state with a high incidence of thrombotic events, which tends to be higher in the third trimester, which is also seen in osteonecrosis in pregnant women. Hypercoagulability contributes to macro and microthromboembolic phenomenon, which leads to vascular occlusion and venous congestion with subsequent ischemic necrosis of bone. With varied etiology of osteonecrosis, it results in common pathway of resulting into the interruption of circulation to the femoral head. Symptoms tend to include vague pain in the region of hip and groin with development of restricted movements and limp only late in the course of disease. Radiographic changes appear late and reveals patchy areas of sclerosis, mottled radiolucency, subchondral lucency and later collapse (Fig. 9.1). Bone scans reveal focal areas of increased uptake in the femoral

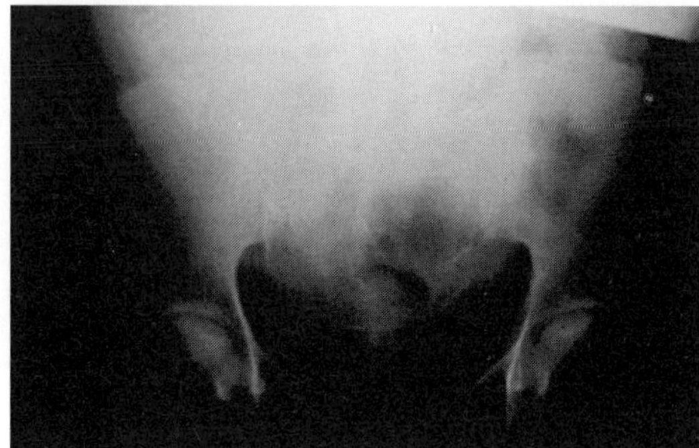

Fig. 9.1 X-ray pelvis showing bilateral femoral osteonecrosis with gravid uterus-fetus

head with classical cold in hot spot appearance. MR images shows classical changes of osteonecrosis, affecting anterolateral segment of femoral head. These demonstrate decreased signal activity on T1 weighted images with classical double-line sign of density on the density sign in T2 weighted images. The natural history of osteonecrosis in association with pregnancy does not differ from other cases of nontraumatic osteonecrosis.

The high prevalence of left sided involvement of pregnant women is mainly because of the high incidence of left sided deep venous thrombosis. This phenomenon can be explained by the anatomy of venous drainage of the left lower extremity within the pelvis.[3,4] The left common iliac vein passes posterior to the right common iliac artery and may be subject to the excessive compression from the weight of developing fetus (Fig. 9.2).

Osteonecrosis in pregnancy may be unilateral, commonly on left side, or bilateral seen in third trimester. Most pregnant women with osteonecrosis have pain in the hip region with antalgic limp, tenderness, and restricted hip movements without any previous history of trauma. Hypervascularity appears very early in the course of disorder, and is consistently observe before osteopenia. Scintigraphy at this early stage shows markedly increased homogeneous uptake in the hip region, before radiolucent radiographic changes of demineralization are seen, in

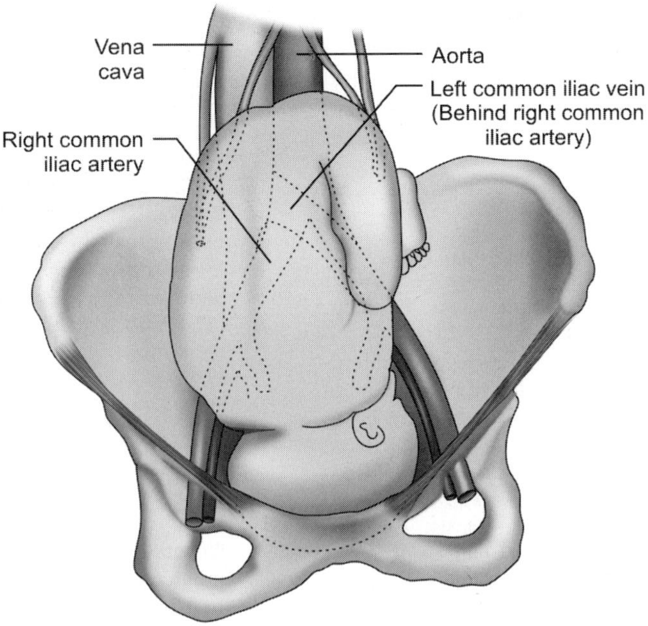

Fig. 9.2 Photograph of pelvis showing anatomy demonstrating the course of the left common iliac vein as it passes posterior to the right common iliac artery

contrast to photopenia, decreased cold spot on scintigraphy, which is seen in early osteonecrosis. MRI reveals increased signal intensity with hip joint effusion, but without a reactive interface of revascularization in the femoral head. Bone marrow edema syndrome has a benign clinical course with preservation of the hip joint space. Clinical and radiological recovery usually occurs within 6 to 12 months, which is confirmed by normal bone scan and MRI studies. Hypercoagulability occurs during late pregnancy with hyperlipemia, depression of fibrinolytic system with increased plasminogen activator inhibitor and decreased protein and antithrombin III. The risk of venous thrombosis in pregnant patients with ATIII deficiency is very high and exposure to multiple factors triggers and activates the intravascular coagulation, which results in bone marrow edema syndrome or osteonecrosis depending upon the reversible or irreversible ischemia.

There is another possibility of hormonal infuences during pregnancy. Estrogen and progesterone produced by placenta alters the metabolism in the liver and results in fat embolism. During pregnancy serum progesterone level increases and approaches that of serum cortisol. Progesterone also induces parathyroid gland hyperplasia, which also may cause development of osteonecrosis. It is likely that underlying pathology of osteonecrosis in pregnancy may be multifactorial.

High clinical suspician of osteonecrosis of hip in association with pregnancy, as well as MRI may lead to early diagnosis and perhaps to better prognosis. Optimal management of this disorder is the topic of ongoing debate. Pronounced bony changes of the femoral head and neck, predisposes to the pathological fracture and hence care should be taken to prevent this complication.[11] The standard treatment consists of analgesic medication with protected and reduced weight-bearing and physical therapy. However, infrequently better results may be achieved by surgical intervention with core decompression and bone grafting.

REFERENCES

1. Pfeifer W. Eine ungewöhnliche form und genese von symmetrischen osteonekrosen beider Femur- und Humeruskopfkappen. Fortschr. Geb. Röntgen. Nuklearmed. 1957;87:346-9.
2. Curtis PH, Kincaid WE. Transitory demineralization of the hip in pregnancy: a report of three cases. J Bone Joint Surg Am. 1959;41A: 1327-33.
3. Montella BJ, Nunley JA, Urbaniak JR. Osteonecrosis of the Femoral Head associated with Pregnancy; In Osteonecrosis: Etiology, Diagnosis and Treatment. Urbaniak JR, Jones JP Jr (Eds); American Academy of Orthopaedic Surgeons, 1st edn; 1997.pp.125-30.
4. Montella BJ, Nunley JA, Urbaniak JR. Osteonecrosis of the Femoral Head associated with Pregnancy: a preliminary report. J Bone Joint Surg Am. 1999;81:790-8.
5. Beaulieu JG, Razzaano CD, Levine RV. Transient osteoporosis of the hip in pregnancy. Clin Orthop. 1976;115:165-8.
6. Curtis PH, Kincaid WE. Transitory demineralization of the hip in pregnancy: a report of three cases. J Bone Joint Surg Am. 1959:41A: 1327-33.
7. Brodell JD, Burns JE Jr, Heiple KG. Transient osteoporosis of the hip of pregnancy. J Bone Joint Surg Am. 1989;71A:1151-7.
8. Samdani A, Lachmann E, Nagler W. Transient osteoporosis of the hip during pregnancy: a case report. Am J Phy Med Rehabil. 1998;77(2): 153-6.
9. Uematsu N, Nakayama Y, Shirai Y, Tamai K, Hashiguchi H, Banzai. Transient osteoporosis of the hip during pregnancy. J Nippon Med Sch. 2000;67(6):459-63.
10. Bezer M, Gokkus K, Kocaoglu B, Erol B, Guven O. Transient osteoporosis of the hip in pregnancy: a report of three cases. Acta Orthop Traumatol Turc. 2004;38(3):229-32.
11. Wood ML, Larson CM, Dahners LE. Late presentation of a displaced subcapital fracture of the hip in transient osteoporosis of pregnancy. J Orthop Trauma. 2003;17(8):582-4.

10

TRANSIENT OSTEOPOROSIS AND OSTEONECROSIS

Transient osteoporosis of the hip is a self-limiting disease of uncertain etiology and pathogenesis that affects young and middle-aged adults, presenting as painful limping, and characterized by osteopenia of the involved joint without pre-existing disease or immobilization. Although this condition was originally described by Curtiss and Kincaid[1] in 1959 in pregnant women of third trimester, but young or middle-aged men are most frequently affected.[2] The syndrome consists of pain in the hip in an adult, lasting for a few months and then subsiding completely, without any exacerbation or residual impairment. Hip pain begins without the significant history of infection or trauma. The pain may be rapid or gradual in onset and is mainly felt on weight-bearing.

The pain may progress within few weeks and may be severe enough to produce marked disability and severe enough to cause a limp. The initial presentation in the hip is dull aching pain in the hip progressing over a period of time; with terminal limitation of movements. This pain is worse on weight-bearing and causes an antalgic gait. At rest the pain is relieved and the range of joint movements of hip joint is slightly restricted. A striking feature of the disease is that, during the period of maximum symptoms, there is disproportionate functional disability.[3] After the onset of symptoms usually X-rays are normal in initial period, but subsequently shows osteopenia. The characteristic X-ray changes do not develop until three to six weeks after the onset of pain. The X-rays of the hip and pelvis show the constant and distinctive feature of rarefaction of the femoral head extending up to the neck and trochanteric region.[4] X-ray characteristically shows profound osteopenia and demineralization of the femoral head and neck. There is striking loss of the cortex of the femoral head, which may progress to complete effacement of the subchondral cortex to nearly total disappearance of the osseous structure, and creates an optical void. This appearance is called "Phantom appearance" of femoral head, which is virtually pathognomic for transient osteoporosis.[5] The osteopenia may be severe and at times may result in subcapital fracture neck femur. The remineralization occurs during the resolution phase of the disease. In severe cases the periacetabular region may also show the porosis. Destruction or arthritic changes are never seen during the course of disease. Hip joint space is never affected regardless of the severity of the condition and duration.[2-4] The hematological tests are within normal limits.[4]

Diagnosis of transient osteoporosis of the hip is important because it simulates osteomyelitis, septic arthritis, neoplasm, or osteonecrosis. Bone scan changes occur earlier than signs of on plain X-rays appear. The change on scan shows homogenously intense increased uptake involving the entire femoral head. Bone scan typically demonstrates increased tracer activity within the femoral head, which may extend to the trochanteric region and acetabulum, and is noted much before osteopenia is seen on the X-rays. In contrast to the findings on plain X-ray, the bone scan are often positive in the first few days after the onset of symptoms, and the findings may return to normal as the symptoms improve. The increased and intense uptake in the femoral head is because of hyperemia, because the demineralization is noted radiographically only later, after the increased uptake. The intensity of activity is greater than seen in osteonecrosis. The CT scan confirms the homogeneous decrease in the bone density of the femoral head and acetabulum.[6] Radiographic changes and evidence of remineralization is paralleled with reduction of pain and other symptoms of the disease. One of the infrequent but significant complications can occur in this disease is development of subcapital fracture neck femur. Patients with subchondral fracture take a longer time to recover. There is often a delay in diagnosis as the X-rays are normal in the initial period, but if suspected an MRI can confirm the diagnosis. Once the disease progresses the proximal femur including the head and neck up to the intertrochanteric area gets demineralized with preserved joint space.[7] MRI is diagnostic, and excludes other causes of hip pain in the adult. MRI shows characteristic features of diffuse bone marrow edema as early as 48 hours after the onset of pain.[5,8,9] On MRI in T1 weighted image transient osteoporosis is seen as replacement of the normal high signal intensity of the bone marrow of the femoral head and neck by an ill-defined area of relatively low signal intensity. On T2 -weighted images this abnormal area displays relatively high signal intensity. The joint effusion is often seen, but there is no evidence of bone erosion, cartilaginous defects or synovial masses. Transient osteoporosis may affect both epiphysis and metaphysis but not the associated soft tissues. No focal changes typical of osteonecrosis are seen.

Until the advent of MRI, disorders of the bone marrow, such as transient osteoporosis, had to be visualized with plain radiography or radionuclide bone scanning. Both these modalities, however, provide only limited information. Radiographs demonstrate only mineralized bone, and a large amount of trabecular bone has to have been lost for an abnormality to be identifiable. Bone scans are more sensitive and provide physiological information which is not noticed by conventional radiography. MRI has the unique ability to image bone marrow and its disorders. It is highly sensitive for the detection of soft-tissue lesions with clarity which neither conventional radiography nor bone scan offers. Early osteonecrosis can mimic transient osteoporosis on MRI, but other focal findings are specific for osteonecrosis. The radiological appearance of transient osteoporosis of the hip and osteonecrosis may be strikingly similar,[5] resulting in unnecessary surgical interventions for this self-limiting condition. It is possible to differentiate transient osteoporosis and osteonecrosis of the head of the femur from the plain X-rays, bone scan and MRI. Bone scan picture of osteonecrosis may be similar, although the increased uptake is usually more limited to the femoral head and less intense. Occasionally, uptake of isotope over the anterosuperior portion of the femoral head is decreased forming a photopenic area or cold spot, which is almost pathognomic of osteonecrosis and is never seen in transient osteoporosis. Classically, it is recognized as focal subchondral signal intensity changes. Appearance of transient osteoporosis on MRI[9] reveals low signal intensity on T1W and high signal intensity from the femoral head to the intertrochanteric region on T2W images. This diffuse, as opposed to focal, homogenous lesion corresponds to the area of increased activity on the bone scan. The lesions that are circumscribed by a rim of low signal intensity on T1-weighted image or double line sign on T2-weighted image, consisting of concentric low and high-signal intensity bands, which represent the interface between osteonecrotic and viable bone. It is noted that low intensity signals in osteonecrosis of the femoral head may take several forms, including homogenous regions of decreased signal intensity, in homogenous areas of low intensity, bands of low intensity, or rings of low intensity around central regions of high-signal intensity.[10] Mitchell et al[11,12] reported that MRI is more sensitive for the early diagnosis of ischemic necrosis of the femoral head than bone scan or CT. The article describes four patterns of ischemic necrosis on MR images.[13]

- ***Homogenous pattern:*** A focal homogenous area of decreased signal intensity that is confined to the anterosuperior subchondral portion of the femoral head.
- ***Inhomogenous pattern:*** Larger irregular areas of decreased signal intensity that occasionally extend into the femoral neck.
- ***Band pattern:*** A band of decreased signal intensity that extends across the femoral neck.
- ***Ring pattern:*** A ring of decreased intensity surrounding an area of relatively normal intensity.

On plain radiography in transient osteoporosis there is diffuse osteopenia of the entire femoral head and neck, without articular erosion or subchondral collapse, unlike in osteonecrosis where the appearance is of a mottled radiolucent area surrounded by an area of sclerosis. There is segmental involvement in the anterosuperior subchondral area of the head of osteonecrosis.[5] MRI shows mottled low-signal lesion in T1W images in osteonecrosis and a high signal lesion in the bone marrow suggesting marrow edema on T2 W images.[5,9]

Transient osteoporosis and osteonecrosis of the hip are two separate clinical entities that have several distinguishing clinical and radiographic features[5] as shown in Table 10.1. Failure to recognize these disorders of unusual cause of pain in the hip can result in delayed or mistaken diagnosis and may lead to unnecessary diagnostic and therapeutic measures.[13,14]

The hip is classically involved, but there are reports of the involvement of the knee, ankle, and the foot.[3] There is a related, similar transient syndrome of osteoporosis that is migratory rather than restricted to the hip and commonly affects the foot and ankle and is associated with swelling of the affected part and is called as regional migratory osteoporosis.[3] A few patients later develop similar changes in the opposite hip or in other joints, then the term regional migratory osteoporosis is used.[15]

There are several recent reports of patients with hip pain, focal loss of radiodensity, positive bone scans and the appearance of bone marrow edema on MRI, without the specific MRI signs of osteonecrosis. This syndrome is called transient marrow edema syndrome and transient osteoporosis.[9,16,17] All the authors regard it as a condition which regresses spontaneously after 6 to 12 months and needs no surgical intervention.[17] However, a few authors consider it as an early phase of osteonecrosis which without surgical treatment, may progress to the full form of osteonecrosis with collapse of the femoral head.[17-19] Turner et al[19] reported five patients who were initially seen with pain in the hip and bone marrow edema pattern on MRI, which subsequently showed focal changes of osteonecrosis which was proved by histopathology. It appears that osteonecrosis occasionally manifests a bone marrow edema pattern on MR images, and there is a slight controversy as to whether transient osteoporosis represents a very early, reversible stage of osteonecrosis.[5] There are reports disproving the relation of transient osteoporosis of the hip and avascular necrosis.[5,8,20] The hypothesis that this condition leads to avascular necrosis of the hip has been disproved by various reports and hence does not warrant any surgical interference. This is a self-limiting condition which needs regular follow-up.

The disease usually lasts for 6 to 12 months and the patient always recovers completely. As the pain gradually diminishes, the limp disappears and hip recovers its full range of movements. The X-ray also shows parallel progressive restoration of the density to normal, and the hip eventually regains its normal appearance within a few months after clinical recovery. The disease is self-limiting and disappears regardless of the treatment.

The clinical and radiological features have been evaluated and three distinct phases of transient osteoporosis have been described.[5,21]

Table 10.1 Distinguishing clinical and radiographic features of transient osteoporosis and osteonecrosis

	Transient osteoporosis	Osteonecrosis
Incidence	Rare	15,000/year
Patient Population Male to Female ratio Age	3 to 1 Men: 40 to 50 years old; Women during last trimester of pregnancy	Equal distribution by sex 20 to 40 years. old
Occurrence in Children	Extremely rare	Equivalent to Legg-Calve-Perthes disease
Predisposing factors	Pregnancy	Known risk factor in 80% of patients
Etiology	Unknown: May be variant of reflex sympathetic dystrophy or avascular necrosis	Mechanical interruption of circulation of femoral head
Laterality	Unilateral, may be recurrent	Bilateral in more than 50% patients
Onset of symptoms	Acute	Insidious
Symptoms	Pain with weight-bearing, antalgic gait, disproportionate functional disability	Pain at rest, limb (late finding)
Imaging finding Radiography	Osteopenia at 4 to 6 weeks	Sclerosis mottled radiolucency, crescent sign, collapse of femoral head
Bone scanning	Diffuse, homogenous lesion; increased uptake of isotope	Lesion more localized, may present with photopenic area
Magnetic resonance imaging	Diffuse bone-marrow-edema pattern, signal intensity decreased on T1- and increased on T2-weighted images	Focal lesion, anterosuperior region of femoral head; decreased signal intensity on both T1- and T2-weighted images; double-line sign
Prognosis	Spontaneously resolves within 6 to 8 months without sequelae; prognosis more guarded in pregnant patients	Progressive in 70–80% of patients, usually leading to collapse of the femoral head and end-stage degenerative joint disease
Treatment	Protect weight-bearing and treatment of symptoms	Early operative intervention generally recommended

- ***Phase One—The initial phase:*** Characterized by a rapid aggravation of pain and functional disability which usually lasts for one to two months, and there is increasing hip pain.
- ***Phase Two—The next phase:*** The symptoms reach a plateau in intensity, which shows osteopenia in the proximal femur, lasts for two to three months and clinical symptoms become more predominant.
- ***Phase Three—The third phase:*** Which extends from four to six months after emergence of symptoms, starts to regress and there is reconstitution of the radiographically visible bone density.[22]

The etiology of idiopathic transient osteoporosis of the hip remains obscure and is unknown. A few authors felt it as one of the forms of bone marrow edema syndrome which can be present in a variable pattern[7] like transient osteoporosis, regional migratory osteoporosis where features migrate from one joint to other-like knee, ankle and foot. However,[15] it has been observed that transient osteoporosis is an unusual but distinct syndrome characterized by self-limiting pain and radiographically evident osteopenia, which distinguishes it from other causes of bone marrow edema pattern, particularly osteonecrosis, on the basis of clinical findings and development of radiographically evident focal osteopenia within eight weeks after the onset of pain. The term transient bone marrow edema syndrome can be used to describe any patient in whom a reversible bone marrow edema pattern is seen on MR images. The bone marrow edema syndrome should be reserved only for patients who do not develop radiographically evident osteopenia.

Mechanical compression of the obturator nerve was considered as a possible cause in pregnant women, but was not proved. Lequesne[3] proposed a non-traumatic form of Sudeck's atrophy, but patients with transient osteoporosis do not show the characteristic trophic changes seen in post-traumatic reflex dystrophy, which shows the evidence of vasomotor dysfunction. Usual diagnostic signs of sympathetic reflex dystrophy, which includes, swelling, skin changes, and typical pathophysiological mechanism are absent.[6] The similarity of idiopathic transient osteoporosis of the hip and regional osteoporosis elsewhere in the skeleton[23] suggest the common etiology and it is classified as a disorder of increased turnover.

Some authors have suggested that transient osteoporosis occurs as a result of transient ischemic insult to the bone.[16,24-26] However, histopathological examination performed in cases where patients were treated by core decompression revealed features consistent with marrow edema without any evidence of ischemic changes,[7,27] though biopsy gave a conclusive diagnosis of transient osteoporosis of the hip. According to a few authors transient osteoporosis is because of the transient ischemic insult[15,17,26] which results in only limited cell death involving only the hemopoietic and fatty elements. However, in osteonecrosis the cell death conventially includes osteocytes. The core biopsy in cases of osteonecrosis shows that osteocyte lacunae in the trabeculae are empty, often enlarged while the surrounding medullary spaces are devoid of viable cells. In addition, the spaces bordering the necrotic areas are filled with dense fibrous tissue.[27,28] There is a possibility that there might be a spectrum of ischemia, from a more limited insult resulting in transient osteoporosis to a more extensive affront progressing to bone death and osteonecrosis.[5] Core decompression may be considered in a few selected cases who do not respond to conservative treatment which gives relief from the intractable pain, but does not alter the course of disease.[5,7]

The mainstay of treatment is conservative, comprising of symptomatic relief with protective weight-bearing, to prevent pathological fractures.[8,29,30] Protective weight-bearing is advised during the period of osteopenia to prevent pathological fracture of the neck of the femur.[31,32] Oral, intravenous bisphosphanates and calcitonin has been used by various authors with beneficial effects.[29,30,33,34] With conservative treatment, the duration of symptoms can be reduced by oral or intravenous bisphosphanates as per various reports.[30,34-38]

Core decompression has been performed to prevent progression to osteonecrosis since many authors believe transient osteoporosis of the hip to be a precursor of avascular necrosis of the head of the femur,[30] but this is an unwarranted procedure as there are various studies which have proved the benign nature of transient osteoporosis.[8,9,19] Patients can be managed conservatively without surgical intervention and need to be followed up periodically with imaging.[30]

■ REFERENCES

1. Curtis PH, Kincaid WE. Transitory demineralization of the hip in pregnancy: a report of three cases. J Bone Joint Surg Am. 1959:41A:1327-33.
2. Pantazopoulos T, Exarchou E, Hartofilakidis-Garofalidis G. Idiopathic Transient osteoporosis of hip. J Bone Joint Surg Am. 1973;55A:315-21.

3. Lequesne M. Transient osteoporosis of hip: a non traumatic variety of Sudeck's atrophy. Ann Rheum Dis. 1968;27:463-71.

4. McCarthy EF. The pathology of transient regional osteoporosis. Iowa Orthop J. 1998;18:35-42.

5. Guerra JJ, Steinberg ME. Distinguishing transient osteoporosis from avascular necrosis of the hip. J Bone Joint Am. 1995;77A:616-24.

6. Kaplan SS, Stegman CJ. Transient osteoporosis of the hip; J Bone Joint Surg Am. 1985;67A:490-3.

7. Gupta P, Sharma S, Gupta S, Singh D, Agarwal A, Chauhan V. Transient osteoporosis of hip: a case report. Indian J Orthop. 2005;39(4):257-2597.

8. Balakrishnan A, Schemitsch EH, Pearce D, McKee MD. Distinguishing transient osteoporosis of the hip from avascular necrosis. Can J Surg. 2003;46(3):187-92.

9. Bloem JL. Transient osteoporosis of the hip: MR imaging. Radiology. 1988;167:753-5.

10. Robinson HJ Jr, Hartleben PD, Lund G, Schreiman J. Evaluation of Magnetic resonance imaging in the diagnosis of osteonecrosis of the femoral head. J Bone Joint Surg Am. 1989;71A:650-63.

11. Mitchell MD, Kundel HL, Steinberg ME, Kressel HY, Alavi A, Axel L. Avascular necrosis of the hip: Comparison of MR, CT and Scintigraphy. Am J Radiol. 1986;147:67-71.

12. Mitchell DG, Rao VM, Dalinka M, Spritzer CE, Axel L, Gefter W, et al. Hematopoietic and fatty bone marrow distribution in normal and ischemic hip. New observation with 1.5-T MR imaging. Radiology. 1986;161:199-202.

13. Seiler JG, Christie MJ, Homra L. Correlation of findings of magnetic resonance imaging with those of bone biopsy in patients who have stage I or II ischemic necrosis of femoral head. J Bone Joint Surg Am. 1989;71A:28-32.

14. Shifrin LZ, Reis ND, Zinman H, Besser MI. Idiopathic transient osteoporosis of the hip. J Bone Joint Surg Br. 1987;69B(5):769-73.

15. Hayes CW, Conway WF, Daniel WW. MR imaging of bone- Marrow edema pattern: transient osteoporosis, transient bone marrow edema syndrome, or osteonecrosis. Radiographics. 1993;13:1001-11.

16. Takatori Y, Kokubo T, Ninomiya S, Nakamura T, Okutsu I, Kamogawa M. Transient osteoporosis of the hip: Magnetic resonance imaging. Clin Orthop. 1991;271:190-4.

17. Hofmann S, Engel A, Neuhold A, Leder K, Kramer J, Plenk Jr H. Bone marrow oedema syndrome and transient osteoporosis of the hip. J Bone Joint Surg Br. 1993;75B:210-3.

18. Mitchell DG. Using MR imaging to probe the pathophysiology of osteonecrosis. Radiology. 1989;171:25-6.

19. Turner DA, Templeton AC, Seizer PM, Rosenberg AG, Petasnick JP. Femoral Capital osteonecrosis: MR finding of diffuse marrow abnormalities without focal lesions. Radiology. 1989;171:135-40.

20. Koo KH, Ahn IO, Song HR, Kim SY, Jones JP. Increased perfusion of the femoral head in transient bone marrow edema syndrome. Clin Orthop. 2002;402:171-5.

21. Schapira D. Transient osteoporosis of the hip. Sem Arthriti and Rheumat. 1992;22:98-105.

22. Ergun T, Lakadamyali H. The relationship between MRI findings and duration of symptoms in transient osteoporosis of the hip. Acta Orthop Turc. 2008;42(1):10-5.

23. Arnstein AR. Regional osteoporosis, Ortho Clin North America. 1972;3:585-600.

24. Chan TW, Dalinka MK, Steinberg ME, Kressel HY. MRI appearance of femoral head osteonecrosis following core decompression and bone grafting. Skeletal Radiol. 1991;20:103-7.

25. Hunder GG, Kelly PJ. Roentgenologic transient osteoporosis of the hip. Ann Intern Med. 1968;68:539-52.

26. Dunstan CR, Evans RA, Somers NM. Bone death in transient regional osteoporosis. Bone. 1992;13:161-5.

27. Plenk H, Hofman S, Eschberger J, G Stettner M, Kramer J, Schneider W, Engel A. Histomorphology and bone morphometry of bone marrow edema syndrome of the hip. Clin Orthop. 1997;334:73-84.

28. Hauzer JP, Pasteels JL, Schoutens A, Hinsenkamp M, Appelboom T, Chochrad I, Perlmutter N. The diagnostic value of Magnetic resonance imaging in nontraumatic osteonecrosis of the femoral head. J Bone Joint Surg Am. 1989;71A:641-9.

29. Diwanji SR, Cho YJ, Xin ZF, Yoon TR. Conservative treatment for transient osteoporosis of the hip in middle-aged women. Singapore Med J. 2008;49(1):17-21.

30. Ma FY, Falkenberg M. Transient osteoporosis of the hip: An atypical case. Clin Orthop. 2006;445:245-9.

31. Wood ML, Larson CM, Dahners LE. Late presentation of a displaced subcapital fracture of the hip in transient osteoporosis of pregnancy. J Orthop Trauma. 2003;178:582-4.

32. Martinez MW, Thomas MR. 54-year-old man with hip pain. Mayo Clin Proc. 2005;80(6):803-6.

33. Varenna M, Zucchi F, Binelli L, Failoni S, Gallazzi M, Sinigaglia L. Intravenous pamidronate in the treatment of transient osteoporosis of the hip. Bone. 2002;31(1):96-101.

34. Kibbi L, Touma Z, Khoury N, Arayssi T. Oral bisphosphonates in treatment of transient osteoporosis. Clin Rheumatol. 2008;27:529-32.

35. Cahir JG, Toms AP. Regional migratory osteoporosis. Eur J Radiol. 2008;67:2-10.

36. Bramlett KW, Killian JT, Nasca RJ, Daniel WW. Transient osteoporosis. Clin Orthop. 1987;222:197-202.

37. Karagkevrekis CB, Ainscow DAP. Transient osteoporosis of the hip associated with osteogenesis imperfecta. J Bone Joint Surg Br. 1998;80B:54-5.

38. Lakhanpal S, Ginsberg WW, Luthra HS, Hunder GG. Transient regional osteoporosis. Ann Intern Med. 1987;106:444-50.

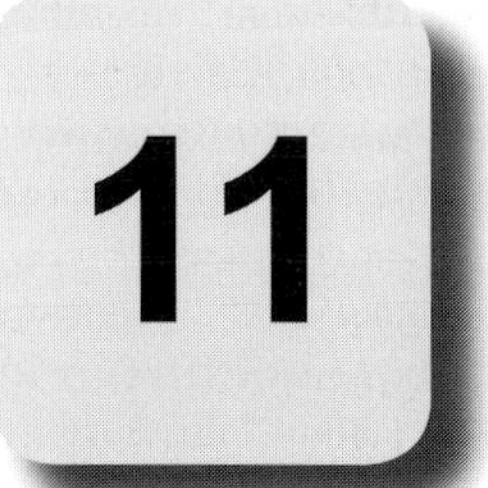

11

TREATMENT: CONSERVATIVE AND SURGICAL

Before entering into a description of some of the treatments available for osteonecrosis, it is important to understand the concept of the risk-benefit ratio. Any surgical procedure has a certain element of risk involved. Even no treatment at all has the risk that the disease will progress, so doing nothing is not risk free. Some procedures may have a lower likelihood of success but have very little risk. Other procedures may have a higher degree of success, but also have a higher degree of risk. The physician must work with the patient in assessing all the factors that evaluate both risk and benefit for the patient in their particular circumstance. What is right for one patient may be absolutely wrong for another. This is particularly true for osteonecrosis because each patient presents with a unique set of factors (age, associated disease, specific joints involved, extent and progression of disease). Any treatment needs to be determined between the patient and the treating surgeon.

The rationale for the treatment of osteo-necrosis of the femoral head requires a lot of consideration.[1,2] Of prime importance in this is the age of the patient, whether both hips are affected, etiology of the associated diseases, demands and requirement of the patient, the stage of the disease when the patient presents for treatment is equally important. The treatment should be planned according to ARCO's classification and Steinberg staging.[3,4]

More than 85 percent patients had collapse of femoral head at two years when symptomatic hips with stage I and II were left untreated. More studies have shown that non-operative treatment yields poor results.

PHARMACEUTICAL TREATMENT

There are no established pharmaceuticals (drugs) for the prevention or treatment of osteonecrosis. In order to treat the disease, we must first understand how the disease develops. In spite of considerable effort by researchers, we still do not know for sure what causes some forms of osteonecrosis (that is, the forms that are not a result of a fracture or radiation). Several risk factors, are defined, but it is not known what effect eliminating or treating the risk factors has on the disease once the disease has begun. However, this is not meant to be a pessimistic outlook for the pharmaceutical treatment of osteonecrosis. Pharmacologic treatment of osteonecrosis remains very limited. Cui et al.[5] demonstrated the effectiveness of antilipid agents in treating steroid-induced osteonecrosis in a chicken model, and Pritchett[6] found that statins were effective in humans receiving steroids. Although osteonecrosis is the result of various conditions, the common final pathway leading to collapse of the femoral head is an uncoupling of the rates of osteoclastic bone resorption and osteoblastic bone regeneration. It is reasoned that by inhibiting the activity of the osteoclasts, collapse of the femoral head might be delayed or even prevented. Alendronate, a bisphosphonate, reduces osteoclast activity and inhibits bone turnover.[7-10]

There are several studies that are being undertaken to evaluate the potential of pharmaceutical treatment. There are several levels of evidence that can be used to support a position by the medical community. They range from the treatment of one patient (a case report) to comprehensive studies evaluating large numbers of patients. Most of the studies concerning the pharmaceutical treatment of osteonecrosis fall somewhere in between—with many being a report of a series of patients treated with a medication with no control group receiving a placebo. It is important to understand this so that you can place the significance of these reports in their proper context. Only a few authors have reported attempts to treat early avascular necrosis with drugs (Hydergine ergoloid mesylates, naftidrofuryl and vincamine), all in studies performed in an uncontrolled manner. Naftidrofuryl reduced bone-marrow pressure in six of nine patients, while systemic pressure was not altered.[11] Eighteen patients with avascular necrosis, who were managed with oral administration of nifedipine had a reduction in pain as determined with the visual-analog scale and as compared with a control group of seven patients who had osteoarthrosis.[12] Preliminary investigation of vasoactive and lipid-lowering agents in the treatment of this disease is ongoing at several centers.[13-15] Early results have shown some diminution in pain in the hip in five patients who were managed with stanozolol, an anabolic steroid that enhances fibninolysis.[13,14]

LIPID-LOWERING AGENTS

Two hypotheses concerning osteonecrosis relate to lipids (fats). One hypothesis proposes that there is an increase in the number of fat cells (lipocytes) in the bone marrow of the diseased joint. Another hypothesis is that there is an increase in the amount of fat contained within cells that eventually causes the cell to malfunction or die.[5,6,15] With this in mind, scientists have investigated whether lipid-clearing agents can be used to prevent the development of osteonecrosis. In a clinical study of 284 patients taking high-dose corticosteroids—the type of steroid used to treat inflammation, a lower incidence of osteonecrosis (1%) was found than is usually reported for this patient population (3–20%).[6,16] Further studies are needed to confirm or disprove these findings.

Anticoagulants

There is increasing evidence that there are abnormal levels of specific factors involved in the coagulation/blood clotting system in some patients with osteonecrosis.[17,18] One study evaluated the use of stanozolol, an anabolic steroid, in five patients.[19] They had variable results with several patients having relief of pain yet progression of the disease as observed by X-rays. In a separate study, 28 patients (35 hips) were treated for 12 weeks with enoxaparin, a drug used to prevent clotting or prevent existing clots from getting larger (an anticoagulant).[14] After two years, most of the hips had not progressed past the early stage of the disease (Ficat Stage I or II) and most (31/35) did not require surgery. Further studies are needed to confirm or disprove these findings.

Hypertensive Medications

Hypertensive medications are drugs used to treat high blood pressure. Several studies have shown that osteonecrosis is associated with an increase in the pressure within the affected bone. The early surgical treatment advocated for osteonecrosis is core decompression. It is believed that a core decompression relieves the pressure and thereby relieves the pain. A similar but another approach to this would be to treat the patient with blood pressure lowering medications. In one study, 17 patients with early stage osteonecrosis underwent treatment with ilioprost, a vasodilator – a drug used to reduce high blood pressure.[20] At one year, function and pain levels improved for these patients. The average clinical assessment scores were significantly improved following treatment. They also found that the amount of bone edema present in the bone was significantly reduced. Similar results were found for another drug, nifedipine. Further studies are needed to confirm or disprove these findings.

Bisphosphonates

Bisphosphonates are a class of drugs that have been used to treat osteoporosis—a disease that is characterized by a low bone mass. Recently, in an effort to reduce bone loss, one bisphosphonate—alendronate has been evaluated in 60 patients diagnosed with osteonecrosis of the hip.[8,9] All patients had symptomatic improvement at one year. Although, the follow-up time ranged from three months to five years, only six patients (ten hips) progressed to the point of needing surgery. It is important to note that these patients were also instructed to avoid bearing weight on their affected hip. Alendronate, a bisphosphonate, reduces osteoclast activity and inhibits bone turnover.[7] It is widely used in the treatment of osteoporosis and has been shown to decrease the prevalence of vertebral compression Alendronate, a bisphosphonate compound, inhibits the resorptive action of mature osteoclasts. It increases apoptosis of osteoclasts and may reduce apoptosis in osteoblasts and osteocytes,[7] thereby reducing the turnover rate of bone. Alendronate appeared to prevent early collapse of the femoral head in hips with Steinberg stage-II or IIIC nontraumatic osteonecrosis. A longer duration of follow-up is needed to confirm whether alendronate prevents or only retards collapse.

Recently, concern has been raised relating to a possible association between bisphosphonate therapy and an increased incidence of osteonecrosis of the jaw. Further study is needed to clarify this possible complication.

Protected Weight-bearing

More than 85 percent patients had collapse of the femoral head at two years when symptomatic hips with Stage I & II were left untreated.[21-26] More studies have shown that nonoperative treatment yields poor results. The only condition for which protected weight-bearing might be effective is a Type A lesion – involvement of the medial aspect of the femoral head. No drugs have been useful and specific in the treatment of osteonecrosis.[27]

Canes, crutches or a walker are useful in alleviating the pain associated with osteonecrosis. They can also be useful in protecting the joint between the time of diagnosis and scheduling of elective surgery. Limiting weight-bearing may also play a role in limiting progression while associated medical conditions are managed. However, protected weight-bearing alone is never an adequate treatment for osteonecrosis nor will it result in cure of the condition, no matter how long it is maintained. Rarely, an associated medical condition may result in a patient not being able to have surgery. In this case, protected weight-bearing may be recommended for pain management.

Electrical Stimulation

Experimentally, electrical stimulation has been shown to enhance osteogenesis and neovascularization, it alters the osseous turnover. Three different methods have been used.

- Noninvasive pulsed electromagnetic field stimulation
- Direct current stimulation of the necrotic area through electrode after core decompression
- Noninvasive direct current stimulation after core decompression.

Eftekhar et al. in 1983, reported the use of pulsed electromagnetic field stimulation.[28] He reported that pain was reduced three to six months after electrical stimulation in

64 percent of hips. Aaron et al. in 1989, reported good to excellent results in 68 percent after pulsed electromagnetic field in Stage II and III disease.[29] These results were superior to those in a matched, retrospectively studied group of 50 hips that had core decompression; 22 (44%) of those hips had clinical success at an average of three years.

Electrical stimulation still remains experimental for osteonecrosis of the femoral head in most of the patients and our institute has no experience of this method.

■ OPERATIVE TREATMENT

Prophylactic Treatment (Stage O and I)

Whenever possible one must prevent the disease from occurring altogether. This can be achieved partially in cases of osteonecrosis of the femoral head by avoiding alcohol abuse, dysbarism and the use of corticosteroids in conditions like renal transplantations, skin manifestations, ulcerative colitis, etc. Sickle cell patients should be monitored closely and at the earliest hint of a crisis, they should be hydrated, oxygenated adequately and acidosis must be corrected. Control of alcoholism will definitely reduce the incidence of osteonecrosis of the femoral head.

A patient with proven unilateral osteonecrosis of the femoral head should be observed closely since 50 to 80 percent of the patients develop bilateral affection.[21,30,31] Any symptoms in untreated hip should be considered as high-risk suspicious of osteonecrosis of the femoral head. If there are no radiographic changes, MRI or bone scanning should be done. If the bone scan is negative, patient should be closely observed and followed. May be sequential MRI has a place in this group of patients for early diagnosis and treatment. A few authors advised only core decompression as treatment for reducing the elevated bone marrow pressure and improvement of the osseous blood flow. It is postulated that core decompression enhances the process of creeping substitution to the necrotic area by stimulating an angiogenic response in the drilled channels.[32] After reviewing multiple reports, the stratification of the hips that had a core decompression according to the stage of osteonecrosis revealed better results in early stages. The average rate of clinical survival was 84 percent for Stage I, 65 percent for Stage II and only 47 percent for Stage III of the disease.[27] The rate of clinical success of core decompression in the largest reported series was 70 percent[33-35] and in the remaining series the rate of clinical success was 53 percent and more than 60 percent of the hips did not need a total hip arthroplasty during the follow-up period.

The results of core decompression were compared with those of conservative treatment by two different prospective studies.[36,37] In both the studies MRI was used as a diagnostic tool and the follow-up period was at least two years. In the case of core decompression performed in precollapse stage 75 percent hips had clinical success with no radiographic progression, whereas in the nonoperative group only 29 percent of hips had clinical success with no radiographic progression. The long-term results of core decompression were evaluated in 128 hips at an average of 11 years by Fairbank et al.[38] for the survival of the hip which did not require additional surgery of hip replacement, had successful clinical result of 88 percent in hips with Stage I disease, and 71 percent for hips with Stage II disease.

From the large previous studies, it can be concluded that core decompression is effective in delaying the need for a total hip replacement and is recommended in moderate size symptomatic lesions of Stage I and II disease.

Treatment in Early Stages (Before Collapse): Stage II and III

The aim of the treatment at the early stage is to reduce the intraosseous tension and perform the procedure, which will achieve early revascularization of the ischemic head.

In the patients in whom changes are evident radiologically before the collapse (II and III), Core decompression and various bone grafting procedures are advised, whereas in late stages III and IV, either osteotomy or various reconstructive procedures like arthroplasty are indicated.

Vascular pedicle grafting, muscle pedicle grafting or free fibular grafting after core decompression are commonly indicated procedures depending upon the stage of the disease. Core decompression and free bone grafting—Free Phemister bone grafting by using long cortical graft from fibula or core decompression and bone grafting using cancellous bone graft from the iliac crest of the same side was advocated in the early stages in the past. However, the results of free fibular grafting are not consistently good and the disease may progress to collapse and deformity of the femoral head, hence its routine use is not recommended. It has been observed that cortical graft adds both to the biomechanical and biological advantages which add to the structural support to the subchondral bone and articular cartilage during the process of healing and revascularization after core decompression. After the technique was popularized by Phemister, cortical strut graft have been used by many workers[30,39-41] which are placed into the core tract in the femoral head. Initially, the authors (Boettcher,[30] Bonfiglio[39]) reported a success rate of 71 percent, ranging from 60 to 80 percent. However, a long-term evaluation showed that only 29 percent had good clinical results after a mean of 14 years. The other workers[32,42] have shown less than satisfactory long-term results.

Whenever the crescent sign had appeared without any collapse, it was taken as an indication of vascular or muscle pedicle grafting in addition to core decompression for early and quick revascularization.[43,44] The use of vascularized grafts was initiated in an effort to enhance revascularization and arrest the process of necrosis. Vascular pedicle grafts have been shown to undergo more incorporation and rapid healing than nonvascularized grafts. There has been considerable variability in the operative technique, where the donor site may be the fibula, ilium.

There has been lot of diversity in the indications for vascularized grafting in the treatment of osteonecrosis. In a few centers it is used for Stage III,[45] whereas others it is reserved for a limited number of hips with Stage II disease.[46,47] Yoo et al.[48] in 1992 analyzed the indications and described the technical considerations where vascularized fibula was anastomosed to a branch of profunda femoris. Urbaniak JR[49] reported the series of 239 hips treated by vascularized fibula to treat Stage II and III osteonecrosis. The initial reports were promising, but 29 percent of hips of stage III had to be operated for replacement arthroplasty at the end of four years. Vascular pedicle graft by anterior approach by using part of the iliac crest with deep circumflex iliac vessel has been used in the treatment of osteonecrosis in Stage II and III with good to excellent results in high percentage of hips.[44] These procedures of vascular pedicle grafting require a lot of technical expertise and a lot of time for operative technique. This procedure is a modality for severe Stage II and early Stage III of osteonecrosis.

Muscle pedicle graft by Meyer's (Quadratus femoris muscle pedicle graft)[47] procedure was performed by posterolateral approach and Sartorius muscle pedicle grafting by anterolateral approach in addition to forage previously, but with unpredicted results. But now we routinely use tensor fascia lata graft (TFL) by lateral approach.[50] However, the use of vascularized pedicle graft is more advantageous since a high percentage of marrow and osteogenic cells survive within a living graft, which helps for early vascularization.

Literature

In 1995, Mont and associates[27] reported the results of a literature search of core decompression. They found 42 reports involving 2025 hips treated by either core decompression (1206 hips) or nonsurgical management (819 hips). In the 24 reports of core decompression, 63.5 percent of the hips had a satisfactory clinical result, compared to only 22.7 percent of the hips in the 21 studies reporting on nonsurgical treatment. There are only two prospective randomized studies on this subject.[25,37] Robinson[25] reported 4/19 radiographic failures noted as progression of the disease and 15/19 clinical successes in the cored group compared to 10/16 radiographic failures and 7/16 clinical successes in the non-surgically managed group. In the cored group, three had proceeded to total hip replacement (THR) compared to seven in the nonsurgical group. Stulberg and associates[37] reported similar results with 8/28-cored hips (Stage I to III) progressing to THR compared to 20/22 conservatively managed hips.

Treatment Following Collapse (Stage IV)

It is believed that once the crescent sign appears and there is a collapse of necrotic bone segment, even if it is minimal on X-ray, further collapse is inevitable and the hip joint is likely to degenerate.[2] Any procedures like core decompression and bone grafting which are likely to revascularize the dead segment is not going to be useful once the collapse of segment occurs. Hence, at this Stage IV, the procedure to change the weight-bearing necrotic segment to nonweight-bearing region by different osteo-tomies are performed.[51-53] The principle of osteotomy is to move necrotic segment away from the major load transmitting area of the acetabulum and to redistribute the weight-bearing forces to articular cartilage that is supported by healthy bone. All these patients of osteotomies require a period of restricted weight-bearing for three to four months till there is radiological evidence of healing of osteotomy.

Transtrochanteric ventral rotational osteo-tomies[51-54] in Stage IV are done primarily in cases with collapse of the femoral head without any degenerative changes. At times instead of ventral rotation, flexion osteotomies are done. Basically, in both these osteotomies the weight-bearing superolateral segment is rotated anteromedially in nonweight-bearing region of acetabulum. Valgus/varus osteotomy is also advised depending upon the situation of collapsed femoral head segment, for proper containment of undamaged femoral head underneath the acetabulum for weight-bearing. McMurray's osteotomy frequently done in earlier days is not considered presently as a suitable operation for osteonecrosis of femoral head. In all these operated patients early mobilization is done but nonweight-bearing is maintained for three to four months.

One possible problem while performing the procedure of osteotomy, is that it may create a difficulty for the surgeon in performing total hip replacement in the future if the need arises. To convert the osteotomy to arthroplasty the surgeon may encounter a difficulty in the removal of implant and implantation of prosthesis since it alters the normal anatomy of the hip, especially during the femoral reaming. Hence, proper selection of patients for angular or rotational osteotomy is essential for the useful outcome of surgery.

Literature

Although a few authors have reported results of either varus or valgus intertrochanteric osteotomy in osteonecrosis,[55,56] Scher and Jakim[57] in 1993 found that valgus osteotomy combined with bone grafting was successful in 80 percent of hips of patients who were not consuming corticosteroids. M Mont et al.[58] in 1994 reported the use of varus osteotomy, which resulted in the preservation of 74 percent hips with Stage III hips at an average follow-up of eleven years.

Sugioka and associates performed rotational osteotomy with excellent results in his hands[51, 52] and other workers reported results of 136 rotational osteotomies in 98 patients followed-up for at least 10 years. Satisfactory clinical results were obtained in 85 percent of hips with Stage II osteonecrosis. Hips that underwent surgery in early stages showed better results than the hips operated on in late stages. The incidence of prosthetic replacement after rotational osteotomy also increased with the advanced stage of the disease with 6.8 percent in Stage II and 24.1 percent in Stage IV osteonecrosis.

Our institution has no experience of osteochondral allograft or spongioplasty or vascular bundle transplantation or electrical stimulation.[59,60]

Treatment in Late Stages (Stage V and VI)

If the patient reports very late in Stage V and VI after degenerative changes have started one is left with no other choice than to do prosthetic replacement (surface replacement, bipolar replacement, hemiarthroplasty; total hip joint replacement), rarely arthrodesis or Girdlestone operation.

It has been observed that there is an early failure of THR in osteonecrosis than in age-matched patients with other diagnoses because of abnormal remodeling of bones, and subsidence of prosthesis because of poor quality of proximal femoral bone. Other contributory factors are—on going systemic disease, defects in mineral metabolism, use of steroids, high level of activity in young patients and increased body weight. Hence, we prefer to delay or eliminate the need for hip replacement by performing head-preserving surgeries, since these methods had less than optimum results.[27]

Results of Total Hip Replacement in Osteonecrosis

Personal experience: It is our institutional preference to use hybrid THR in young patients with osteonecrosis. Though long-term results are not available, early results at two years follow-up have shown a remarkable change in the Harris hip score in these patients.

Literature

Early reports on the use of THR for osteonecrosis showed a high incidence of unsatisfactory results. Stauffer[61] reported a 50 percent failure with a follow-up of 10 years whereas; Salvati and Cornell[62] reported a 37 percent failure with eight years of follow-up. In both these studies, cemented prostheses were used.

The results using cementless prostheses have been mixed. Brinker and associates[63] reported 80 percent excellent results at a follow-up of four to six years with a revision rate of 10 percent. The revision rate in patients younger than 35 years of age was 24 percent. Thigh pain was noted in 25 percent of patients after THR using porous coated anatomic (PCA) prostheses at a follow-up of four to six years.[64] Another study using porous coated THR in 78 cases reported a failure rate of 20.5 percent and an incidence of acetabular and femoral osteolysis of 20.5 percent at a follow-up of 7.2 years (Kim et al.). [65]

Surgical procedures of arthroplasty and arthrodesis are indicated in late stages. Following procedures may be indicated:
1. Hemiarthroplasty
2. Bipolar hip replacement
3. Surface replacement
4. Total joint replacement
5. Arthrodesis
6. Excision head neck femur (Girdlestone operation).

Discussion

The need to treat ischemia of the femoral head is becoming more common since many

Table 11.1 Procedure of head-preserving surgery

Sr no	Name of surgery
1.	Only core-decompression—rarely indicated
2.	Core decompression with bone grafting • Phemister fibular grafting • Cancellous iliac crest • TFL muscle pedicle graft • Meyer's muscle pedicle graft • Sartorius muscle pedicle graft • Vascular pedicle bone grafting
3.	Osteotomy • Ventral rotation osteotomy • Flexion osteotomy • Valgus/varus osteotomy • Mac Murray's osteotomy

cases are detected in early stages in young patients. One must consider the possibility of osteonecrosis if the individual has pain in the vicinity of the hip that had history of associated disease like Sickle cell, Gaucher's, Gout etc.[66-71] Early diagnosis prior to the appearance of radiological changes is essential in the treatment of ischemic necrosis. Its diagnosis is based on bone scan, MRI or functional bone investigations, as osteonecrosis is the response to the vascular impairment of the bone marrow circulation. X-ray examination is of limited value in early diagnosis but has importance in staging since it helps in planning the treatment and the prognosis. The X-rays become positive late in the condition after the process of repair has started. Elevated bone marrow pressure is a useful investigation where the X-ray is of little or no value.[47,70,72] It is also useful in early diagnosis of hip at risk in patient with unilateral disease with high index of suspicion especially when bone scans is negative. Core decompression offers the opportunity to study histological changes of early bone ischemia. It also achieves reduction in the symptoms of the precollapse stage of ischemic necrosis. Core decompression is the effective treatment in the preradiological and pre-collapse stage of osteonecrosis of the femoral head[70,72,73] especially if coupled with bone grafting. Certainly, early diagnosis is the key to the success of head-preserving operations. However, the invasive procedure of functional bone investigation (FBI) is no longer done in our institution and has been replaced by bone scan and MRI. Once the crescent sign appears it is desirable to couple the bone grafting procedure with the core decompression preferably by vascular pedicle grafting. In patients with ischemic necrotic segment without crescent sign, Stage I and stage IIA, one may consider core decompression and Phemister bone grafting, since it provides biochemical and biological graft, whereas once the crescent sign appears without any collapse vascular or muscle pedicle graft is a good procedure especially in stage IIB, C and stage III. Once the collapse of ischemic segment occurs all the procedures of core decompression and bone grafting are not expected to do any more good, and at this stage osteotomies amongst head preserving operative groups are indicated.[51,54,74] In such a situation one must analyze the possible future development in osteonecrosis, so that a failed osteotomy does not affect or worsen the situation for performing total hip joint replacement. However, this does not reduce the importance of the effectiveness of osteotomies, since at this stage this is the only type of operation in which relatively young patients do not undergo joint replacement and a benefit of 10 to 15 years can be easily drawn from an osteotomy. Different types of intertrochenteric osteotomies, which preserve the joint, are important and efficient methods to treat the cases of ischemic necrosis of the femoral head, which usually threatens younger patients by its rampant destruction of the joint, which may result in sever disability. Basically in osteonecrosis of the femoral head, which is common in the young age group a conservative surgical approach is chosen[1] rather than a radical approach of reconstructive surgery.

Essentially the result depends on the preoperative condition of the joint and the site of necrotic focus. From our experience, if the ischemic necrosis of the femoral head is diagnosed early in Stage 0 and I, core decompression by and large gives very good results. However, only core decompression should be avoided and it must be coupled with bone grafting in the tract of the core to avoid iatrogenic fractures.

Core decompression may be effective in symptomatic relief, but is of no greater value than conservative management in preventing collapse in early osteonecrosis of the femoral head.[75] Jones[76] in 1993 analyzed nine studies and showed that in 218 of 369 patients where 59 percent core decompression performed in the precollapse stage the prevention of progressive collapse failed. Steinberg et al.[77,78] in 1991, concluded that core decompression provided more predictable pain relief and changed the indications for THR more consistently than conservative management.

It has been observed that there is an early failure of THR in osteonecrosis than in age-matched patients with other diagnoses because of abnormal remodeling of bones, and subsidence of prosthesis because of poor quality of proximal femoral bone. There are various cause of failure of THR in osteonecrosis mainly because of on-going systemic disease, defects in mineral metabolism, use of steroids, high level of activity in young patients and increased body weight. Hence, we prefer to delay or eliminate the need for hip replacement by performing head-preserving surgeries.

Head-preserving operations certainly gives satisfactory results in Stage II, III and IV (Table 11.1). The prognosis of Stage II and III is fairly good whereas in Stage IV it is satisfactory since about one-third of this group are likely to progress further and may require joint resurfacing or total hip joint replacement.[79] For more advance disease hemiarthroplasty, bipolar replacement, total hip joint replacement and arthrodesis are the surgical options. Arthrodesis for ischemic necrosis of the femoral head should only be considered rarely since in a large percentage of cases, the opposite hip is likely to be involved.

Recommendations for Treatment as per MMont et al.[27]

We offer recommendations for the treatment of avascular necrosis of the femoral head that can be used as a general guide and then individualized to the specific patient (Table 11.2).[27] After it has been determined whether a patient has precollapse or postcollapse stage disease, there are many factors to consider that may alter the prognosis and that will influence the treatment process. The extent of the lesion has been found to be important prognostically, with hips that have a mild lesion (involving less than 15 percent of the head) faring better with all treatment methods than those that have moderate or severe larger lesions. Osteosclerotic changes in the femoral head have been shown in several studies to respond better to most types of treatment than cystic changes. Medial (Type-A) lesions have been found to have a much better prognosis than central (Type-B) or lateral (Type-C) lesions of the head. Patients who had systemic lupus erythematosus were reported to have poorer results after treatment than did matched patients who did not have systemic lupus erythematosus.

Our approach[43,44] to the management of osteonecrosis in young adults can be summarized in the Flow chart 11.1.

Table 11.2 Recommended treatment based on radiographic and clinical findings as per Michael Mont et al. 1995

Radiographic evidence of collapse of femoral head	Criteria								
	Involvement of femoral head (percent)	Location of lesion	Radiographic changes	Age (Yrs)	Level of activity	General health	Use of corticosteroids	Systemic lupus erythematosus	Method of treatment
None	<15	Type A	Osteosclerotic	< 50	Active	Good	None	Absent	Core decompression or electrical stimulation or both
Mild	15-30	Type B					Intermittent or <20 mg prednisolone/ day		Osteotomy, vascularized or non-vascularized bone graft
Severe	>30	Type C	Cyst formation	>50	Inactive	Poor	Continuous or >20 mg prednisolone/ day	Present	Total hip replacement

Flow chart 11.1 Algorithm for the management of osteonecrosis of the femoral head

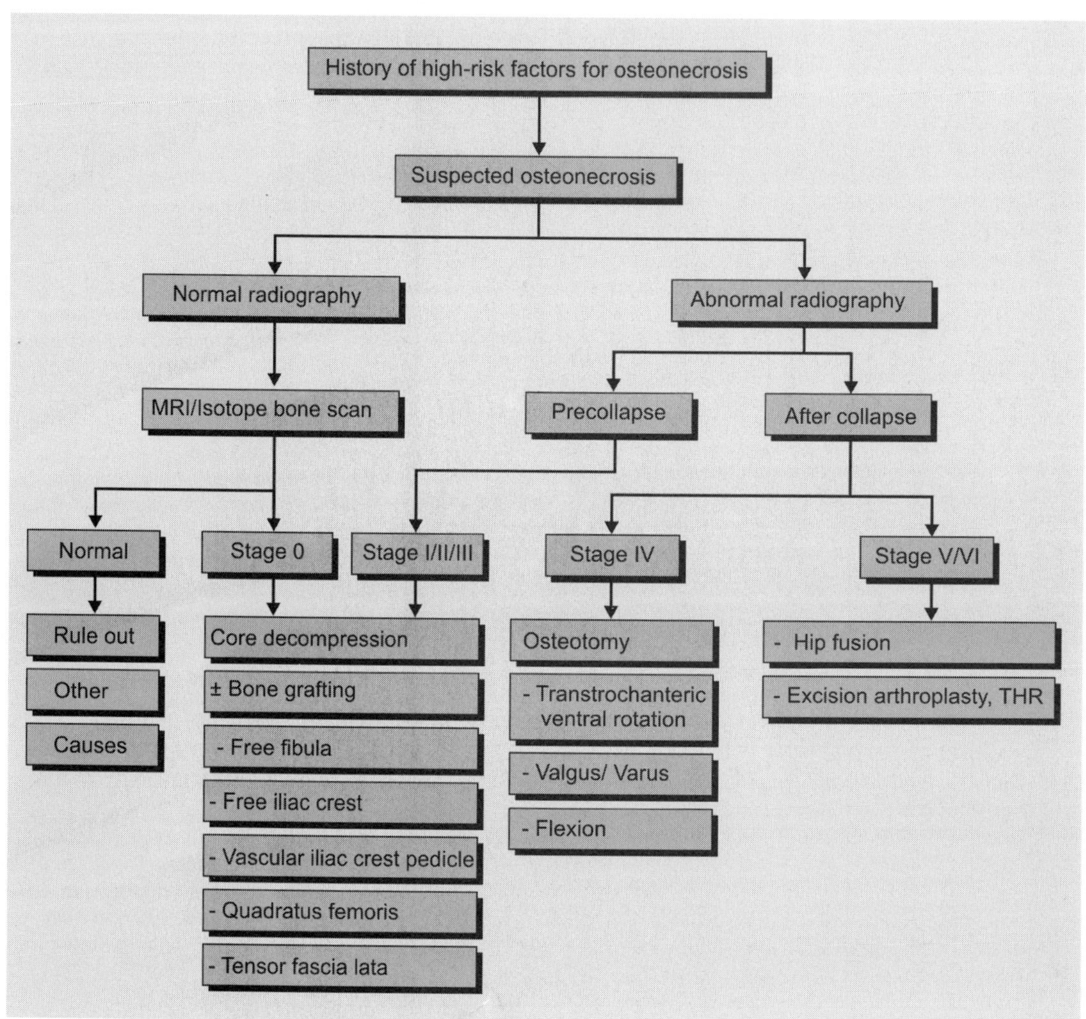

REFERENCES

1. Kerboul M, Thomine J, Postel M, et al. The conservative surgical treatment of idiopathic aseptic necrosis of the femoral head. J Bone Joint Surg Br. 1974;56B:291-6.

2. Kenzora JE, Glimcher MJ. Pathogenesis of idiopathic osteonecrosis: The ubiquitous crescent sign. Orthop Clin North Am. 1985;16: 681-96.

3. Gardeniers JWM. ARCO international classi- fication of osteonecrosis. ARCO News. 1993; 5:79-82.

4. Steinberg ME, Hayken GD, Steinberg DR. A quantitative system for staging avascular necrosis. J Bone Joint Surg Br. 1995;77B: 34-41.

5. Cui Q, Wang GJ, Su CC, Balian G. Lovastatin prevents steroid induced adipo- genesis and osteonecrosis. Clin Orthop. 1997;344:8-19.

6. Pritchett JW. Statin therapy decreases the risk of osteonecrosis in patients receiving steroids. Clin Orthop. 2001;386:173.

7. Rodan GA, Fleisch HA. Bisphosphonates: mechanisms of action. J Clin Invest. 1996; 97:2692-6.

8. Agarwala S, Jain DK, Joshi VR, Sule A. Efficacy of alendronate, a bisphosphonates, in the treatment of AVN of the hip. A prospective open-label study. Rheumatology (Oxford). 2005;44:352-9.

9. Agarwala S, Shah S, Joshi VR. The use of alendronate, in the treatment of avascular necrosis of the femoral head. of the hip. J Bone Joint Surg Br. 2009;91B:1013-8.

10. Lai KA, Shen WJ, Yang CY, Shao CJ, Hsu JT, Lin RM. The use of alendronate to prevent early collapse of the femoral head in patients with nontraumatic osteonecrosis. J Bone Joint Surg Am. 2005;87:2155-9.

11. Arlet J, Mazieres B, Thiechert M, Vallieres G. The effect of I V injection of nafidrofuryl (Praxilene). In intramedullary pressure in patients with osteonecrosis of the femoral head. Bone circulation and bone necrosis. Edited by Arlet J, Mazieres B, Berlin, Springer. 1990;pp.405-6.

12. Laroche M, Jacquemier JM, Montane de la Rogue P, Arlet J, Mazieres B. La nifedepine per os ameliore les douleurs de losteonecrose de la tete femorale. Rev rhumat. 1990;57:669-70.

13. Glueck CJ, Freiberg R, Glueck HI, Tracy T, Stroop D, Wang Y. Idiopathic osteonecrosis, hypofibrinolysis, high plasminogen activator inhibitor, high lipoprotein and therapy with Stanozolol. Am J Hematol. 1995;48:213-20.

14. Glueck CJ, Freiberg RA, Sieve L, Wang P. Enoxaparin prevents. Progression of stages I and II osteonecrosis of the hip. Clin Orthop. 2005;435:164-70.

15. Petri M, Mont MA, Hungerford DS. Pharmacological agents for the treatment of early stages of avascular necrosis. Unpublished data.

16. Wang GJ, Cui Q, Balian G. The pathogenesis and prevention of steroid induced osteonecrosis. Clin Orthop. 2000;370:295-310.

17. Gluek CJ, Freiberg R, Tracy T, Stroop D, Wang P. Thrombophilia and hypofibrinolysis: Pathophysiologies of osteonecrosis. Clin Orthop. 1997;334:43-56.

18. Jones LS, Mont MA, Le Tb, et al. Procoagulants and Osteonecrosis. J Rheumatology. 2003;30(4):783-91.

19. Glueck CJ, Freiberg RA, Wang P. Role of Thrombosis in Osteonecrosis; Current Hematol Rep. 2003;2:417-22.

20. Disch MaC, Matziiolis G, Perka C. The management of necrosis-associated and idiopathic bone marrow oedema of the proximal femur by intravenous iloprost. J Bone Joint Surg Br. 2005; 87B:560-4.

21. Merle d' Aubigne R, Postel M, Mazabraund A, Massias P, Gueguen J. Idiopathic necrosis of the femoral head. In adults. J Bone Joint Surg Br. 1965;47B:612-33.

22. Musso ES, Mitchell SN, Schink-Ascani M, Bassett CAL. Results of conservative management of osteonecrosis of the femoral head. A retrospective review. Clin Orthop. 1986; 207:209-15.

23. Ohzono K, Saito M, Takaoka K, Ono K, Saito S, Nishina T, Kadowaki T. The natural history of nontraumatic avascular necrosis of the femoral head. J Bone Joint Surg Br. 1991;73B:68-72.

24. Patterson RJ, Bickel WH, Dahlin DC. Idiopathic avascular necrosis of the head of the femur. A study of fifty two cases. J Bone and Joint Surg Am. 1964;46A:267-82.

25. Robinson HJ Jr, Springer JA. Success of core decompression in the management of early stages of avscular necrosis: a four year prospective study. Orthop Trans. 1992-1993;16: 707.

26. Takatori Y, Kokubo T, Niniomiya S, Nakamura S, Morimoto S, Kasuba L. Avascular necrosis of the femoral head. Natural history and magnetic resonance imaging. J Bone Joint Surg Br. 1993; 75B:217-21.

27. Mont MA, Hungerford DS. Non-traumatic avascular necrosis of the femoral head: J Bone Joint Surg Am. 1995;77A:459-74.

28. Eftekhar NS, Schink-Ascani MM, Mitchell SN, Bassett CAL. Osteonecrosis of the femoral head treated by pulsed electromagnetic fields: a preliminary report. In the Hip: Proceedings of eleventh open scientific meeting of the hip society St Louis. CV Mosby. 1983;306-30.

29. Aron RK, Lennox D, Bunce GE, Ebert T. The conservative treatment of osteonecrosis of femoral head. A comparison of core decompression and pulsing electromagnetic fields. Clin Orthop. 1989;249:209-18.

30. Boettcher WG, Bonfiglio M, Smith K. Non-traumatic necrosis of the femoral head. II. Experiences in treatment. J Bone Joint Surg Am. 1970;52:322-9.

31. Ficat RP. Idiopathic bone necrosis of the femoral head. Early diagnosis and treatment. J Bone Joint Surg Br. 1985;67:3-9.

32. Springfield DS, Enneking WJ. Surgery for aseptic necrosis of the femoral head. Clin Orthop. 1978;130:175-85.

33. Hungerford DS. Response: The role of core decompression in the treatment of ischemic necrosis of the femoral head. Arthrit and Rheumat. 1989;32:801-6.

34. Steinberg ME, Brighton CT, Bands RE, Hartman KM. Capacitive coupling as an adjunctive treatment for avascular necrosis. Clin Orthop. 1990;261:11-8.

35. Steinberg ME, Hosick WB, Hartman K. 300 cases of core decompression with bone grafting for avascular necrosis of the femoral head. (Abstract) ARCO News. 1992;4:120-1.

36. Dutton RO, Amstuz HC, Thomas BJ, Hedley AK. Tharies surface replacement for osteonecrosis of femoral head J Bone Joint Surgery Am. 1982; 64:1225-37.

37. Stulberg BN, Davis AW, Bauer TW, et al. Osteonecrosis of the femoral head: A prospective randomised treatment protocol. Clin Orthop. 1991;268:140-51.

38. Fairbank AC, Bhatia D, Jinnah RH, Hungerford DS. Long term results of core decompression for ischemic necrosis of the femoral head. J Bone joint Surg Br. 1995;77:42-9.

39. Bonfiglio M, Voke EM. Aseptic necrosis of the femoral head and non-union of the femoral neck. Effect of treatment by drilling and bone grafting (Phemister technique). J Bone and Joint Surg Am. 1968;50A:48-66.

40. Dunn AW, Grow T. Aseptic necrosis of the femoral head. Treatment with bone grafts of doubtful value. Clin Orthop. 1977;122:249-54.

41. Smith KR, Bonfiglio M, Montogomery WJ. Nontraumatic necrosis of the femoral head treated with tibialbone grafting. A follow-up note. J Bone Joint Surg Am. 1980;62A:845-7.

42. Marcus ND, Enneking WF, Massam RA. The silent hip in idiopathic aseptic necrosis. Treatment by bone grafting. J Bone and Joint Surg Am. 1973;55A:1351-66.

43. Babhulkar SS. Osteonecrosis of the femoral head (in young individuals) Indian Journal of Orthopedics. 2003;37(2):77-86.

44. Babhulkar SS. Osteonecrosis of femoral head: Treatment by core decompression and vascular pedicle grafting. Indian Journal of Orthopaedics, January Issue 1, March. 2009;43:27-35.

45. Iwata H, Torii S, Hasegawa Y, Itoh H, et al. Indications and results of vascularised pedical iliac bone graft in avascular necrosis of femoral head. Clin Orthop. 1993;295:281.

46. Meyers MH. The treatment of osteonecrosis of the hip with fresh osteochondral allografts and with the muscle-pedicle graft technique. Clin Orthop. 1978;130:202-9.

47. Meyers MH. Osteonecrosis of the femoral head treated with the muscle-pedicle graft. Ortho clinic of North America. 1985;16:741-5.

48. Yoo MC, Chung DW, Hahn CS. Free vascularised fibula grafting for the treatment of osteonecrosis of the femoral head. Clin Orthop. 1992;277:128-38.

49. Urbaniak JR, Aitken GSE, Nunley JA, Goldner RD. Treatment of aseptic necrosis of the femoral head by free vascularized fihular graft. Ortliop Trans. 1988;12:191.

50. Baksi DP. Treatment of osteonecrosis of the femoral head by drilling and muscle-pedicle bone grafting. J Bone Joint Surg Br. 1991;73B: 241-5.

51. Sugioka Y. Transtrochanteric anterior rotational osteotomy of the femoral head in the treatment of osteonecrosis affecting the hip in a new osteotomy operation, Clin Orthop. 1978; 130:191-201.

52. Sugioka Y, Katsuki I, Hotokebuchi T. Transtrochanteric rotational osteotomy of the femoral head for the treatment of osteonecrosis. Follow-up statistics. Clin Orthop. 1982;169:115-26.

53. Sugoika Y, Katsuki I, Tsutsui H. Transtrochanteric anterior rotational Osteotomy for idiopathic and steroid induced necrosis of the femoral head; indications and long term results, Clin Orthop. 1992;277:111-20.

54. Kempt I, Karger C. Associates: Post rotational osteotomy of femoral head in avascular necrosis. Rev Chir Ortho. 1984;70:271-82.

55. Giunti A, Vicenzi G, Toni A, et al. Intertrochanteric osteotomy in the treatment of idiopathic osteonecrosis of the head of the femur in adults: A study of 76 cases with a follow up of 3-16 years. Ital J Orthop Traumatol. 1984; 10:31-7.

56. Saito S, Ohzono K, Ono K. Joint preserving operations for idiopathic avascular necrosis of the femoral head. J Bone Joint Surg Br. 1988; 70B: 78-84.

57. Scher MA, Jakim I. Intertrochanteric osteotomy and autogenous bone grafting for avascular necrosis of the femoral head. J Bone Joint Surg Am. 1993;75A:1119-33.

58. Mont MA, Fairbank AC, Jinnah RH, Krackow KA, Hungerford DS. Varus osteotomy for avascular necrosis of the femoral head: results of long-term follow-up. Read at the annual meeting

of The American Academy of Orthopaedic Surgeons. New Orleans Lousiana. Feb 26, 1994.

59. Steinberg ME, Hayken GD, Steinberg DR. The conservative management of avascular necrosis of the femoral head. In Bone Circulation. Arlet A, Ficat RP, Hungerford DS (Eds). Baltimore; Williams and Wilkins; 1984.pp.334-7.

60. Steinberg ME, Brighton CT, Hayken GD, et al. Electrical stimulation in the treatment of osteonecrosis of the femoral head–a 1 year follow-up. Orthop. Clin North Am. 1985;16: 747-56.

61. Stauffer RN. Ten-year follow-up study of total hip replacement. J Bone Joint Surg Am. 1982; 64A:983-90.

62. Salvati EA, Cornell CN. Long-term followup of total hip replacement in patients with avascular necrosis. In Bassett FH III (Ed): Instructional Course Lectures XXXVII. Park Ridge, IL, American Academy of Orthopaedic Surgeons; 1988.pp.67-73.

63. Brinker MR, Rosenberg AG, Kull L, et al. Primary total hip arthroplasty using uncemented porous-coated femoral components in patients with osteonecrosis of the femoral head. J Arthroplasty. 1994;9:457-68.

64. Lins RE, Barnes BC, Callaghan JJ, et al. Evaluation of uncemented total hip arthroplasty in patients with avascular necrosis of the femoral head. Clin Orthop. 1993;297:168-73.

65. Kim YH, Oh JH, Oh SH. Cementless total hip arthroplasty in patients with osteonecrosis of the femoral head. Clin Orthop. 1995;320:73-84.

66. Hunder GG, Warthington JW, Bickel NH. Avascular necrosis of the femoral head in a patient of Gout: JAMA. 1968;203(1):47-9.

67. Jones JP Jr, Jameson RM, Engleman EP. Alcoholism, Fat embolism, and avascular necrosis. J Bone Joint Surg Am. 1968;50A:1065.

68. Fisher DE, Bickel WH. Corticosteroid induced avascular necrosis. A clinical study of seventy-seven patients. J Bone Joint Surg Am. 1971;53A: 859-73.

69. Fisher DE, Bickel WH, Holley KE, et al. Corticosteroid induced aseptic necrosis II. Experimental study. Clin Orthop. 1972;84:200-6.

70. Hungerford DS, Jones LC. Diagnosis of osteonecrosis of the femoral head. In Schoutens A, Arlet J , Gardeniers JWM, et al (Eds). Bone Circulation and Vascularisation in Normal and Pathological Conditions. New York, NY, Plenum Press; 1993.pp.265-75.

71. Solomon L. Drug induced arthropathy and necrosis of femoral head. J Bone Joint Surg Br. 1973;55B:246-61.

72. Ficat RP. Idiopathic bone necrosis of the femoral head: Early diagnosis and treatment. J Bone Joint Surg Br. 1985;67B:3-9.

73. Camp JF, Calwelf CW. Core decompression of the femoral head for osteoncerosis. J Bone Joint Surg Am. 1986;68:1313-9.

74. Simonnet JH, Aubaniac JM. The results of intertrochanteric flexion osteotomy in idiopathic avascular necrosis of femoral head - 52 cases - Rev. Chir. Ortho. 1984;70:219-29.

75. Koo KH, Kim R. Quantifying the extent of osteonecrosis of the femoral head: A new method using MRI. Bone Joint Surg Br. 1995; 77B:875-80.

76. Jones JP Jr Fat embolism, intravascular coagulation, and osteonecrosis. Clin Orthop. 1993;(292):294-308.

77. Steinberg ME, Brighton CT, Corces A, Hayken GD, Steinberg DR, Strafford B, Tooze SE, Fallon M. Osteonecrosis of the femoral head. Results of core decompression and grafting with and without electrical stimulation. Clin Orthop. 1989;249:199-208.

78. Steinberg ME. Core decompression of the femoral head for avascular necrosis: indications and results. Canadian J Surg. 1995;38 (Supplement 1):S18-S24.

79. Dutton RO, Amstuz HC, Thomas BJ, Hedley AK. Tharies surface replacement for osteonecrosis of femoral head. J Bone Joint Surgery Am. 1982; 64:1225-37.

12

ROLE OF CORE DECOMPRESSION AND BONE GRAFTING

A consistently satisfactory operative treatment for osteonecrosis of the femoral head in young patients remains to be demonstrated. Nonoperative treatment before the stage of collapse results in a high rate of radiographic progression, particularly in symptomatic patients. Ohzono et al.[1] reported a 68 percent rate of progression to collapse of the articular surface of the femoral head in 1 to 15 hips that had been treated nonoperatively. Stulberg et al.[2] reported similar results, demonstrating progression to collapse of the articular surface in eight of twelve hips that had been randomized to nonoperative treatment before the development of a subchondral fracture.

ROLE OF CORE DECOMPRESSION

Core decompression offers the opportunity to study histological changes of early bone ischemia. It also achieves reduction in the symptoms of the precollapse stage of ischemic necrosis. Core decompression is the effective treatment in preradiological and precollapse stage of avascular necrosis of the femoral head.[3-7] The aim of the treatment at an early stage is to reduce the intraosseous tension and perform the procedure, which will cause early revascularization of ischemic head. In the patients in whom the changes are evident radiologically before the collapse (II and III), core decompression and various bone grafting procedures are advised (Figs 12.1 to 12.6). Presently core decompression and stem cell injection into the necrotic region is advocated by many workers.[8-12]

Core decompression may be effective in symptomatic relief, but is of no greater value than conservative management in preventing collapse in early osteonecrosis of the femoral head (Figs 12.1 and 12.2).[13,14] Jones (1993) analyzed nine studies and showed that in 218 of 369 patients where, 59 percent core decompression performed in the precollapse stage, the prevention of progressive collapse failed.[14] Steinberg et al. (1989, 1995) concluded that core decompression provided more predictable pain relief and changed the indications for total hip replacement (THR) more consistently than conservative management.[15,16]

Once the crescent sign appears, it is desirable to couple the bone grafting procedure with the core decompression preferably, by vascular pedicle grafting. In patients with ischemic necrotic segment without crescent sign, Stage I and Stage IIA Phemister[17] bone grafting appears to be a good choice, since it provides biochemical and biological graft, where as once the crescent sign appears without any collapse, vascular or muscle pedicle graft is a good procedure especially in Stages IIB, IIC and Stage III.[18-20]

However, only core decompression should be avoided and it must be coupled with bone grafting in the tract of the core to avoid iatrogenic fractures.

VARIOUS BONE GRAFTING PROCEDURES

In the patients in whom changes are evident radiologically before the collapse (II and III), core decompression and various bone

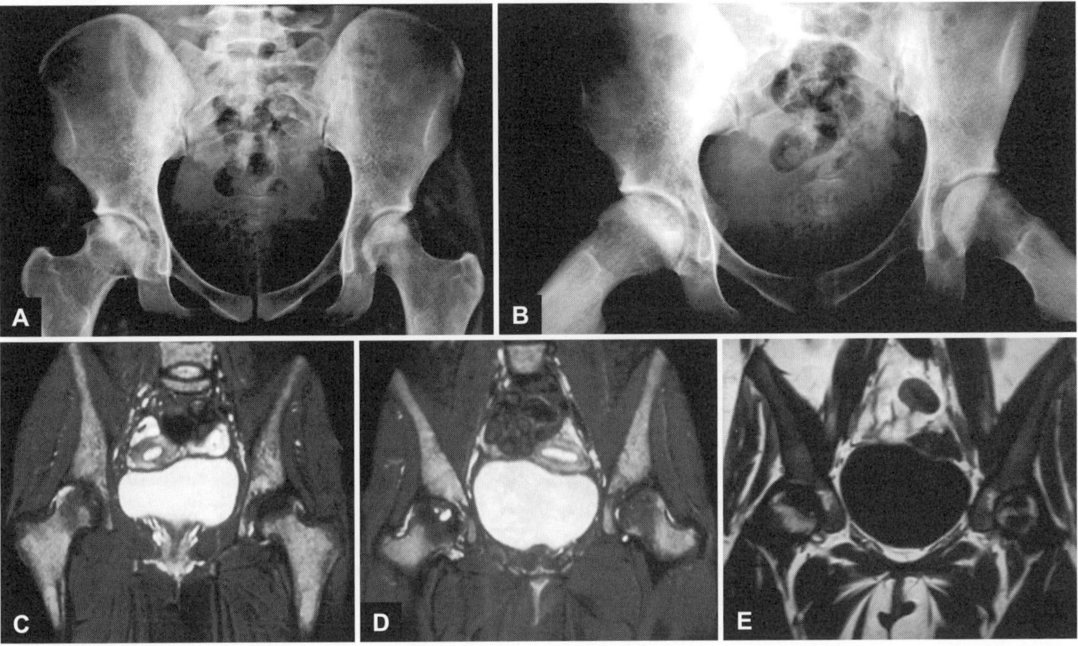

Figs 12.1A to E X-ray pelvis of a young girl of sickle cell disease with Stage III/IV osteonecrosis right femoral head classically seen in plain X-ray with no changes on left side. MRI shows Stage III right side with Stage II on left side (which was not detected on plain X-ray)

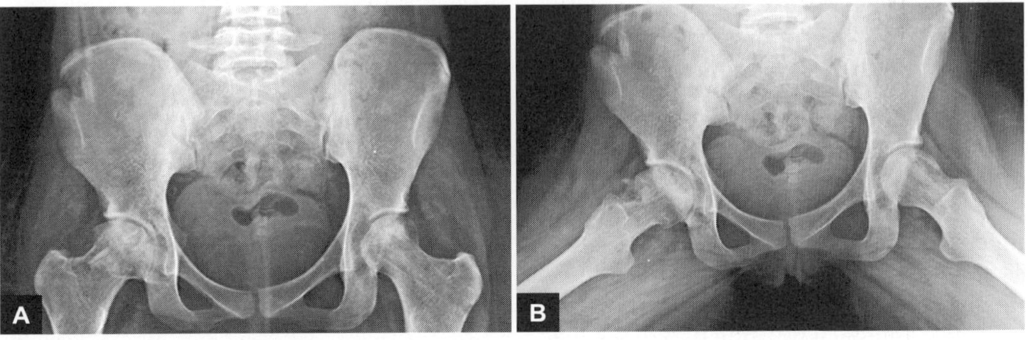

Figs 12.2A and B X-rays of same patient, three months after only core decompression on left side and core decompression and tensor fascia lata (TFL) grafting on right side

grafting procedures are advised. Vascular pedicle grafting, muscle pedicle grafting or free fibular grafting after core decompression are commonly indicated depending upon the stage of the disease. Core decompression and free bone grafting-free Phemister bone grafting by using long cortical graft from fibula or tibia are indicated in Stages I and IIA in-patients with ischemic necrotic segment (without crescent sign), which appears to be a better choice, since it provides biochemical and biological graft. It is observed that cortical graft adds both to the biomechanical and biological advantages during the process of revascularization and the progressive collapse of femoral head.

Core decompression and bone grafting using cancellous bone graft from the iliac crest of the same side is advocated in early stages. Whenever the crescent sign had appeared without any collapse, especially in Stage III, it was taken as an indication for vascular or muscle pedicle grafting in addition to core decompression for early and quick revascularization. Meyer's (Quadrates femoris muscle pedicle graft) procedure by posterolateral approach (Figs 12.3 to 12.5) and Sartorius muscle pedicle grafting (Figs 12.6A to C) by anterolateral approach in addition to forage was done previously, but had unpredictable outcome.[21,22] Now, we routinely use TFL muscle pedicle graft as advocated by DP Baksi.[18] However, use of vascularized pedicle graft is more advantageous since a high percentage of marrow and osteogenic cells survive within a living graft, which helps for early vascularization.[19,20] This is done by the anterior approach by using part of the iliac crest with deep circumflex iliac vessels.

The following bone grafting procedures are advocated after core decompression depending upon the stage of disease and expected outcome:

A. Core decompression only—Rarely indicated
B. Core decompression with bone grafting

i. Phemister fibular grafting (described in next chapters)
ii. Cancellous iliac crest
iii. TFL muscle pedicle graft (described in next chapters)
iv. Meyer's muscle pedicle graft (Figs 12.3 to 12.5)
v. Sartorius muscle pedicle graft (Figs 12.6A to C)
vi. Vascular pedicle bone grafting (described in next chapters)

Various bone grafting techniques have been described, including the addition of cancellous bone grafting to core decompression and the use of structural strut autogenous grafts and allografts, osteochondral allografts, and muscle-pedicle bone grafts.[13-23]

Techniques that are the most similar to free vascularized fibular grafting include the use of structural strut cortical autogenous grafts and the use of allografts. Boettcher et al.[23] in 1970, reported good or fair results after a mean duration of follow-up of six years, in 21 of 28 hips that had been treated with a nonvascularized cortical strut graft after collapse of the subchondral bone, as well as in 9 of 10 hips treated with grafting before collapse. Buckley et al.[24] reported apparent arrest of clinical and radiographic aspects of the disease in 18 of 20 hips that had been treated with nonvascularized autogenous grafts and allografts. Comparison of the results in our patients with those reported by Buckley et al[24] is difficult because of the small number of hips. In addition, their study involved only asymptomatic patients who had Stage I or II disease, whereas all our patients were symptomatic preoperatively and none had Stage I disease: in most hips (84 of 103), the disease had advanced past Stage II at the time of the operation. The vascularized graft may be used either from Iliac crest[18,19, 25-29] or free vascular fibula may be transferred at the site of the osteonecrotic femoral head.[30-38]

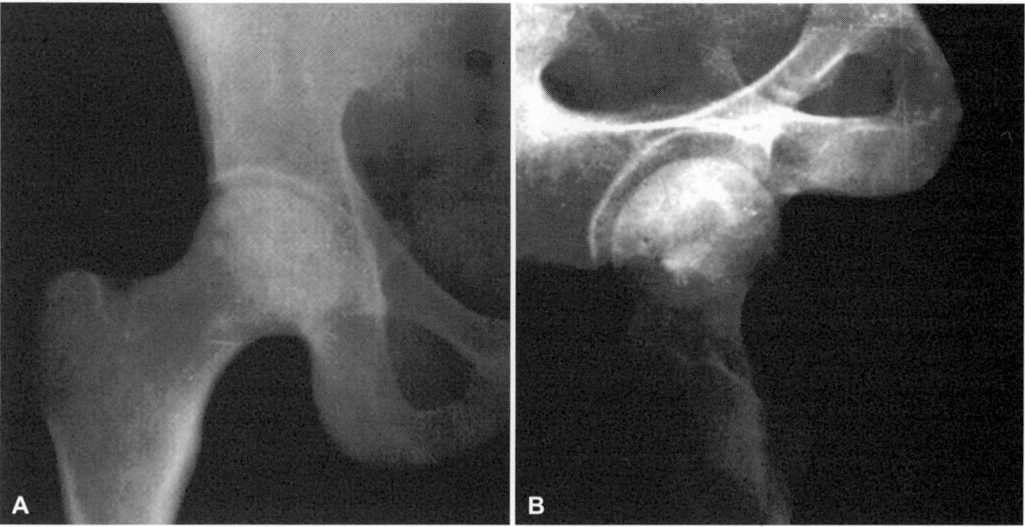

Figs 12.3A and B X-ray right hip showing changes of Stage III osteonecrosis following chronic renal disease

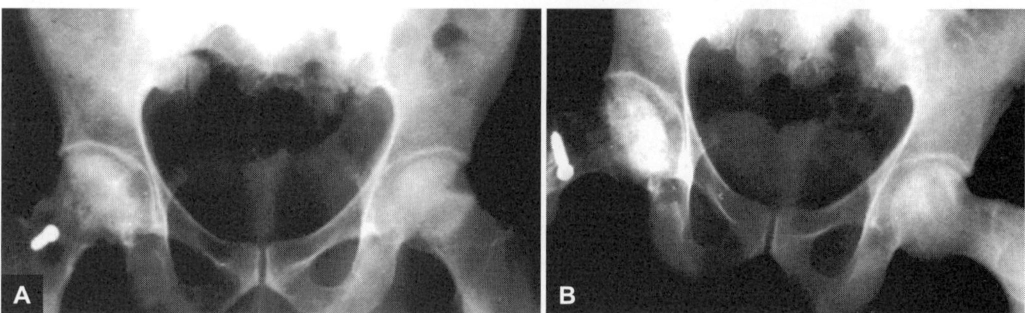

Figs 12.4A and B X-rays of same patient (Fig. 12.3A) right hip two years after Meyer's muscle pedicle grafting, showing good revascularization, no deformation of femoral head

The rationale for vascularized bone grafting is based on four aspects of the operation and postoperative care:

1. Decompression of the femoral head, which may interrupt the cycle of ischemia and intraosseous hypertension that is thought to contribute to the disease.
2. Excision of the sequestrum that might inhibit revascularization of the head.
3. Filling of the defect that is created with osteoinductive cancellous graft.
4. A viable cortical strut to support the subchondral surface and to enhance the revascularization process; and protection of the healing construct by a period of limited weight-bearing. Both intra-articular and extra-articular techniques of implanting the vascularized fibular grafting for osteonecrosis of the femoral head are in vogue.

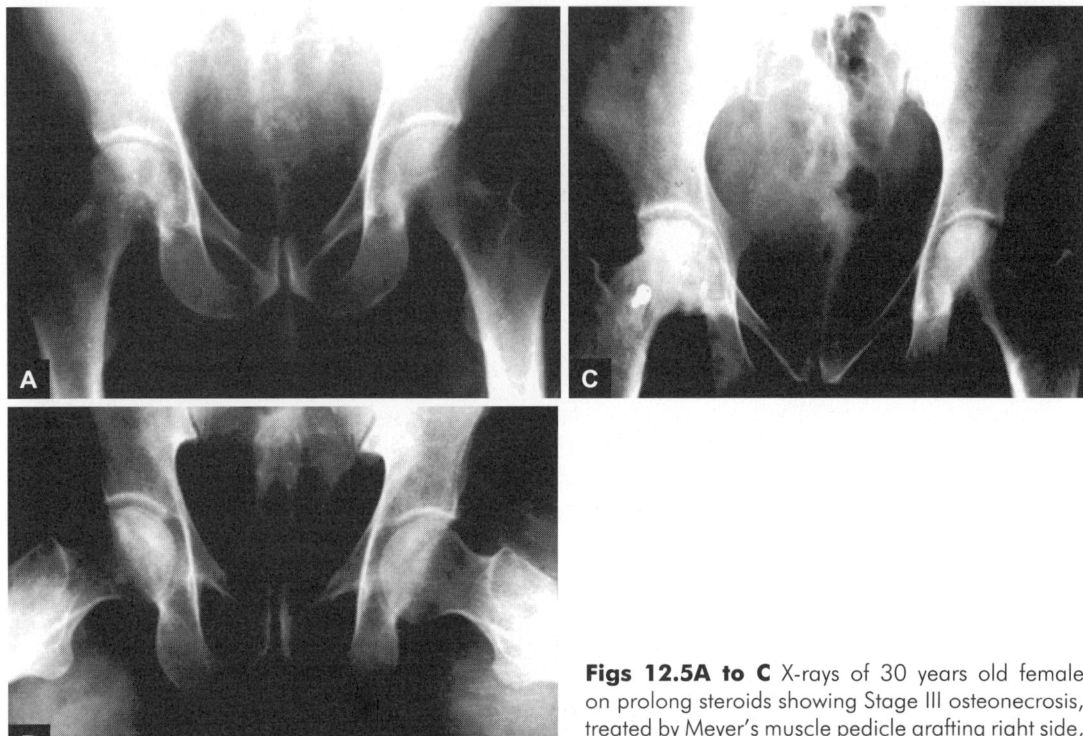

Figs 12.5A to C X-rays of 30 years old female on prolong steroids showing Stage III osteonecrosis, treated by Meyer's muscle pedicle grafting right side, showing good revascularization of femoral head

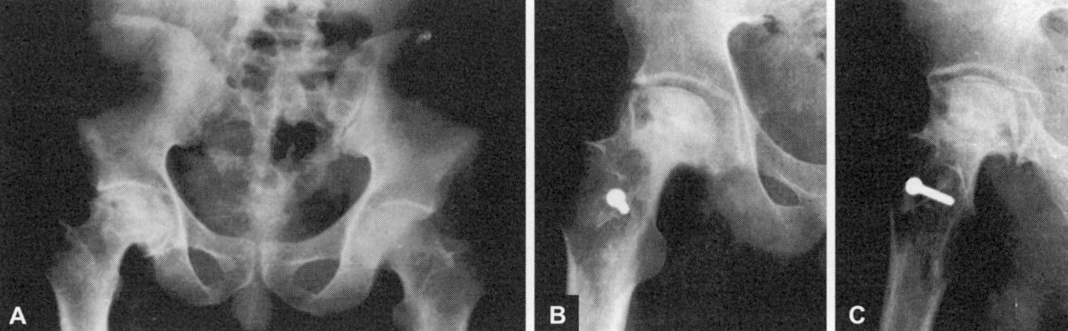

Figs 12.6A to C X-rays of 42 years alcoholic male showing Stage IV osteonecrosis, treated by Sartorius muscle pedicle grafting right side, showing fairly good revascularization of femoral head

■ REFERENCES

1. Ohzono K, Saito M, Takaoka K, Ono K, Saito S, Nishina T, Kadowaki T. Natural history of non-traumatic avascular necrosis of the femoral head. J. Bone and Joint Surg Br. 1991;73B(1):68-72.
2. Stulberg BN, Davis AW, Bauer TW, Levine M, Easley K. Osteonecrosis of the femoral head. A prospective randomized treatment protocol. Clin. Orthop. 1991;268:140-51.
3. Hungerford DS. Bone marrow pressure. venography and core decompression in ischemic necrosis of the femoral head. In The Hip Proceeditigs oft/ic Seventh open Scientific Meeting of The Hip Society. St Louis, CV Mosby; 1979.pp.218-37.
4. Hungerford DS, Zizic TM. Alcoholism associated ischemic necrosis of the femoral head. Early diagnosis and treatment. Clin Ortthop. 1978; 130:144-53.
5. Ficat RP, Arlet J. Ischemia and Necroses of Bone, DS Hungerford (Ed). Baltimore, Williams and Wilkins, 1980.
6. Ficat RP. Idiopathic bone necrosis of the femoral head: Early diagnosis and treatment. J Bone Joint Surg Br. 1985;67B:3-9.
7. Camp JF, Calwelf CW. Core decompression of the femoral head for osteonecrosis. J Bone Joint Surg Am. 1986;68:1313-9.
8. Hernigou P, Poignard, Manicom O, Mathieu G, Rouard H. The use of percutaneous autologous bone marrow transplantation in nonunion and avascular necosis of bone. J Bone Joint Surg Br. 2005;87B:896-902.
9. Hernigou P, Poignard A, Zilber S, Rouard H. Cell therapy of hip osteonecrosis with autologous bone marrow grafting. Indian Journal of Orthopaedics. 2009;43(1):40-5.
10. Gangji V, Hauzeur P, Matos C, Maertelaer VD, Toungouz M, Lambermont M. Treatment of osteonecrosis of the femoral head with implantation of autologous bone-marrow cells. A Pilot study. J Bone Joint Surg Am. 2004;86A: 1153-60.
11. Gangji V, Hauzeur P. Treatment of osteonecrosis of femoral head with implantation of autologous bone–marrow cells; Surgical technique. J Bone Joint Surg Am. 2005;87A: 106-12.
12. Sen Ramesh kumar. Management of avascular necrosis of femoral head at pre-collapse stage. Indian Journal of Orthopaedics. 2009;43(1):6-16.
13. Koo KH, Kim R. Quantifying the extent of osteonecrosis of the femoral head: A new method using MRI. J Bone Joint Surg Br. 1995;77B:875-80.
14. Jones JP Jr. Fat embolism, intravascular coagulation, and osteonecrosis. Clin Orthop. 1993;292:294-308.
15. Steinberg ME, Brighton CT, Corces A, Hayken GD, Steinberg DR, Strafford B, Tooze SE, Failon M. Osteonecrosis of the femoral head. Results of core decompression and grafting with and without electrical stimulation. Clin Orthop. 1989;249:199-208.
16. Steinberg ME. Core decompression of the femoral head for avascular necrosis: indications and results. Canadian J Surg. 1995;38 (Supplement 1):S18-S24.
17. Phemister IB. Treatment of the necrotic head of the femur in adults. J Bone and Joint Surg Am. 1949;31A:55-66.
18. Baksi DP. Treatment of osteonecrosis of the femoral head by drilling and muscle-pedicle bone grafting. J Bone Joint Surg Br. 1991;73B: 241-5.
19. Babhulkar SS. Osteonecrosis of the femoral head (in young individuals) Indian Journal of Orthopaedics. 2003;37(2):77-86.
20. Babhulkar SS. Osteonecrosis of femoral head: Treatment by core decompression and vascular pedicle grafting Indian Journal of Orthopaedics. 2009;43(1):27-35.
21. Meyers MH. The treatment of osteonecrosis of the hip with fresh osteochondral allografts and with the muscle-pedicle graft technique. Clin Orthop. 1978;130:202-9.
22. Meyers MH. Osteonecrosis of the femoral head treated with the muscle-pedicle graft ;Ortho clinics of North America. 1985;16:741-5.
23. Boettcher WC, Bonfiglio M, Smith K. Non-traumatic necrosis of the femoral head. Part II. Experiences in treatment. I Bone and Joint Surg Am. 1970;52A:322-9.
24. Buckley PD, Gearen PF, Petty RW. Structural bone-grafting for early atraumatic avascular necrosis of the femoral head.I Bone and Joint Surg Am. 1991;73A:1357-64.
25. Leung PC, Chow YY. Reconstruction of proximal femoral defects with a vascular-pedicle graft J Bone Joint Surg Br. 1984;66B:32-7.
26. Leung PC. Vascular bone grafts from iliac crest Microsurgical technique in Orthopaedics Pho Robert WH, Butterworths; 135-44.

27. Plakseychuk AY, Bogov AA, Plakseychuk YA. vascularised Iliac crest Graft in the treatment of aseptic necrosis of femoral head; Reconstructive Microsurgery Current Trends Proceedings 12th Symposium International Society of Reconstructive Microsurgery, Singapore; 1996.pp.85-7.

28. Plakseychuk AY, Kim SY, Park BC, Varitimidis SE, Rubash HE, Sotereanos DG. Vascularised compared with nonvascularised fibular bone grafting for the treatment of osteonecrosis of the femoral head. J Bone Joint Surgery Am. 2003;85:589-96.

29. Iwata H, Torii S, Hasegawa Y, Itoh H, et al. Indications and results of vascularised pedical iliac bone graft in avascular necrosis of femoral head. Clin Orthop. 1993.pp.295:81.

30. Brunelli G. Free microvascular fibular transfer for idiopathic femoral head necrosis: long-term follow-up. J Reconstr. Microsurg. 1991;7: 285-95.

31. Fujimaki A, Yamauchi Y. Vascularized fibular grafting for the treatment of aseptic necrosis of the femoral head—preliminary results in four cases. Microsurgery. 1983,4:17-22.

32. Gilbert A, Judet H, Judet J, Ayatti A. Microvascular transfer of the fibula for necrosis of the femoral head. Orthopedics. 1986;9:885-90.

33. Gonzalez del Pino, J, Knapp K, Gomez Castresana F, Benito M. Revascularization of femoral head ischemic necrosis with vascularized bone graft: a CT scan experimental study. Skel. Radiolog. 1990;19:197-202.

34. Tamai S, Hori Y, Fujiwara H. Treatment of avascular necrosis of lunate and other bones by vascular bundle transplantation. In Microsurgery for Major Limb Reconstruction, JR Urbaniak (Ed). St Louis, CV Mosby. 1987. pp.209-19.

35. Urbaniak JR. Aseptic necrosis of the femoral head treated by vascularized fibular graft. In Microsurgery fir Major I.imb Reconstruction, Edited by JR Urbaniak. St Louis CV Mosby; 1987.pp.178-84.

36. Urbaniak JR, Aitken GSE, Nunley JA, Goldner RD. Treatment of aseptic necrosis of the femoral head by free vascularized fibular graft. Orthop. Trans. 1988;12:191.

37. Yoo MC. Free vascularized fibular graft in treatment of osteonecrosis affecting the hip. In The Hip: Clinical Studies and Basic Research: Proceedings of the 1st Western Pacific Area Conference on the Hip, R Ueno N Akamatsu. Y Itami H Tagaiva and S Yoshino. Amsterdam (Eds). Elsevier; 1984.pp.189-92.

38. Yoo MC, Chung DW, Hahn CS. Free vascularized fibula grafting for the treatment of osteonecrosis of the femoral head. Clin Orthop. 1992;277:128-38.

13

CORE DECOMPRESSION AND FREE FIBULAR GRAFTING

Core decompression and free bone grafting–free Phemister type bone grafting by using long cortical graft from fibula was practiced in the early days, before the excellent results of vascular fibular grafting were achieved. However, the results of free fibular grafting are not consistently good and the disease may progress to collapse and deformity of the femoral head, hence its routine use is not recommended. It is observed that cortical graft adds both to the biomechanical and biological advantages during the process of revascularization. It is commonly indicated in Stage I, rarely in Stage II and Stage III, especially when both hips need surgical treatment, which is planned in one sitting (Figs 13.1 to 13.4). Whenever the crescent sign had appeared without any collapse, it was taken as the indication for vascular or muscle pedicle grafting in addition to core decompression for early and quick revascularization and free fibular cortical grafting should be avoided.

The use of a nonvascularized bone graft, as originally described by Phemister,[1] has had variable success in the treatment of osteonecrosis. Marcus et al.[2] reported satisfactory clinical results in 7 of 11 hips at the time of short-term follow-up (range, two to four years). Dunn and Grow[3] reported only 4 good results in 23 patients treated with nonvascularized bone grafting. Nelson and Clark[4] treated 52 hips with Phemister bone grafting and concluded that the technique is not effective once collapse has occurred. Boettcher et al.[5] reported success in 27 (71%) of 38 hips six years after nonvascularized tibial strut grafting. However, in a longer-term evaluation (performed at a mean of 14 years postoperatively) that included the original 38 hips in the study by Boettcher et al.[5] Smith et al.[6] found that only 16 (29%) of 56 hips still had a good result.

We are aware of only one report comparing the clinical results of vascularized fibular

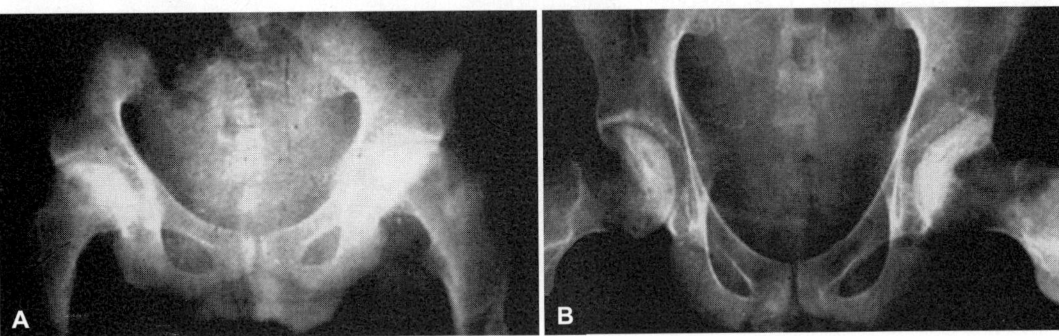

Figs 13.1A and B Young patient of 20 years with steroid induced osteonecrosis: X-ray showing stage III osteonecrosis on the both sides

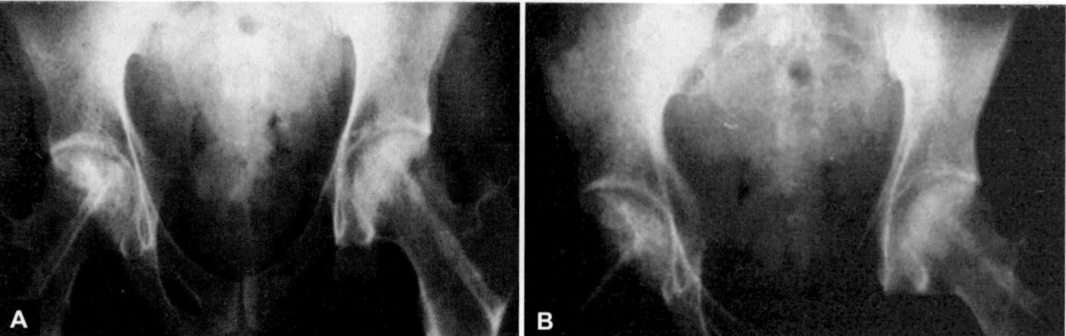

Figs 13.2A and B X-rays of the same patient as Figures 13.1A and B treated by core decompression and free fibular graft. X-rays after two and half years showing good revascularization and incorporation of free fibular graft on both sides

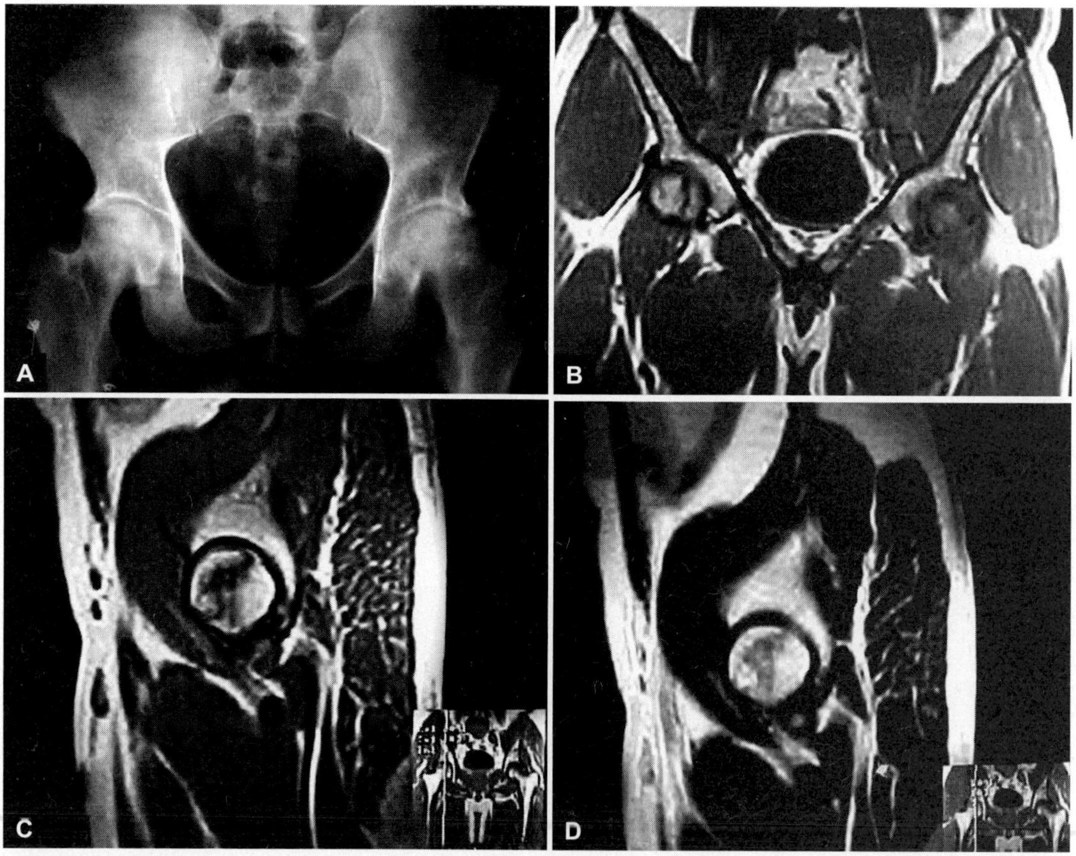

Figs 13.3A to D Plain X-ray and MRI in 45 years sickler showing bilateral osteonecrosis of femoral head, stage III

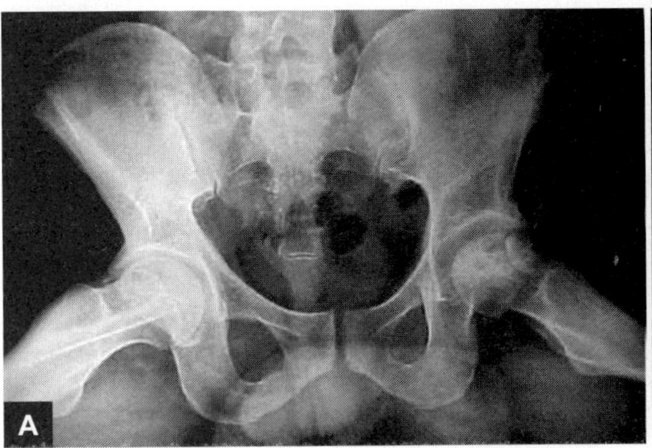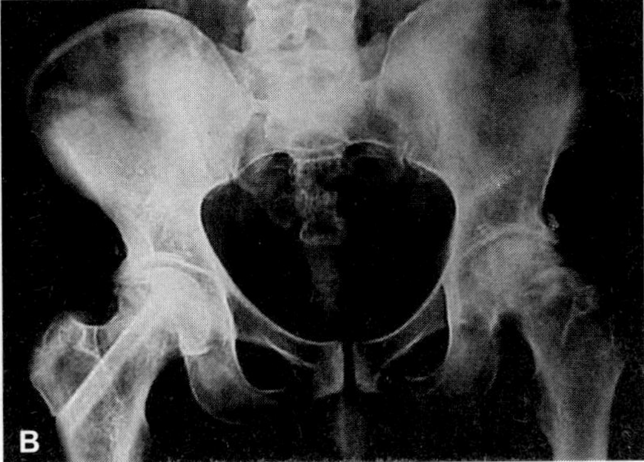

Figs 13.4A and B X-rays one year after surgery—Core decompression and free fibular graft on right side, core decompression and TFL grafting left side, showing good vascularization on both sides

grafting with those of nonvascularized fibular grafting for femoral head osteonecrosis.[7] Plakseychuk et al.[7] evaluated the results of vascularized fibular grafting (220 hips) and nonvascularized fibular grafting (123 hips) in a retrospective cohort study from two institutions in different countries. They matched 50 hips by the stage, size, and etiology of the lesion and by the mean preoperative Harris hip score and they reported the results at a minimum of three years postoperatively. The mean Harris hip score improved for 70 percent of the hips treated with vascularized fibular grafting and 36 percent of the hips treated with non-vascularized fibular grafting. The seven-year rate of survival of the stages I and II hips (pre-collapse) was 86 percent after treatment with vascularized fibular grafting compared with 30 percent after nonvascularized fibular grafting. The authors concluded that vascularized fibular grafting is associated with better clinical and radiographic results, especially when it is performed prior to collapse of the femoral head.

Operative Procedure

With the patient in the supine position on a fracture table, a 5 cm straight lateral skin incision was made in the trochanteric region and centered over the proximal femoral metaphysis. The proximal margin of the incision was at the level of the vastus lateralis ridge of the greater trochanter. The entry site of the core track was located just proximal to the level of the lesser trochanter. The iliotibial band was incised longitudinally, and the origin of the vastus lateralis was elevated in a T-shape to expose the lateral portion of the proximal part of the femur. For the nonvascularized fibular grafting, a 12 to 15 mm diameter core was cut, under fluoroscopic control, with cannulated cutting reamers over the guidewire. The reamers were advanced to the center of the lesion, within 5 to 10 mm of the subchondral plate of the femoral head. The procedure involved removal of a 12 to 15 mm diameter cylindrical core of bone from the femoral head and neck (Figs 13.5 and 13.6). Curettes were employed under fluoroscopic control to remove necrotic bone from the superoanterior aspect of the femoral head. Cancellous bone graft was harvested from the greater trochanter and was carefully packed into the femoral head. The nonvascularized graft was harvested from the ipsilateral leg, according to the surgical technique described by Phemister,[1] inserted into the core, and may or may not be fixed with a 1.5 mm Kirschner wire.

Discussion

Strut grafting procedures, as originally des-cribed by Phemister,[1] had encouraging clinical

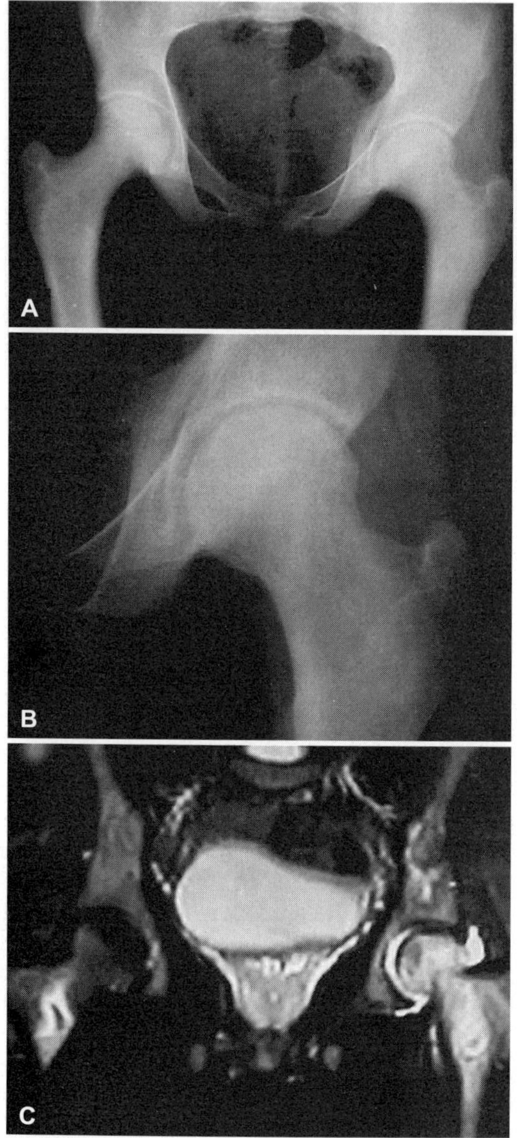

Figs 13.5A to C X-rays and MRI showing osteonecrosis of the left femoral head in young patient of sickle cell disease

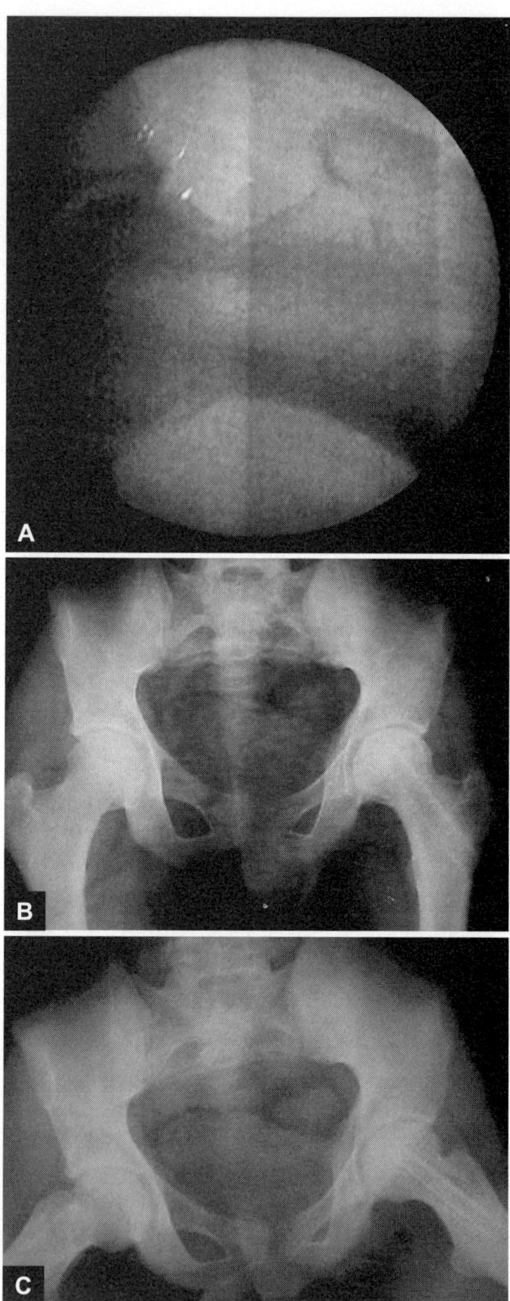

Figs 13.6A to C X-rays of same patient as figures 13.5A to C showing the operative procedure of core decompression and free fibular grafting. (A) Picture showing image picture of core tract which is filled by fibular graft (B and C)

results in early reports.[5,6,8-21] At a mean of eight years, Buckley et al.[15] reported excellent results in 18 (90%) of 20 hips in which a Ficat stage I or II lesion had been treated with core decompression combined with tibial autografting and fibular grafting (both autogenous and allogenic). Boettcher et al.[5] initially reported success in 27 (71%) of 38 hips 6 years after the use of cortical tibial strut grafts. However, a long-term evaluation of a larger cohort of patients, at a mean of 14 years, showed that only 16 (29%) of 56 hips had a good result.[16] Later studies demonstrated a high rate of radiographic signs of progression even in hips with a precollapse stage of osteonecrosis. Nelson and Clark[4] evaluated the results of 52 hips treated with Phemister bone grafting and concluded that it was not effective in arresting progression and its role in the treatment of osteonecrosis is uncertain. Malizos et al.[22] evaluated the effects of free vascularized fibular grafting, nonvascularized fibular grafting, and core decompression in an experimental canine model. Histomorphometric evaluation demonstrated that core decompression and nonvascularized fibular grafting provided poor healing potential, whereas the implantation of a free vascularized fibular graft induced primary callus formation within the necrotic host bone, profound revascularization, and increased osteoinductive potential. Kane et al[23] compared the results of free vascularized fibular grafting and core decompression for the treatment of femoral head osteonecrosis (Ficat Stage II or III) in a group of 40 patients followed for a minimum of two years. Fifty-eight percent of the hips treated with core decompression had failed and had been converted to total hip arthroplasty, whereas only 20 percent of the hips treated with free vascularized fibular grafting had been converted to total hip arthroplasty. The authors concluded that free vascularized fibular grafting had significantly better results ($p = 0.025$) and provided structural support, concomitant circulation, and osteogenic potential. Scully et al.[24] performed survival analysis of 98 hips treated with core decompression and 614 hips treated with vascularized fibular grafting and demonstrated that core decompression had as good an outcome as vascularized fibular grafting in hips with Ficat stage I disease. However, hips with stage II or III disease had a significantly better outcome after vascularized fibular grafting

($p < 0.0001$). Whenever both hips are involved and one hip procedure requires longer time, one can consider free fibular grafting if surgery has to be performed in one sitting, especially to reduce the morbidity. Such examples will be shown in next chapter of TFL grafting and vascular pedicle grafting chapter.

Several groups of surgeons have performed free vascularized fibular grafting in large series of patients with reproducibly high rates of satisfactory results.[25-27] However, the complexity of the procedure, the need for microsurgical anastomosis, and the operative duration have raised questions regarding its efficacy.

The literature suggest that free vascularized fibular grafting provides better clinical results and prevents radiographic signs of progression and collapse of the femoral head more frequently than does nonvascularized fibular grafting.[25-36] A marked difference with regard to signs of radiographic progression and collapse was noted between the A and B subgroups in the precollapse groups (Stages I and II). All hips with >30 percent involvement of the femoral head treated with non-vascularized grafting had radiographic signs of progression, and 15 of the 18 hips had collapsed by the time of the most recent follow-up. Of the 18 hips with >30 percent involvement treated with vascularized grafting, only three had radiographic signs of progression and three had collapsed.

Nonvascularized Bone Grafting

Cortical bone grafts have been used in the treatment of avascular necrosis of the femoral head to provide structural support to the subchondral bone and articular cartilage during the process of healing after core decompression. With a technique popularized by Phemister,[1] Boettcher et al.[5] and Bonfiglio et al.[8] cortical strut grafts are harvested from the ilium, fibula, or tibia and are placed into a core track in the femoral head. These authors suggested that a period of three to six months of protected weight-bearing is needed until there is radiographic evidence of healing. Boettcher et al.[5] initially reported success in 27 (71%) of 38 hips six years after use of cortical tibial strut grafts. Success rates have ranged from 60 to 80 percent in reports with short-term follow-ups. However, a long-term evaluation that included the original patients of Boettcher et al.[5] showed that only 16 (29%) of 56 hips had a good clinical result after a mean of 14 years (range, 4 to 27 years). Other reports have also shown less than satisfactory long-term results. Reporting on a slightly modified procedure, Buckley et al.[15] described the results after core decompression combined with tibial autogenous grafts (three hips), fibular autogenous grafts (seven hips) or fibular allografts (ten hips) at an average of eight years (range, 2 to 19 years). They reported an excellent result in 18 (90%) of 20 hips that had Stage I or II disease. More complex procedures for nonvascularized bone grafting include methods for addition of graft through a cortical window in the femoral neck. As far as we know, Ganz and Buchler[37] first reported the use of cancellous bone grafts through a window in the femoral neck combined with an osteotomy; however, because of inadequate follow-up, their results cannot be evaluated. This procedure was modified by Yamamoto et al.[38] and by Itoman and Yamamoto,[39] who used corticocanellous iliac strut autogenous grafts. Itoman and Yamamoto[39] reported a good or excellent clinical result in 23 (61%) of 38 Stage II or III hips at an average of 9 years (range, 2 to 15 years). Scher and Jakim[40] combined this procedure with a valgus osteotomy in patients who were not taking corticosteroids. They reported a good or excellent clinical result in 36 (80%) of 45 hips at an average of 5 years (range, 3 to 11 years). In a group of 13 patients who had avascular necrosis of the femoral head and who did not use corticosteroids. Rosenwasser et al.[41] combined complete evacuation of the femoral head through a window at the head-neck junction of the femur with grafting with cancellous bone from the iliac crest. They reported an excellent result in 13 of 15 hips with Stage II or III disease at an average of 12 years (range, 9 to 15 years). Another approach

consists of bone grafting through a so-called trapdoor that is made through the articular cartilage in the femoral head. This procedure was reported by Merle d'Aubigne et al.[42] Judet et al.[43] and Ganz and Buchler,[37] and it was later described in detail by M Mont[44] and Meyers et al.[45] Meyers and Conveny[46] have reported a good or excellent clinical result in eight of nine Stage III hips at an average of 3 years (range, 1 to 9 years). The use of an osteochondral allograft to replace the femoral head was described by Meyers et al.[45] in Stages III and IV hips. In one study Meyers and Convery[46] reported a good result in 34 (74%) of 46 hips at an average of four years (range, 1 to 12 years) in patients who did not take corticosteroids. In future bone grafting may become more useful in the treatment of avascular necrosis of the femoral head as methods to enhance the growth of bone through the use of cytokines or improved methods of electrical stimulation which might become the part of orthopedic practice. The enhancement of healing that may be possible with these techniques could shorten the period of restricted weight-bearing and make the procedures more attractive, ensure better compliance, and, it is hoped, lead to more successful outcomes. At present, we reserve these techniques for severe stage II pre-collapse lesions, early stage III lesions, or hips that have been unsuccessfully treated with core decompression.

■ REFERENCES

1. Phemister IB. Treatment of the necrotic head of the femur in adults. J Bone and Joint Surg Am. 1949;31A:55-66.
2. Marcus ND, Enneking WF, Massam RA. The silent hip in idiopathic aseptic necrosis: treatment by bone grafting. J Bone Joint Surg Am. 1973;55A:1351-66.
3. Dunn AW, Grow T. Aseptic necrosis of the femoral head. Treatment with bone grafts of doubtful value. Clin Orthop. 1977;122:249-54.
4. Nelson LM, Clark CR. Efficacy of Phemister bone grafting in nontraumatic aseptic necrosis of the femoral head. J Arthroplasty. 1993;8: 253-8.

5. Boettcher WC, Bonfiglio M, Smith K. Non-traumatic necrosis of the femoral head. Part II. Experiences in treatment. J Bone and Joint Surg Am. 1970;52A:322-9.

6. Smith KR, Bonfiglio M, Montogomery WJ. Nontraumatic necrosis of the femoral head treated with tibial bone grafting. A follow-up note. J Bone Joint Surg Am. 1980;62A:845-7.

7. Plakseychuk AY, Kim SY, Park BC, Varitimidis SE, Rubash HE, Sotereanos DG. Vascularised compared with nonvascularised fibular bone grafting for the treatment of osteonecrosis of the femoral head. J Bone Joint Surgery Am. 2003;85:589-96.

8. Bonfiglio M, Voke EM. Aseptic necrosis of the femoral head and non-union of the femoral neck. Effect of treatment by drilling and bone-grafting (Phemister technique). Bone and Joint Surg Am. 1968;50A:48-66.

9. Warner JJ P, Philip JH, Brodsky CL, Thornhill TS. Studies of nontraumatic osteonecrosis. The role of core decompression in the treatment of nontraumatic osteonecrosis of the femoral head. Clin Orthop. 1987;225:104-27.

10. Ficat RP. Idiopathic bone necrosis of the femoral head. Early diagnosis and treatment. J Bone Joint Surg Br. 1985;67:3-9.

11. Springfield DS, Enneking WJ. Surgery for aseptic necrosis of the femoral head. Clin Orthop. 1978;130:175-85.

12. Hungerford DS. Response: The role of core decompression in the treatment of ischemic necrosis of the femoral head. Arthrit and Rheumat. 1989;32:801-6.

13. Steinberg ME, Brighton CT, Bands RE, Hartman KM. Capacitive coupling as an adjunctive treatment for avascular necrosis. Clin Orthop. 1990;261:11-8.

14. Steinberg ME, Hosick WB, Hartman K. 300 cases of core decompression with bone grafting for avascular necrosis of the femoral head. (Abstract) ARCO News. 1992;4:120-1.

15. Buckley PD, Gearen PF, Petty RW. Structural bone grafting for early atraumatic avascular necrosis of the femoral head. J Bone Joint Surg Am. 1991;73A:1357-64.

16. Dunn AW, Grow T. Aseptic necrosis of the femoral head. Treatment with bone grafts of doubtful value. Clin Orthop. 1977;122:249-54.

17. Smith KR, Bonfiglio M, Montogomery WJ. Nontraumatic necrosis of the femoral head treated with tibial bone grafting. A follow-up note. J Bone Joint Surg Am. 1980;62A:845-7.

18. Marcus ND, Enneking WF, Massam RA. The silent hip in idiopathic aseptic necrosis. Treatment by bone grafting. J Bone and Joint Surg Am. 1973;55A:1351-66.

19. Babhulkar SS. Osteonecrosis of the femoral head (in young individuals) Indian Journal of Orthopaedics. 2003;37(2):77-86.

20. Saito S, Ohzono K, Ono K. Joint preserving operations for idiopathic avascular necrosis of the femoral head. J Bone Joint Surg Br. 1988;70B:78-84.

21. Camp JF, Calwelf CW. Core decompression of the femoral head for osteoncerosis. J Bone Joint Surg Am. 1986;68:1313-9.

22. Malizos KN, Seaber AV, Glisson RR, Quarles LD, Rizk WS, Urbaniak JR. The potential of vascularized cortical graft in revitalizing necrotic cancellous bone in canines. In: Urbaniak JR, Jones JP (Eds). Osteonecrosis: etiology, diagnosis, and treatment. 1st edn Rosemont, IL: American Academy of Orthopaedic Surgeons. 1997.pp.361-71.

23. Kane SM, Ward WA, Jordan LC, Guilford WB, Hanley EN Jr. Vascularized fibular grafting compared with core decompression in the treatment of femoral head osteonecrosis. Orthopedics. 1996;19:869-72.

24. Scully SP, Aaron RK, Urbaniak JR. Survival analysis of hips treated with core decompression or vascularized fibular grafting because of avascular necrosis. J Bone Joint Surg Am. 1998; 80:1270-5.

25. Gilbert A, Judet H, Judet J, Ayatti A. Micro-vascular transfer of the fibula for necrosis of the femoral head. Orthopedics. 1986;9:885-90.

26. Malizos KN, Soucacos PN, Beris AE. Osteo-necrosis of the femoral head. Hip salvaging with implantation of a vascularized fibular graft. Clin Orthop. 1995;314:67-75.

27. Sotereanos DG, Plakseychuk AY, Rubash HE. Free vascularized fibula grafting for the treatment of osteonecrosis of the femoral head. Clin Orthop. 1997;344:243-56.

28. Plakseychuk AY, Bogov AA, Plakseychuk YA. Vascularised iliac crest graft in the treatment of aseptic necrosis of femoral head; Reconstructive Microsurgery Current Trends Proceedings 12th Symposium International Society of Reconstructive Microsurgery, Singapore. 1996. pp.85-7.

29. Brunelli G, Brunelli G. Free microvascular fibular transfer for idiopathic femoral head necrosis: long-term follow-up. J Reconstr Microsurg. 1991;7:285-95.

30. Fujimaki A, Yamauchi Y. Vascularized fibular grafting for the treatment of aseptic necrosis of the femoral head – preliminary results in four cases. Microsurgery. 1983;4:17-22.

31. Gonzalez del Pino J, Knapp K, Gomez Castresana F, Benito M. Revascularization of femoral head ischemic necrosis with vascularized bone graft: a CT scan experimental study. Skel Radiolog. 1990;19:197-202.

32. Tamai S, Hori Y, Fujiwara H. Treatment of avascular necrosis of lunate and other bones by vascular bundle transplantation. In Microsurgery for Major Limb Reconstruction, JR Urbaniak (Eds). St Louis, CV Moshy. 1987. pp.209-19.

33. Urbaniak JR. Aseptic necrosis of the femoral head treated by vascularized fibular graft. In Microsurgery fir Major Limb Reconstruction, JR Urbaniak (Eds). St Louis; CV Mosby. 1987. pp.178-84.

34. Urbaniak JR, Aitken GSE, Nunley JA, Goldner RD. Treatment of aseptic necrosis of the femoral head by free vascularized fihular graft. Orthiop. Trans. 1988;12:191.

35. Yoo MC. Free vascularized fibular graft in treatment of osteonecrosis affecting the hip. In The Hip: Clinical Studies and Basic Research: Proceedings of the 1st Western Pacific Area Conference on the Hip, R Ueno, N Akamatsu, Y Itami, H Tagaıva, S Yoshino, Amsterdam, Elsevier (Eds). 1984.pp.189-92.

36. Yoo MC, Chung DW, Hahn CS. Free vascularized fibula grafting for the treatment of osteonecrosis of the femoral head. Clin Orthop. 1992;277:128-38.

37. Ganz R, Buchler U. Overview of attempts to revascularise the dead head in aseptic necrosis of the femoral head: Osteotomy and revascularization. Hip. 1983.pp.296-305.

38. Yamamoto M, Itoman M, Sagamoto N, Moritza M. Strut bone graft for aseptic necrosis of the femoral head: Theory and surgical technique. Orthop Surg. 1983;34:902-8.

39. Itoman M, Yamamoto M. Pathogenesis and treatment of idiopathic aseptic necrosis of the femoral head. Clin Immunol. 1989;21:713-25.

40. Scher MA, Jakim I. Intertrochanteric osteotomy and autogenous bone grafting for avascular necrosis of the femoral head. J Bone Joint Surg Am. 1993;75A:1119-33.

41. Rosenwasser MP, Garino JP, Kiernan HA, Michelsen CB. Long-term follow-up of thorough debridement and cancellous bone grafting of the femoral head for avascular necrosis. Clin Orthop. 1994;306:17-27.

42. Merle d'Aubigne R, Postel M, Mazabraud A, Massias P, Gueguen J. Idiopathic necrosis of the femoral head in adults. J Bone and joint Surg Br. 1965;47B(4):612-33.

43. Judet R, Judet J, Launois B, Gubler JP. Trial of experimental revascularization of the femoral head. Rev Chir Orthop Reparatrice Appar Mot. 1966;52:277-303.

44. Mont MA, Hungerford DS. Non-traumatic avascular necrosis of the femoral head. J Bone Joint Surg Am. 1995;77A:459-74.

45. Meyers MH, Jones Re, Bucholz RW, Wenger DR. Fresh autogenous grafts and osteochondral allografts for the treatment of segmental collapse in osteonecrosis of the hip. Clin Orthop. 1983;174:107-12.

46. Meyers MH, Convery FR. Grafting procedures in osteonecrosis of the hip. Sem Arthroplasty. 1991;2:189-97.

14

CORE DECOMPRESSION AND TFL MUSCLE PEDICLE GRAFTING

◼ INTRODUCTION

Osteonecrosis of the femoral head is a painful disabling condition seen in association with many disorders like corticosteroid consumption, alcohol abuse, hemoglobinopathy (sickle cell disease, coagulopathies), and renal, hepatic and skin disorders commonly affecting young patients ranging in age from 20 to 40 years.[1-3] It is now recognized as a major musculo-skeletal problem mostly affecting the young people in their productive years of life. It is often characterized by relentless progression despite treatment, resulting in subchondral fracture, collapse and painful arthrosis.[4] Hence it is essential to diagnose and treat the patients of osteonecrosis early to prevent any further disintegration and collapse of the femoral head. Advanced osteonecrosis with secondary osteoarthritis is reported in 5 to 18 percent of total patients undergoing total hip replacement in the US.[4-7] The aim of the treatment in osteonecrosis is to reduce the intraosseous pressure and to perform the head-preserving procedure, which will cause early revascularization of the ischemic head. Various types of muscle pedicle grafting after core decompression are indicated early in the disease, depending upon the stage of the disease and have shown excellent results in revascularization of the femoral head and prevention of collapse.

Once diagnosed it is desirable to subject the patient to early surgical intervention. The rationale for the treatment of osteonecrosis of the femoral head requires a lot of consideration. Of prime importance is the age of patients. Whether both hips are affected, etiology of the associated diseases, demands and requirement of the patients, and the stage of the disease when the patient presents for treatment are equally important. The treatment is planned according to ARCO's classification[8] (Table 14.1) and Steinberg staging.[9] Only core decompression may relieve the pain but it does not achieve revascularization of the femoral head. Hence, core decompression should always be supplemented by one of the procedures of bone grafting. To achieve early vascularization, vascular pedicle grafting using deep circumflex iliac vessel with iliac crest is very useful, but preoperative femoral angiography is mandatory to confirm the presence of deep circumflex iliac artery pedicle.[10] This procedure is technically demanding, tedious and time-consuming and may not be feasible bilaterally in one sitting. However, muscle pedicle graft using tensor fascia lata (TFL) graft is very easy and is commonly performed whenever both hips need simultaneous surgery in one sitting. In the past, muscle pedicle graft using quadratus femoris (Meyer's procedure)[11] was propagated in the treatment of osteonecrosis, but it did not achieve satisfactory early revascularization and came in to disrepute since the results were not encouraging. Dr DP Baksi[12] reported treatment of osteonecrosis by multiple drilling and muscle pedicle grafting by use of TFL graft with relief of pain and improvement in the hip movements. Though vascularized pedicle graft by using part of the iliac crest with deep circumflex iliac vessels is more advantageous since a high percentage of marrow and osteogenic cells survive within a living graft, it is difficult to perform this surgery on both hips in one sitting. As per our Institutional philosophy we prefer to operate both hips in the same sitting since it reduces the hospital stay, the cost of drugs and in many cases patient may not turn up for surgery on the opposite hip, especially the poor compliance group of patients. Hence, use of muscle pedicle graft of TFL along with iliac crest after core decompression is commonly advocated when bilateral hips are involved and surgery is recommended early in a single sitting.

The natural history of osteonecrosis of the femoral head before the development of the crescent sign or before the collapse of the femoral head has never been well defined. The possibility of progression to collapse is thought to increase after the development of an abnormality that can be seen on plain radiographs and such a possibility and the course of collapse may be highly variable and unknown.[7] It is generally agreed that symptomatically and radiographically abnormal hip will progress to collapse of the femoral head when treated nonoperatively.[7] To avoid these complications and to avoid early replacement arthroplasty in a group of young patients many operative procedures to salvage the femoral head are in vogue.

Head preserving operation of core decompression and various types of bone grafting procedures certainly gave excellent results in the early stage of osteonecrosis. Despite the many reports on the utility of various

Table 14.1 ARCO Classification

Finding	0	1	2	3	4
Finding	All present techniques normal or non-diagnostic	X-ray and CT are normal At least ONE of the below is positive	No crescent sign: X-ray abnormal: Sclerosis, lysis, focal porosis	Crescent Sign on the X-ray and/or flattening of articular surface of femoral head	Osteoarthritis joint space narrowing, acetabular changes, joint destruction
Finding	X-ray CT Scintigraph MRI	Scintigraph MRI Quantitate on MRI	X-ray, CT Scintigraph MRI *Quantitate MRI and X-ray	X-ray, CT only Quantitate on X-ray	X-ray only
Finding	No	Medial	Central	Lateral	No
Finding	No	Quantitation % Area Involvement Minimal A<15% Moderate B 15–30% Extensive C>30%	Length of crescent A<2 mm B 2–4 mm C>4 mm	% surface collapse dome depression A<15% B-15–30% C>30%	No

operative procedures, no single method has uniformly demonstrated the arrest of disease or prevention of collapse of the femoral head effectively. Core decompression only gave good clinical results initially (Ficat and Arlet)[13,14] but the long-term results were poor.[11] The use of nonvascularized tibial (Phemister) or fibular bone graft (Boettcher and Bonfiglio)[15] is useful only in the early stages but in later stages, the results were very poor. Subarticular curettage and cancellous bone grafting failed to relieve pain and prevent progressive collapse of the femoral head.[16,17] Meyers[11] reported use of fresh cancellous graft combined with quadratus femoris muscle pedicle graft which gave good results in stage I and II, but was unsatisfactory in stage III and IV. Though pain and deformity improved initially, vascularization of the femoral head was poor.

The vascularized fibular grafting is associated with better clinical and radiographic results than is nonvascularized fibular grafting in precollapse hips.[7] However, the successful use of free vascularized bone grafts requires a meticulous process of procuring the vascular fibula with microanastomosis to the recipient site. The microsurgical procedure requires specialized training, equipment and expertise. The TFL muscle pedicle graft by using part of the iliac crest described in this article is easy to perform and does not require any special equipment or technique, and still has the advantages of increased vascularity like vascularized bone graft (Figs 14.1A to H). We have analyzed and report a series of patients of osteonecrosis of the femoral head treated by core decompression and TFL muscle pedicle graft of part of the iliac crest.

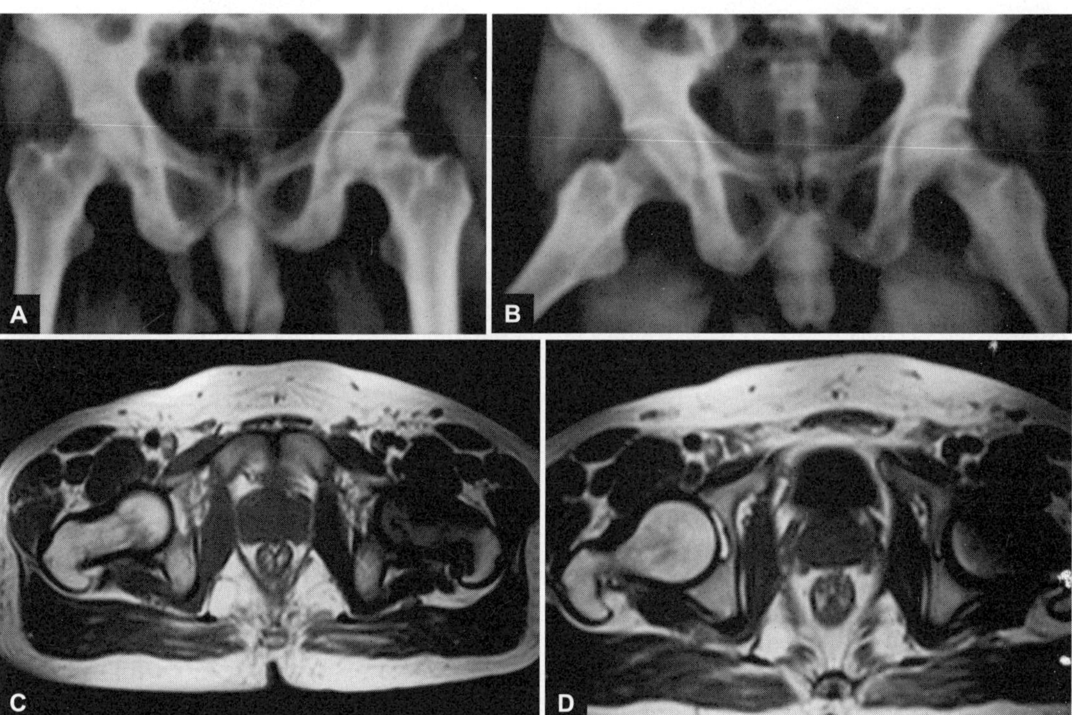

Figs 14.1A to D (A and B) Preoperative X-ray 52 years male steroid induced osteonecrosis of the femoral head left side; (C and D) Preoperative MRI showing classical changes of osteonecrosis left side

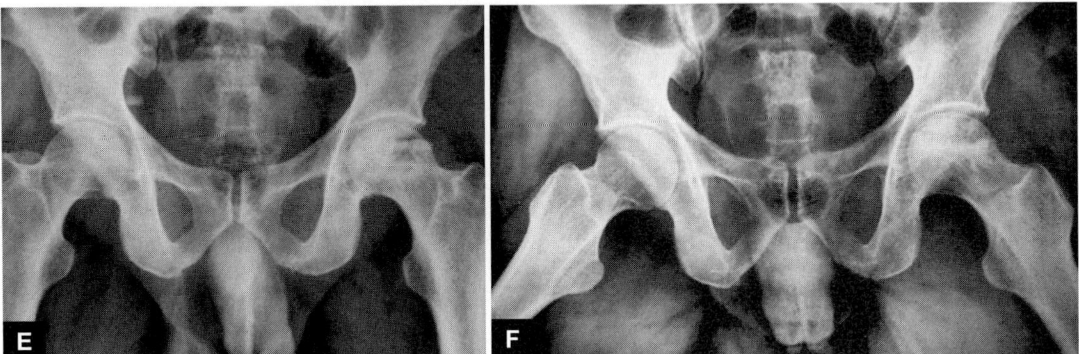

Figs 14.1 E and F Immediate postoperative X-ray after core decompression and TFL grafting

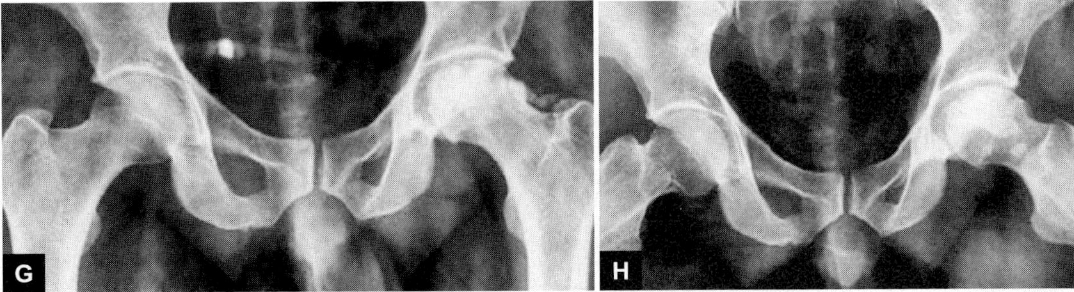

Figs 14.1G and H X-ray—Postoperative three years follow-up after core decompression and TFL grafting showing good revascularization and restoration of contour of the femoral head left side

Ninety hips of osteonecrosis of the femoral head in 68 young patients of different etiology with stages II and III were treated by core decompression and TFL muscle pedicle graft with iliac crest. Patients with a mean age of 30 years (16–52 years) with a minimum follow-up of three years were included in the analysis. Forty-four patients with involvement of one hip, and 22 patients with bilateral involvement were operated in one sitting. Two patients with bilateral involvement had core decompression and TFL grafting on one side and free fibular grafting on the opposite side. The surgery of core decompression and TFL muscle grafting with iliac crest have shown excellent results in preventing the collapse of the femoral head. Core decompression and TFL grafting is an easy procedure and this article describes the series of patients of

osteonecrosis treated by this method. Of the 68 patients (90 hips), 47 were males and 21 females. Thirty-three hips were in stage II and 57 had stage III involvement. Twenty-eight patients (42%) were following alcohol abuse, twenty-one patients (30%) were following consumption of corticosteroids and ninteen patients had sickle cell hemoglobinopathy (28%). Almost all patients had substantial relief from pain with good improvement in the range of movements. The radiological improvement was judged by diminisheing of density and attempt at revascularization as seen by healing of cystic changes, disappearance of crescent sign and restoration of normal trabecular pattern and shape of the femoral head.

In stage II, all patients had completely improved without any deterioration and had complete relief from pain, whereas 11 patients of stage III had residual pain for about 30 weeks. Three patients of stage III (8%) proceeded to further collapse and femoral head got deformed requiring THR. As per Harris Hip Score results, there was improvement in the score of > 25 points in 70 percent cases while 50 percent showed improvement in the score of >28 points in both the stages. Postoperatively bone scan and digital substraction arteriogram was done in 20 patients, 10 in each in stage II and III, at the end of 12 weeks, and findings showed hundred percent patency and viability of the TFL muscle pedicle graft.

■ MATERIAL AND METHODS

This article reports the study of 68 patients of osteonecrosis of the femoral head, affecting 92 femoral heads in stage II and III, wherein 90 hips were treated with core decompression and iliac crest-TFL muscle pedicle grafting by using part of the iliac crest with TFL muscle pedicle over a duration of 16 years, from January 1995 to December 2010 with a minimum follow-up for three years. All patients were young 16 to 52 years of age with a mean age of 30 years.

Forty-four patients had unilateral affection where as 24 patients had bilateral involvement, but on 22 occasions bilateral TFL

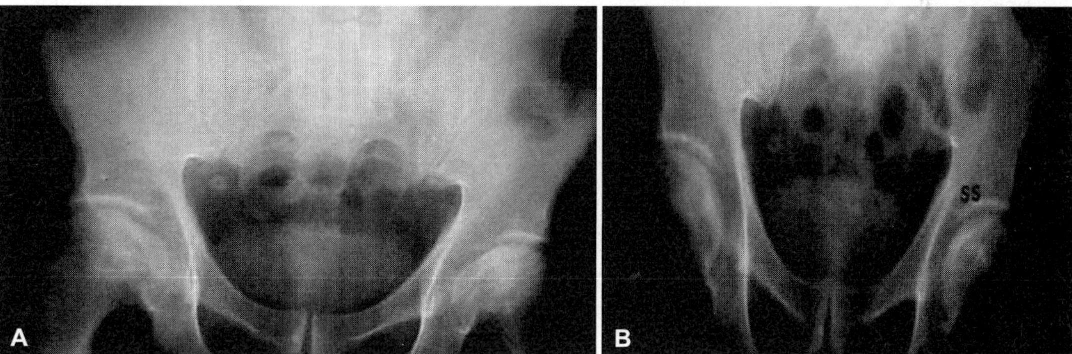

Figs 14.2A and B Preoperative X-ray 50 years male steroid induced osteonecrosis of the femoral head both sides

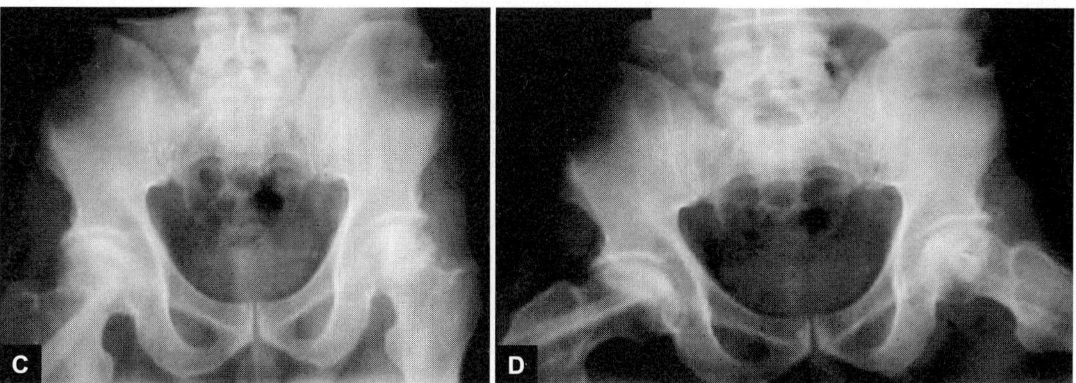

Figs 14.2C and D Postoperative 1.5 years follow-up X-ray after core decompression and TFL grafting on left side and free fibular graft on right side showing good revascularization and restoration of contour of the femoral head

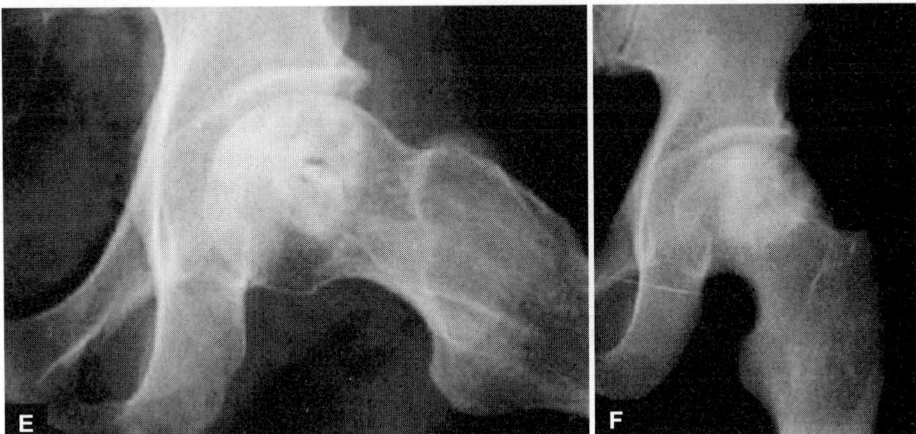

Figs 14.2E and F X-ray 1.5 years postoperative showing good revascularization and restoration of contour of the femoral head on left side after core decompression and TFL grafting

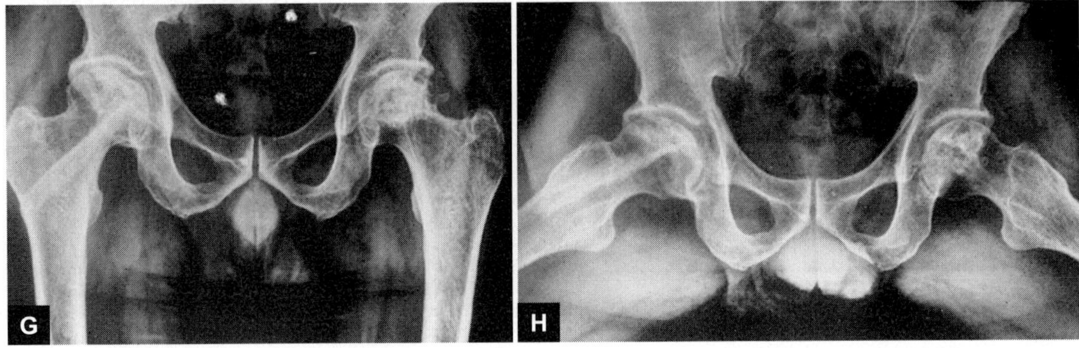

Figs 14.2G and H X-ray nine years postoperative showing good revascularization and restoration of contour of the femoral head on left side after core decompression and TFL grafting with good hip joint space

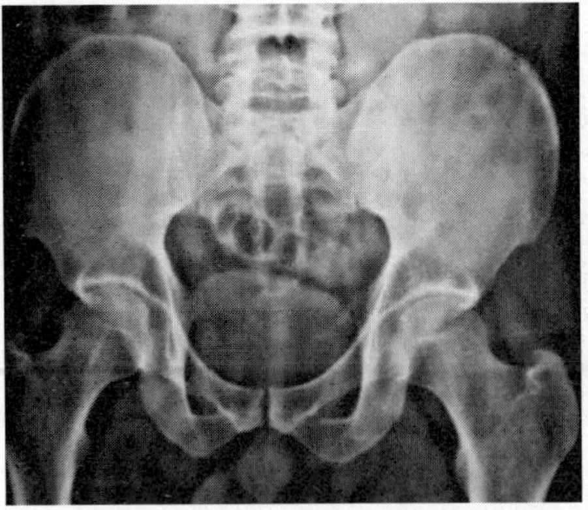

Fig. 14.3A X-ray showing alcohol induced osteonecrosis both sides in 31 years male

grafting was done in one sitting, whereas two patients in the bilateral group were operated by TFL muscle pedicle graft on one side and free fibular grafting on the opposite side in a single sitting (Figs 14.2 and 14.3). Thus the TFL grafting procedure was performed on total of 90 hips in 68 patients. At our Institute many patients of sickle cell disease with osteonecrosis are studied and treated, where the procedure of vascular pedicle grafting is not performed on any patient, because of the possibility of high prevalence of thrombosis in the vascular pedicle in this disease. Similarly, in patients with bilateral involvement, surgery of TFL grafting in one sitting is preferred to

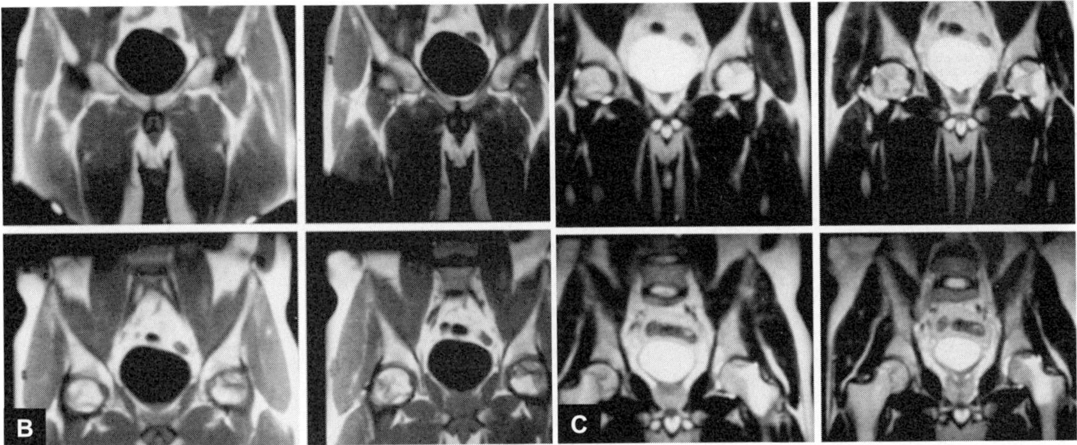

Figs 14.3B and C MRI showing bilateral osteonecrosis of the femoral heads

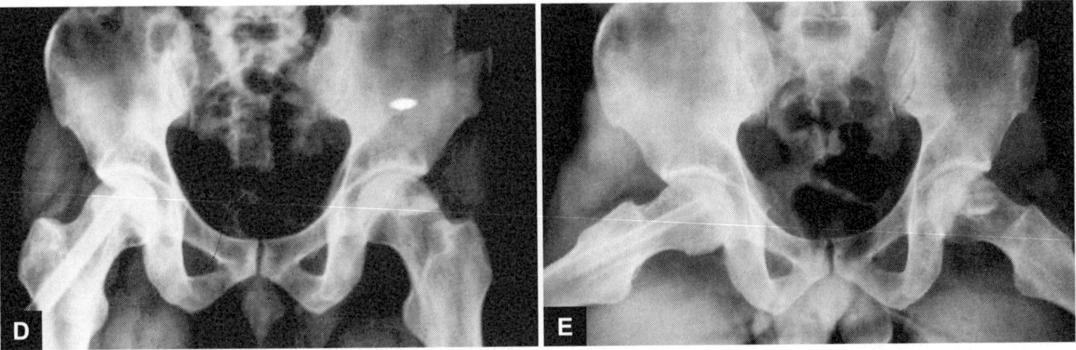

Figs 14.3D and E X-ray 12 weeks postoperative after core decompression and TFL graft left side and free fibular graft right side

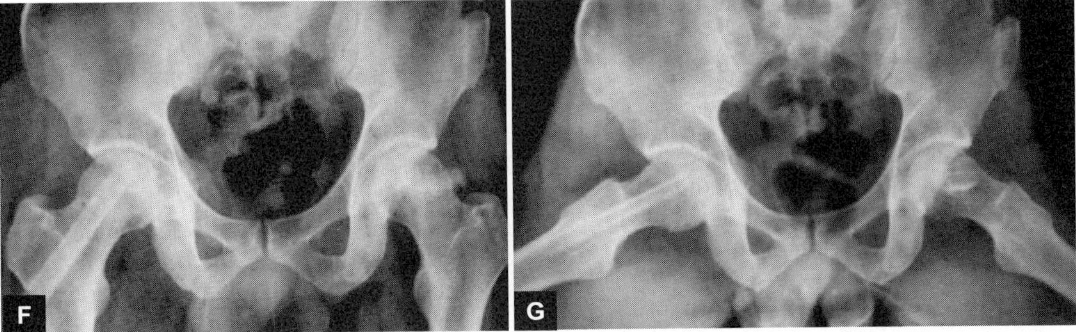

Figs 14.3F and G X-ray 1 year postoperative after core decompression and TFL graft left side and free fibular graft right side showing good consolidation of TFL grafting left side with restoration of the normal femoral head contour

Table 14.2 Demography of patients affecting 90 hips operated by TFL grafting showing stages, age and sex

Stage of Disease	Number of Hips	Male Hips	Female Hips	Age of the patient			
				16–20	21–30	31–40	41 and Above
Stage II	33	20	13	2	11	16	4
A	-						
B	15						
C	18						
Stage III	57	36	21	4	18	22	13
A	6						
B	36						
C	15						

vascular pedicle grafting, mainly because of the long time required for the vascular pedicle procedure. Amongst 68 patients, 28 patients (42%) were following alcohol abuse, 21 patients (30%) were following consumption of corticosteroids and 19 patients had sickle cell hemoglobinopathy (28%). The demography of patients is shown in Table 14.2. Amongst 24 bilateral hips, 17 patients had stage III on one side and stage II on the other side. Seven patients had stage III in both hips.

OPERATIVE TECHNIQUE

After administering spinal anesthesia, patient is put in supine position with the sandbag underneath the gluteal region on the operative side. A curvilinear incision is taken on the lateral side of the hip extending from the iliac crest about 5 cm posterior to the anterior superior iliac spine and to the greater trochanter and extending downwards about 2 cm below the base of the greater trochanter in the subtrochanteric region. The iliac crest is exposed, freed from the inner lip by erasing three abdominal muscles till one just reaches about 2 cm. Similarly, the iliac crest with attached tensor fascia lata on the external surface is exposed. The cleavage between the Sartorius and tensor fascia lata is identified. An incision is made between the anterior and middle fibers of the TFL and clearly 2 to 3 cm width of TFL middle fibers are separated up to the iliac crest. With pneumatic saw osteotomy of the iliac crest is done superiorly, and about 2 to 3 cm distally and medially with isolation of the TFL graft externally. This isolated iliac crest graft with TFL pedicle is best done by subperiosteal separation of muscles on either side of the lip of the ilium without disturbing the vascular supply. The desired size of the TFL with full width of the iliac crest is raised and retracted downwards with attached fibers of the TFL. The TFL muscle pedicle graft just prepared gets its vascular supply from the superior gluteal artery and the ascending branch of the lateral circumflex femoral artery. The reflected pedicle of the TFL with fibers of the gluteus minimus muscle is erased from the outer surface of the ilium and is retracted downwards and brought down up to the anterior capsule of the involved hip joint. The hip capsule is opened with a T-shaped incision. The anterior capsule and thickened synovium is excised. The ischemic necrotic segment is exposed and examined for its deformation and change in the contour. A small window is made anteriorly at the junction of articular surface of the femoral head and anterior surface of the neck of the femur by a pneumatic drill. Under image intensifier, through this window, serial reaming is done in the ischemic segment of the femoral head right up to the subchondral region in all the directions. Care is taken not to perforate the articular surface. Subsequently, the entire necrotic tissue is removed by curette which creates a big void in the head of the femur usually in the upper quadrant of the femoral head, wherein the inferior quadrant is usually not disturbed. With the special instrument and punch-impactor the deformed femoral head with articular cartilage is raised superiorly to match its original shape under image intensifier in all the directions. The created void is partially filled and packed with little cancellous bone removed from the iliac crest after performing the osteotomy. Subsequently, the retracted and raised pedicle of the TFL with the iliac crest is prepared nicely to repose through the window defect at the head-neck junction. Two holes are made superiorly and inferiorly in the femoral neck by 2-mm drill bits. Similarly, two holes are prepared in the pedicle of the iliac bone with TFL graft. Subsequently, the TFL pedicle is impacted into the head under image control right up to the subchondral region of the femoral head and the graft tied by No.1 Vicryl to the femoral head and neck. Additionally, the muscle belly is also stitched to the capsule inferiorly and superiorly. The suction drain is kept at the hip and iliac crest site and the wound is closed in layers. In bilateral cases, a similar procedure is performed in the same sitting on the opposite side.

■ POSTOPERATIVE PROTOCOL

Postoperatively the limb-hip is kept in 20 degree abduction and 30 degree flexion and 10 degree of internal rotation to avoid tension on the TFL pedicle. The patient is mobilized after 15 days in bed and after four to six weeks patient can be mobilized out of bed on nonweight-bearing crutch walking if only one hip is operated. Whereas in bilateral cases, the patient is advised bed rest with mobilzation of hips after four weeks and weight-bearing is started after only 10 weeks. The patient is allowed partial weight-bearing after 10 weeks and full weight-bearing after 14 to 16 weeks.

Follow-up

Follow-up by clinical and radiological examination was done every three months for one year, every six months for the next five years and then yearly follow-up thereafter. Harris hip score system was used for assessment of the results. The follow-up period varied from three to sixteen years. Postoperatively bone scan and digital subtraction arteriogram was done in 20 patients, ten each in stage II and III, at the end of 12 weeks, which showed hundred percent patency and viability of the TFL muscle pedicle graft.

Results

The patients had good clinical improvement with relief from pain and improvement in the range of movements. The radiological improvement was judged by diminishment of density and attempt at revascularization as seen by healing of cystic changes, disappearance of crescent sign and restoration of normal trabecular pattern and shape of femoral head. Almost all patients had good relief from pain with good improvement in the range of movements. As per Harris hip score results, there was improvement in the score of > 25 points in 70 percent cases while 50 percent had improvement in the score of >28 points in both the stages. The mean +SD improvement in Harris hip score at three year's follow-up was 27.6 + 6.4. The difference in the preoperative and postoperative score across the whole sample was significant ($P < 0.05$).

Stage II: Seventy percent of stage II hips completely improved without any deterioration and had complete relief from pain. No patient progressed to stage III postoperatively.

Stage III: About 20 percent patients of stage III had residual low-intensity pain for about 30 weeks. About 30 percent patients had painless limp for 24 to 30 weeks with restriction of flexion beyond 100 degrees. Eight percent patient (five patients) progressed to further collapse, got deformed but without any progression to arthrosis. Out of this, in 4 percent patients (three patients) surgery of the total hip joint was advised.

DISCUSSION

The need to treat ischemia of the femoral head is becoming more common since many cases are detected in early stages in young patients. One must consider the possibility of osteonecrosis if individual has pain in the vicinity of the hip, and has history of chronic alcoholism, corticosteroid consumption, or associated diseases like sickle cell disease, Gauchers, Gout, etc.[18-21] Early diagnosis prior to the appearance of radiological changes is crucial in the treatment of ischemic necrosis. Its diagnosis is based on clinical examination and by bone scan, CT, and MRI, as osteonecrosis is the response to the vascular impairment of the bone marrow circulation. X-ray examination is of limited value in the early stage, but has importance in staging since it helps in planning the treatment and the prognosis. The X-rays become positive late in the condition after the process of repair has started. The ischemic death of bony and marrow tissues occurs in osteonecrosis. Different imaging modalities provide different information on the mineralized and nonmineralized component of the bone. Though bone scan is also important, MRI has dramatically improved the diagnosis of osteonecrosis, and in about 30 to 70 percent cases of femoral head osteonecrosis, the other hip is affected in due course of time.[18,22] Hence, it is necessary to rule out early involvement of the contralateral hip, which is asymptomatic by either bone scan or MRI. MRI is the most accurate imaging modality for the diagnosis of osteonecrosis of the femoral head, especially in the early stages when there are only bone marrow changes.[23] Characteristic MRI signal alterations in the anterosuperior portion of the femoral head surrounded by a band of low signal intensity on T1- and T2-weighted images represent the diagnostic criteria of osteonecrosis.[25-27] The occurrence of a double-line sign on the T2-weighted image represents a pathognomonic sign, but its absence does not rule out the diagnosis of osteonecrosis. Marcus et al. Steinberg et al. Ficat and Arlet, and ARCOs classification[7,8-29] are the various staging systems in vogue for the diagnosis of osteonecrosis, but with inherent problems of low reliability. The Association Research Circulation Osseous (ARCO) has proposed a new international classification system including radiographs, CT, bone scans, and MRI.[8] This classification system incorporates the lesion size and the location of the lesion. Quantitation (% area involvement of the femoral head, length of crescent sign, percent surface collapse, and dome depression) and location of the lesion (medial, central or lateral) represent important prognostic factors. This ARCO's classification has been proposed as the preferred system for the future, which is used in this study.

Core decompression offers the opportunity to study histological changes of early bone ischemia. It also achieves reduction in the symptoms of the pre-collapse stage of ischemic necrosis because of reduction of pressure in the compartment. Barring exceptional circumstances, there is hardly any role for conservative treatment of osteonecrosis of the femoral head and surgery is rendered inevitable.

Steinberg et al. reported that progression occurred in 92 percent of 48 hips that had undergone nonoperative management.[30,31] While observing the patients with protected weight-bearing, more than 85 percent patients had collapse of the femoral head at two years when symptomatic hips with stage I and II were left untreated. Many studies have shown that nonoperative treatment yields poor results. The only condition for which protected weight-bearing might be effective is a Type A lesion, i.e. involvement of the medial aspect of the femoral head. No drugs have been useful and specific in the treatment of osteonecrosis, though recently the use of Alendronate has been advised. Once diagnosed, it is desirable to subject the patient to early surgical intervention. The rationale for the treatment of osteonecrosis of the femoral head requires a lot of consideration. Prime consideration should be given to the age of the patient, whether both hips are affected, etiology of the associated diseases, functional demands of the patients, and the stage of the disease when the patient presents for treatment. Only core decompression may relieve the pain but is not useful for revascularization of femoral head; hence, core decompression should always be supplemented by one of the procedures of bone grafting. Core decompression is an effective treatment in the pre-radiological and pre-collapse stage of avascular necrosis of the femoral head,[18,32,33] especially if coupled with bone grafting. Jones analyzed nine studies and showed that in 218 of 369 patients (59%), in whom core decompression was performed in the pre-collapse stage, failed to prevent the progressive collapse.[34-36] Steinberg et al.[19,30,31] concluded that core decompression provided more predictable pain relief and changed the indications for arthroplasty more consistently than conservative management. However, only core decompression should be avoided, and it must be coupled with bone grafting in the tract of the core to avoid iatrogenic fractures.[10,37] Despite many reports on salvage procedures, no method has clearly demonstrated the arrest of disease before subchondral fracture or slow down of the progression of the collapse of the femoral head and arthrosis. The use of a nonvascularized bone graft, as originally described by Phemister, has had variable success in the treatment of osteonecrosis. Marcus et al.[28] reported satisfactory clinical results in seven out of eleven hips at the time of short-term follow-up (range: 24 years). The other workers concluded that Phemister bone-grafting technique is not effective once collapse has occurred. Boettcher et al.[15] reported success in 27 (71%) of 38 hips six years after non-vascularized tibial strut grafting. However, a longer term evaluation (performed at a mean of 14 years postoperatively) that included the original 38 hips in the study by Boettcher et al. found that only 16 (29%) of the 56 hips still had a good result.[38] Once the crescent sign appears without collapse, it is desirable to couple the bone grafting procedure with the core decompression, preferably vascular or muscle pedicle grafting, to achieve early revascularization.[38,39,10,12]

Vascularized pedicle graft by using part of the iliac crest with deep circumflex iliac vessels is more advantageous since a high percentage of marrow and osteogenic cells survive within a living graft, which helps for early vascularization.[10,40-43] However, muscle pedicle graft using TFL graft is very easy and is commonly performed whenever both hips need simultaneous surgery.[44] Muscle pedicle graft using quadratus femoris (Meyers procedure)[11] was also propagated in the treatment of osteonecrosis, but it did not achieve satisfactory early revascularization and went into disrepute since the results were not encouraging, though Meyers reported a success rate of 57 percent and Baksi[12] reported 93 percent good results. Use of TFL graft is commonly advocated when bilateral hips are involved and surgery is performed in a single sitting.[44] The study by Plakseychuk et al.[42,43] on free vascular fibular grafting showed better clinical results and prevention of radiographic signs of progression and collapse of the femoral head more frequently than does nonvascularized fibular grafting. A marked difference with regard to signs of radiographic progression and collapse was noted between the A and B subgroups in the pre-collapse groups (stages I, and II). The potential disadvantages of vascularized fibular grafting are a longer operation time, need of microvascular technique, a longer operative scar, and the fact that it is associated with more donor site morbidity such as ankle instability, toe-clawing, subtrochanteric fracture, and heterotopic ossification. To achieve early vascularization TFL muscle pedicle grafting along with the iliac crest is very useful. This procedure is easy and is technically not demanding (Figs 14.4 and 14.5).

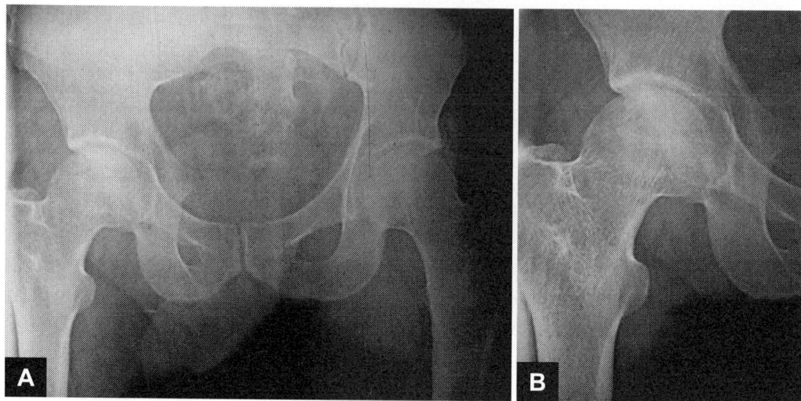

Figs 14.4A and B X-ray pelvis AP view showing alcohol induced osteonecrosis right side in 36 years male

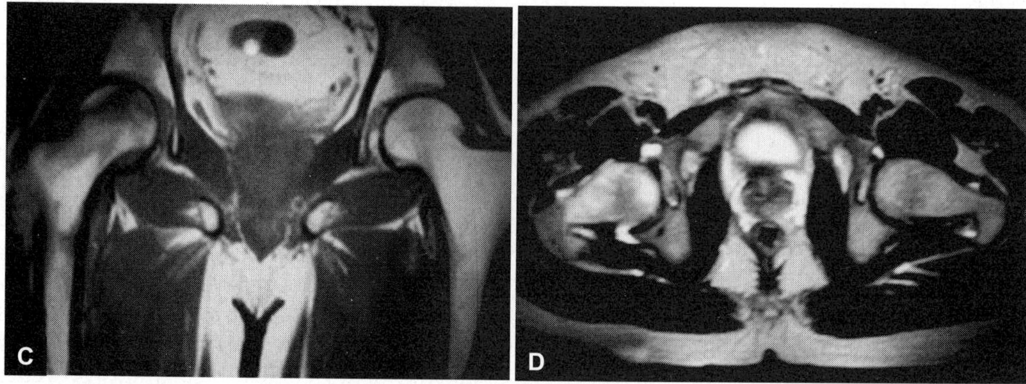

Figs 14.4C and D MRI showing osteonecrosis of the femoral head right side

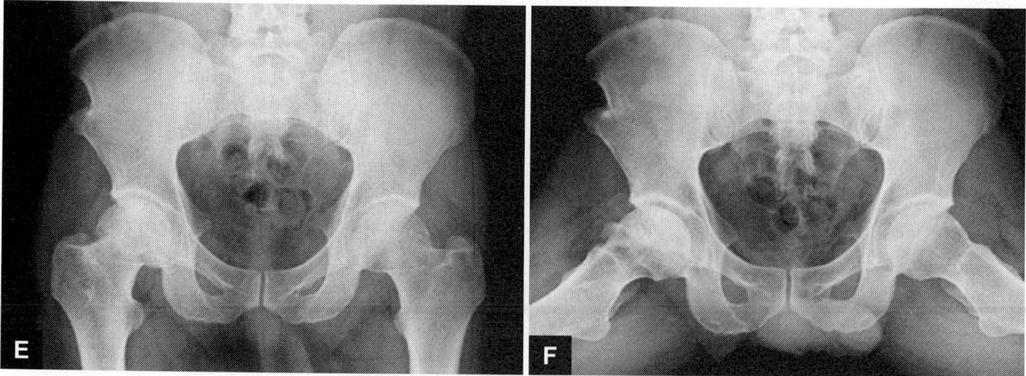

Figs 14.4E and F X-ray showing good incorporation of TFL graft maintenance of articular surface of femoral head at the end of 2 years follow-up

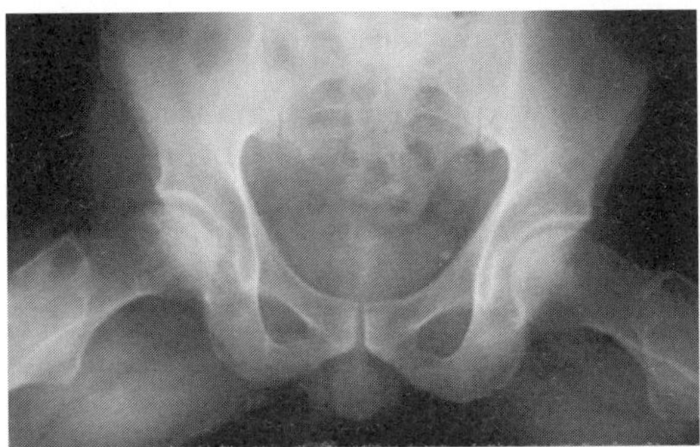

Fig. 14.5A X-ray showing alcohol induced osteonecrosis of the femoral head on both sides in 45 years male

The TFL grafting provides a significant benefit for hips in stages II and III. The rationale of this procedure (Figs 14.4 and 14.5) of TFL pedicle bone grafting is based on the following three points:

1. Decompression of the femoral head, which acts as compartment syndrome following increased intraosseous pressure, and interrupts the circulation that is thought to contribute to the disease.

2. Excision of the necrotic tissue, which inhibits revascularization of the head.

3. Filling of the defect that is created after core and filled with TFL muscle pedicle

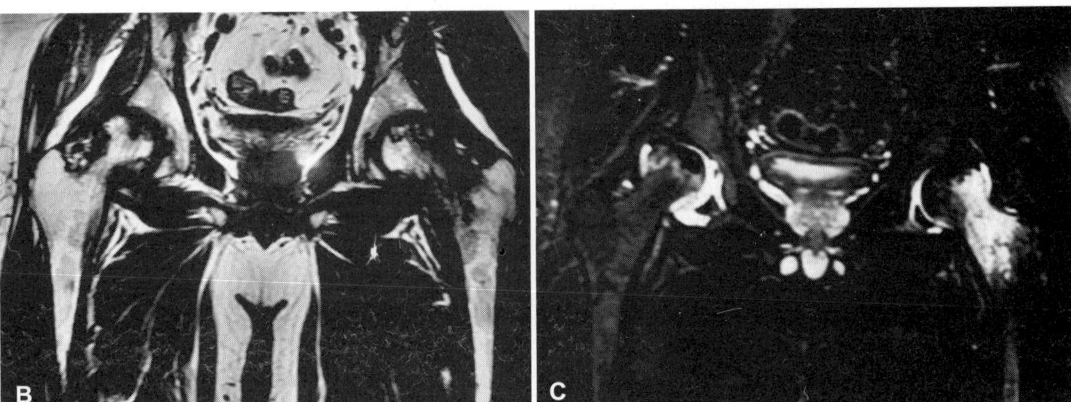

Figs 14.5B and C MRI showing classical changes of osteonecrosis of both the femoral heads

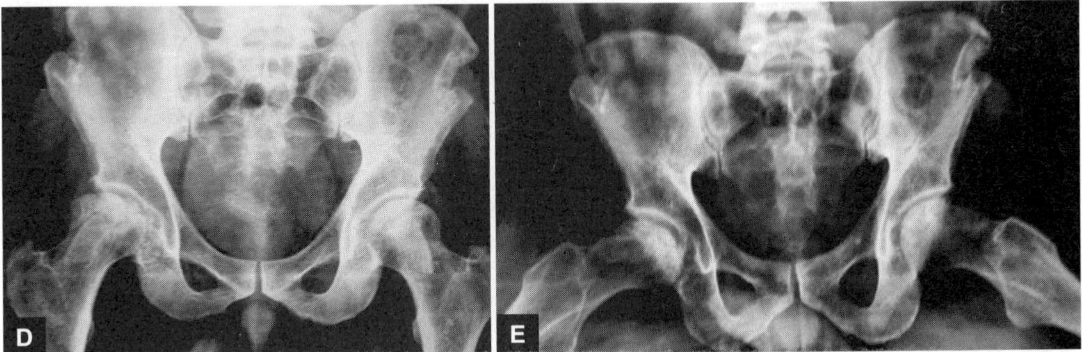

Figs 14.5D and E X-ray 12 months postoperative after core decompression and TFL grafting in one sitting showing good incorporation of graft and showing good restoration of articular surface

with iliac crest, acts, an osteoinductive cancellous graft, which is viable and supports the subchondral surface and enhances the revascularization process.

It does not require advanced training of microsurgical technique nor any special equipment and can be performed by any average orthopedic surgeon. Morbidity of the donor site is minimal and operative time required is comparable to total hip arthroplasty, and all problems and obstacles associated with vascularized fibular graft are avoided by this technique. Head-preserving operation of core decompression and TFL pedicle grafting certainly gives excellent results in stages II and III. The prognosis of stages II and III is fairly good, whereas in stage IV, it is not satisfactory since about one-third of the stage IV group are likely to progress further and may require total hip joint replacement or resurfacing operations. Prosthetic replacement is frequently an unappealing option for patients who have osteonecrosis because many patients are young and the etiological factors associated with the disease are also associated with complications after total hip arthroplasty, hemiarthroplasty, and surface replacement. At our institute, many patients of sickle cell disease with osteonecrosis are studied and treated, by this procedure of TFL muscle pedicle grafting. Out of 103 patients treated by Urbanaiak et al.[7] by free vascular fibular grafting, total hip replacement was performed in 34 percent cases in stages II and III within five years. There was survivorship and the probability of conversion within 5 years to THR rate of 11 percent in Stage II and 23 percent survival for Stage III. In the study by Shin Yoon Kim,[38] the rate of conversion to total hip replacement was 13 percent (3 of 23 hips) in the vascularized graft group and 22 percent (5 of 23 hips) in the nonvascularized graft group in comparison only 3 patients out of 68 of TFL muscle pedicle grafting were advised total hip replacement in the present series at the end of 16 years (Figs 14.6A to F).

The hips treated with TFL muscle pedicle grafting seemed to have less dome depression of the femoral head and the retention of sphericity, probably because of more rapid revascularization and increased osteoinductive potential of the pedicle graft (Figs 14.6G and H). It has been observed that there is an early failure of total hip replacement in osteonecrosis than in age-matched patients with other diagnoses because of abnormal remodeling of bones and subsidence of prosthesis because of poor quality of proximal femoral bone.[42] Other contributory factors for failure are ongoing systemic disease, defects in mineral metabolism, use of steroids, and high level of activity in young patients and increased body weight. Hence, we prefer to delay or

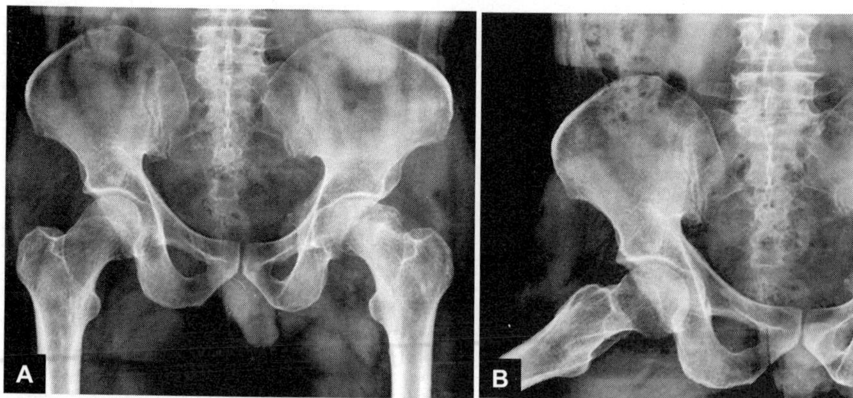

Figs 14.6A and B X-ray showing alcohol induced osteonecrosis of the femoral heads both sides, Stage II—right side, and Stage III—left side in 52 years male

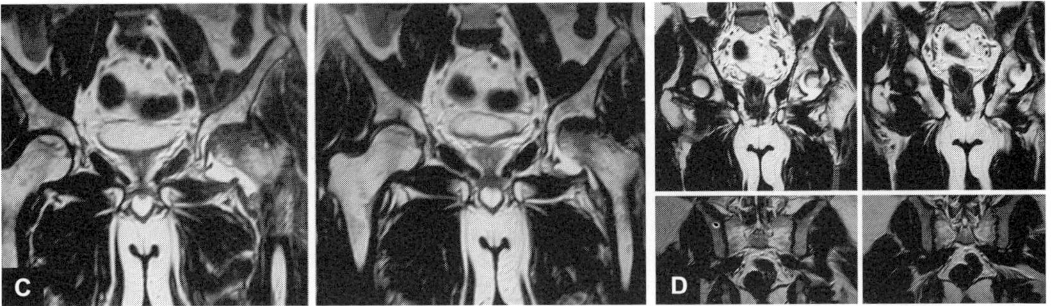

Figs 14.6C and D MRI showing bilateral osteonecrosis of the femoral heads in 52 years male

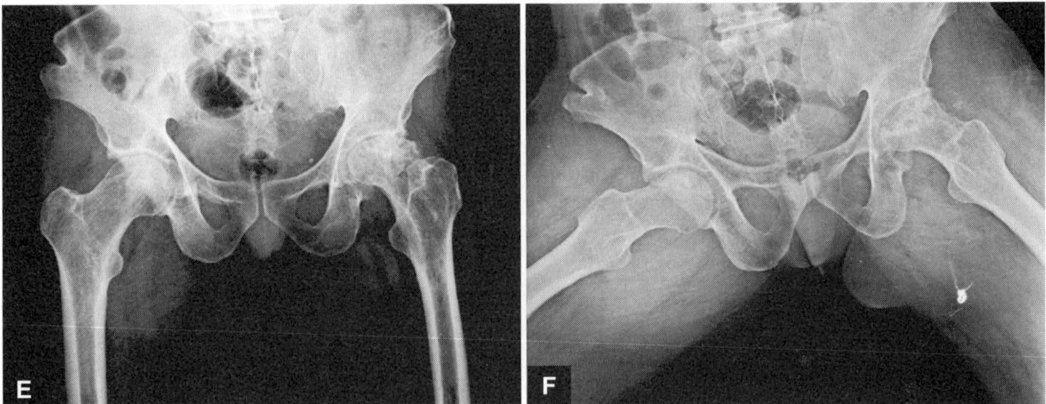

Figs 14.6E and F X-ray, one year postoperative showing collapse of femoral head with arthritic changes left side, good incorporation of graft right side with good joint space. Patient is advised THR left side

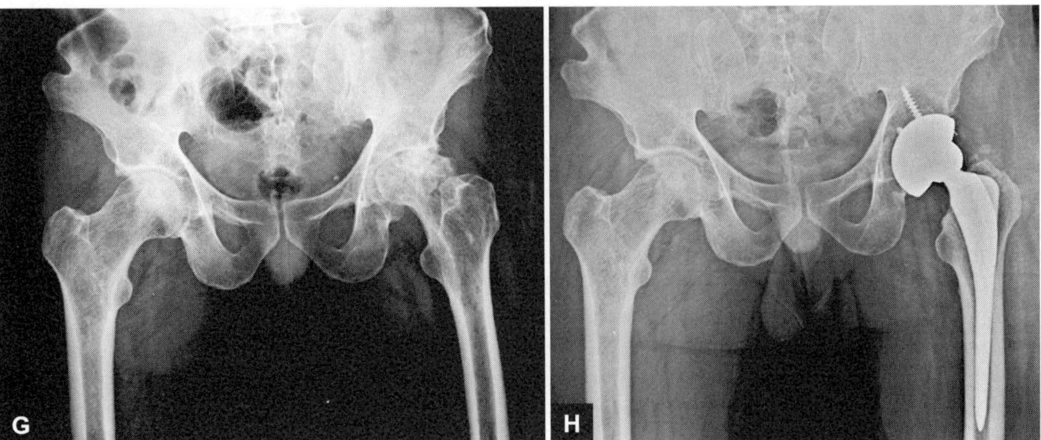

Figs 14.6G and H Preoperative X-ray showing collapse of femoral head with arthritic changes left side, good incorporation of graft right side with good joint space. X-rays 4 months postoperative:Uncemented THR done on left side

eliminate the need for hip replacement by performing head-preserving surgeries,[10,37,44] of which core decompression and TFL muscle pedicle grafting are the choice of surgery, especially in bilateral cases and patients with sickle cell disease with stages II and III. Out of 68 patients, only 5 patients progressed to collapse, and surgery of joint replacement was advised in 3 patients.

CONCLUSION

Basically, osteonecrosis of the femoral head is a multifactorial, heterogeneous group of disorder that leads to a final common pathology of mechanical failure of the femoral head. In this study more than 70 percent patients had osteonecrosis because of alcohol abuse (42%) and steroid consumption (30%) and in 28 percent cases belonged to sickle cell disease. It is common in young age group where a conservative surgical approach is chosen, rather than a radical approach of reconstructive surgery. If diagnosed early head preserving operation of core decompression and TFL muscle pedicle bone grafting yields an excellent result.[45] Essentially the result depends on the preoperative condition of the joint and the site of the necrotic focus and the associated disease, which may be the cause of osteonecrosis. From our experience, if the ischemic necrosis of the femoral head is diagnosed early in stages II, and III core decompression and TFL muscle pedicle grafting gives very good results. In stage III, even if there is slight collapse with deformation, the depressed segment can be elevated and deformity corrected after elevation and bone grafting. Out of 68 patients with 90 hips only 5 patients progressed to collapse and surgery of joint replacement was advised in 3 patients of stage III. The long standing effect of surgery was excellent with great improvement in the Harris hip score, achieving improvement in the score between 70 and 80 points in the majority of patients at the final follow-up period.

REFERENCES

1. Glimcher MJ, Kenzora JE. The biology of osteonecrosis of the human femoral head and its clinical implications: Part III. Discussion of the etiology and genesis of the pathological sequelae; comments on treatment. Clin Orthop. 1979;140:273-312.
2. Herndon JH, Aufranc OE. Avascular necrosis of the femoral head in the adult. A review of its incidence in a variety of conditions. Clin Orthop. 1972;86:43-62.
3. Glimcher MJ, Kenzora JE. The biology of osteonecrosis of the human femoral head and its clinical implications: Part II. The pathological changes in the femoral head as an organ and in the hip joint. Clin Orthop. 1979;139:283-312.
4. Kenzora JE, Glimcher MJ. Pathogenesis of idiopathic osteonecrosis: The ubiquitous crescent sign. Orthop Clin North Am. 1985;16:681-96.
5. Mankin HJ. Nontraumatic necrosis of bone (osteonecrosis). N Eng J Med. 1992;326:1473-9.
6. Mont MA, Hungerford DS. Non-traumatic avascular necrosis of the femoral head. J Bone Joint Surg. 1995;77A:459-74.
7. Urbaniak JR, Coogan PG, Gunneson EB, et al. Treatment of osteonecrosis of the femoral head with free vascularised fibular grafting: A long-term follow-up study of one hundred and three hips. J Bone Joint Surg. 1995;77A:681-94.
8. Gardeniers JWM. ARCO international classi-fication of osteonecrosis. ARCO News. 1993;5:79-82.
9. Steinberg ME, Hayken GD, Steinberg DR. A quantitative system for staging avascular necrosis. J Bone Joint Surg Br. 1995,77B:34-41.
10. Babhulkar SS. Osteonecrosis of femoral head. Treatment by core decompression and vascular pedicle grafting. Indian J fournal of Orthopaedics. 2009;43(1):27-35.
11. Meyers MH. The treatment of osteonecrosis of the hip with fresh osteochondral allografts and with the muscle-pediclegraft technique. Clin Orthop. 1978;130:202-9.
12. Baksi DP. Treatment of osteonecrosis of the femoral head by drilling and muscle-pedicle bone grafting. J Bone Joint Surg Br. 1991;73-B:241-5.
13. Ficat P, Arlet J, Hungerford DS (Eds). Ischaemia and Necrosis of Bone. Baltimore, MD, Williams and Wilkins, 1980.

14. Ficat RP. Idiopathic bone necrosis of the femoral head. Early diagnosis and treatment. J Bone Joint Surg. 1985;67B:3-9.

15. Boettcher WG, Bonfigilo M, Smith K. Non-traumatic necrosis of the femoral head: II. Experiences in treatment. J Bone Joint Surg. 1970;52A:322-9.

16. Steinberg ME, Brighton CT, Hayken GD, et al. Electrical stimulation in the treatment of Osteonecrosis of the femoral head—a 1year follow-up. Orthop. Clin North Am. 1985;16: 747-56.

17. Steinberg ME, Hayken GD, Steinberg DR. The conservative management of avascular necrosis of the femoral head. In Bone Circulation. Edited by Arlet A, Ficat RP, Hungerford DS. Baltimore; Williams and Wilkins; 1984.pp.334-7.

18. Hungerford DS, Jones LC. Diagnosis of osteo-necrosis of the femoral head. In Schoutens A, Arlet J, Gardeniers JWM, et al. (Eds): Bone Circulation and Vascularisation in Normal and Pathological Conditions. New York, NY, Plenum Press; 1993.pp.265-75.

19. Steinberg ME, Hayken GD, Steinberg DR. A quantitative system for staging avascular necrosis. J Bone Joint Surg. 1995;77B:34-41.

20. Arlet J, Ficat P. Forage-biopsie de la tete femorale dans l'osteonecrose primitive. Obser-vations histo-pathologiques portant sur huit forgaes. Rev Rhumat. 1964;31:257-64.

21. Bradway JK, Morrey BF. The natural history of the silent hip in bilateral atraumatic osteonecrosis. J Arthroplasty. 1993;8:383-7.

22. Mitchell DG, Steinberg ME, Dalinka MK, et al. Magnetic resonance imaging of the ischaemic hip: Alterations within the osteonecrotic, viable, and reactive zone. Clin Orthop. 1989;244:60-77.

23. Shimizu K, Moriya H, Akita T, et al. Prediction of collapse with magnetic resonance imaging of avascular necrosis of the femoral head. J Bone Joint Surg Am. 1994;76A:215-23.

24. Beltran J, Knight CT, Zuelzer WA, et al. Core decompression for avascular necrosis of the femoral head: Correlation between long-term results and preoperative MR staging. Radiology. 1990;175:533-6.

25. Robinson HJ Jr. Success of core decompression in the management of early stages of avascular necrosis: A four-year prospective study. Proceedings of the American Academy of Orthopaedic Surgeons 59th Annual Meeting, Washington DC, Park Ridge, IL, American Academy of Orthopaedic Surgeons; 1992. p.177.

26. Norman A, Bullough P. The radiolucent crescent line. An early diagnostic sign of avascular necrosis of the femoral head. Bull Hosp Joint Dis. 1963;24:99-104.

27. Harris WH Traumatic arthritis of the hip, J Bone Joint Surg Am. 1969;51A:738-43.

28. Marcus ND, Enneking WF, Massam RA. The silent hip in idiopathic aseptic necrosis. treatment by bone grafting. J Bone Joint Surg Am. 1973;55A:1351-66.

29. Kerboul M, Thomine J, Postel M, et al. The conservative surgical treatment of idiopathic aseptic necrosis of the femoral head. J Bone Joint Surg Br. 1974;56B:291-6.

30. Steinberg ME, Brighton CT, Hayken GD, et al. Electrical stimulation in the treatment of Osteo-necrosis of the femoral head–a 1 year follow-up. Orthop. Clin North Am. 1985;16: 747-56.

31. Steinberg ME, Hayken GD, Steinberg DR. The conservative management of avascular necrosis of the femoral head. In Bone Circulation. Edited by Arlet A, Ficat RP, Hungerford DS. Baltimore; Williams and Wilkins; 1984.pp.334-7.

32. Ficat P, Arlet J, Hungerford DS (Eds). Ischaemia and Necrosis of Bone. Baltimore, MD, Williams and Wilkins, 1980.

33. Ficat RP. Idiopathic bone necrosis of the femoral head. Early diagnosis and treatment. J Bone Joint Surg Br. 1985;67B:3-9.

34. Jones JP Jr. Intravascular coagulation and osteonecrosis. Clin Orthop. 1992;277:41-53.

35. Jones JP Jr Fat embolism, intravascular coagula-tion, and osteonecrosis. Clin Orthop. 1993;292: 294-308.

36. Jones JP Jr. Concepts of etiology and early pathogenesis of osteonecrosis. In Schafer M (Ed). Instructional Course Lectures 43. Rosemont, IL, American Academy of Ortho-paedic Surgeons; 1994.pp.499-512.

37. Babhulkar SS. Osteonecrosis of the femoral head (in young individuals) Indian Journal of Orthopaedics. 2003;37(2):77-86.

38. Yoon S, Goo Y, Kim PT, Ihn JC, Cho BC, Koo KH. Vascularized compared with nonvascularized fibular grafts for large osteonecroic lesion of the femoral head. J Bone Joint Surg Am. 2005; 87:2012-8.

39. Dutton RO, Amstuz HC, Thomas BJ, Hedley AK. Tharies surface replacement for osteonecrosis of femoral head. J Bone Joint Surgery Am. 1982; 64:1225-37.

40. Leung PC, Chow YY. Reconstruction of proximal femoral defects with a vascular-pedicled graft. J Bone Joint Surg Br. 1984;66B:32-7.

41. Leung PC. Vascular bone grafts from iliac crest microsurgical technique in orthopaedics. Pho Robert WH, Butterworths; 135-44.
42. Plakseychuk AY, Bogov AA, Plakseychuk YA. vascularised Iliac crest Graft in the treatment of aseptic necrosis of femoral head; Reconstructive Microsurgery Current Trends Proceedings 12th Symposium International Society of Reconstructive Microsurgery, Singapore; 1996. pp.85-7.
43. Plakseychuk AY, Kim SY, Park BC, Varitimidis SE, Rubash HE, Sotereanos DG. Vascularised compared with nonvascularised fibular bone grafting for the treatment of osteonecrosis of the femoral head. J Bone Joint Surgery Am. 2003; 85:589-96.
44. Iwata H, Torii S, Hasegawa Y, Itoh H, et al. Indications and results of vascularised pedical iliac bone graft in avascular necrosis of femoral head. Clin Orthop. 1993;295:281.
45. Babhulkar Sudhir. Osteonecrosis femoral head treatment by core decompression and iliac crest TFL muscle pedicle grafting: In bone grafting, edited by Dr Alessandro zorzi (Ed) Intech 2012, ISBN: 978-953-51-0324-0, Chapter-7, page no. 107-124.

TREATMENT BY CORE DECOMPRESSION AND VASCULAR PEDICLE GRAFTING

The principles of this treatment are to reduce the intraosseous tension and perform the procedure, which will achieve early revascularization of the ischemic head. Use of vascularized pedicle graft is more advantageous since a high percentage of marrow and osteogenic cells survive within a living graft, which helps for early vascularization. The operation is performed by the anterior approach by using part of the iliac crest with deep circumflex iliac vessels. Nine patients were stage IIB, C and 22 patients were stage IIIC according to Association Research Circulation Osseous (ARCO's) system. In a period of 15 years in this Institute 31 patients were treated by this technique in which, 16 patients had osteonecrosis following alcohol abuse, 12 patients following corticosteroid consumption, three patients had idiopathic osteonecrosis. Out of 31 patients only one patient progressed to collapse and surgery of joint replacement was advised. Digital substraction arteriography performed in nine patients at the end of 12 weeks showed the patency of the deep circumflex artery in all cases and bone scan performed in six other patients showed high uptake in the grafted area of the femoral head proving the efficacy of the operative procedure. At the final follow-up period of five to eight years there was mean ± SD improvement in Harris Hip Score of 28.2 ± 6.4 (p<0.05). Forty-eight percent of patients had an improvement of more than 28 points in the Harris Hip Score.

INTRODUCTION

Osteonecrosis of the femoral head is a disabling condition frequently seen in association with many disorders like corticosteroids consumption, alcohol abuse, hemoglobinopathy (sickle cell disease, coagulopathies), and certain renal, hepatic and skin disorders commonly affecting young group of patients around the age 20 to 40 years.[1,2] It is often characterized by relentless progression despite treatment, resulting in subchondral fracture, collapse and painful disabling arthrosis.[3] Hence, it is essential to diagnose and treat the patients of osteonecrosis early to prevent the disintegration and collapse of the femoral head. The true prevalence of the disease is difficult to ascertain. In 5 to 18 percent of patients undergoing total hip replacement in the US, the indication was reported to be advanced osteonecrosis with secondary osteoarthritis. [4-6]

The average age of patients in a large series was found to be 38 years, with only 20 percent of patients being older than 50 years of age.[5] In another study, the mean age was reported to be 34 years.[6] Osteonecrosis is usually associated with one or more risk factors, approximately two-thirds of these are related to alcohol abuse and corticosteroid intake. The remaining third are associated with diverse conditions like sickle cell hemoglobinopathy, storage disorders like Gauchers disease, pregnancy, coagulopathies and decompression sickness. Other groups of patients prone to developing osteonecrosis include organ transplant recipients, patients with inflammatory bowel disease, and lupus erythematosus. Patients with history of pain in the groin, radiating pain in the thigh and symptoms mimicking prolapsed intervertebral disk, should be evaluated properly. All these patients should be grouped as high index of suspicion examined properly and kept under constant follow-up. They should be properly screened and observed. The reported incidence of bilaterality ranges from 6 to 72 percent.[7-9] Despite a high incidence of bilaterality only about 15 percent of patients report bilateral symptoms on initial presentation.[9] The difficulty in estimating the prevalence of osteonecrosis arises because the condition is asymptomatic in the early stages. The term 'Silent Hip' is applied to the asymptomatic hip in patients who present for the management of the contralateral painful hip.[7]

The natural history of osteonecrosis of the femoral head before the development of crescent sign or before the collapse of the femoral head has never been well defined. The possibility of progression to collapse is thought to increase after the development of a abnormality that can be seen on plain radiographs and such a possibility and the course of collapse may be highly variable and unknown.[6] It is generally agreed that symptomatic, radiographically abnormal hip will progress to collapse of the femoral head when treated nonoperatively.[6] To avoid these complications and to avoid early replacement arthroplasty in young patients, many operative procedures to salvage the femoral head are in vogue.[19-30]

Head-preserving operation of core decompression and various types of bone grafting certainly gives excellent results in the early stage of osteonecrosis. Despite the many reports on the utility of various operative procedures, no single method has uniformly demonstrated the arrest of disease or prevention of collapse of the femoral head effectively. The study performed by James Urbanaiak et al.[6] strongly suggests that vascularized fibular grafting is associated with better clinical and radiographic results than nonvascularized fibular grafting in precollapse hips. However, the successful use of free vascularized bone grafts requires a meticulous process of procuring the vascular fibula with microanastomosis to the recipient site. The microsurgical procedures require specialized training, equipment and expertise. The vascular pedicle bone graft by using part of the iliac crest with the deep circumflex iliac vessel described in this article is easy to perform and does not require any special equipment or technique, and still has the advantages of the vascularized bone graft. A vascularized bone graft remains viable and is incorporated more rapidly in to the surrounding bone than a free graft.

MATERIAL AND METHODS

This retrospective study comprised of 31 patients of osteonecrosis of the femoral head treated with core decompression and vascular pedicle grafting by using part of the iliac crest with the deep circumflex iliac vessels in a duration of 15 years, from January 1990 to December 2005 with a minimum follow-up of five years and average follow-up of eight years. All 31 patients had positive important clinical signs highly suggestive of osteonecrosis of the femoral head and were investigated by X-rays, bone scan, computed tomography (CT) and magnetic resonance imaging (MRI) to confirm the diagnosis.[10] Early diagnosis and proper staging of the disease was important criteria for planning the treatment and improving clinical outcome.[11-14] For this study a new international classification system proposed by the Association Research Circulation Osseous (ARCO) has been used which includes radiographs, CT, bone scans, and MRI.[15] The diagnosis of osteonecrosis was considered as established if any of the following criteria were found:

- Pathognomonic radiographic changes (collapse of the femoral head, Anterolateral sequestration, and crescent sign). [16,17]
- A double line on T2-weighted MRI.[18]
- Increased uptake surrounding a photo-penic area of bone scan (cold in hot).[18]
- Positive finding on bone biopsy—showing empty lacunae involving multiple adjacent trabeculae.[15]

Whenever bone scan was negative in such a high-risk group of patients with strong clinical suspicion, the patients were subjected to sequential MRI, especially on the contralateral side. In this study all patients were young in the age group of 18 to 52 years, with a mean age of 32 years. Seven patients had bilateral involvement, where only one hip was operated with vascular pedicle graft and the other hips with early involvement (Stage I) was treated with core decompression and free fibular graft. Hematological investigations for hepatic, renal function and coagulopathy to assess the hepatorenal function were carried out in each individual. Nine patients were stage IIB, C and twenty-two patients were stage IIIC according to ARCO's system (Table 15.2). Out of 31 patients 16 patients had osteonecrosis following alcohol abuse, 12 patients following corticosteroid consumption, and 3 patients had idiopathic osteonecrosis. There were 26 males and 5 females with large majority (22) in stage III of osteonecrosis (Table 15.3). Once the surgery of vascular pedicle graft was planned, preoperative angiography was performed on each patient to confirm the presence of deep circumflex iliac artery (Fig. 15.2B). Follow-up by clinical assessment and radiological examination was done every three months for one year, every six months for next five years and then there was yearly follow-up thereafter. Initially in 15 patients, digital substraction arteriography was performed at the end of 12 weeks which showed the patency of deep circumflex artery, and bone scan showed high uptake in the grafted area of the femoral head proving the efficacy of the operative procedure. However, this investigation was not performed routinely after proving the efficacy in early cases. Harris Hip Score system[19] was used for assessment of the results.

Operative Technique of Core Decompression and Vascular Pedicle Grafting

Harvesting the vascular iliac crest graft requires careful isolation of the deep circumflex iliac vessel from its origin, as described by Leung PC and Chow YYN (1984).[25,26] After necessary (? spinal) anesthesia the patient is placed in a supine position. A curvilinear incision is taken at the midinguinal region extending along the inguinal ligament from the point of femoral pulsations proximally to the uppermost convexity of the iliac crest and distally it should be turned anterolaterally up to the subtrochanteric region. Subsequently the inguinal ligament is properly exposed and retracted upwards to expose the femoral artery, which is traced above the inguinal ligament where it becomes the external iliac artery. Then the most important landmark is the origin of the inferior gastric artery on the medial side of the external iliac artery which is identified and opposite to it is the origin of the deep circumflex iliac artery which can be easily identified laterally, as shown in Figure 15.1A. Once the deep circumflex iliac artery is identified which is constantly found, is traced upwards and laterally toward the anterior superior iliac spine and iliac crest (Fig. 15.1B). The iliac crest should be freed from the inner lip by erasing three abdominal muscles till you just reach the top of the iliacus muscle. Similarly the iliac crest should be freed by stripping the tensor fascia and gluteus medius on the external surface. This isolation of the iliac crest graft is best done by subperiosteal separation of muscles on either side of the lip of the ilium without disturbing the vascular supply. The desired size of free vascularized iliac bone is now marked on the external surface and osteotomy of the iliac crest is performed with a sharp osteotome or pneumatic saw. Properly planned free iliac crest graft along with vascular pedicle of the deep circumflex iliac artery is now ready for transfer (Figs 15.1B to D).

Now the inferior part of the curvilinear incision is extended from the medial side to anterolaterly up to the subtrochanteric region. Subsequently the hip joint is exposed by retracting gluteus medius laterally and by erasing vastus lateralis from the anterior portion of the subtrochanteric femur, which will expose the hip joint capsule anteriorly. The hip capsule is cut in a T shaped manner and

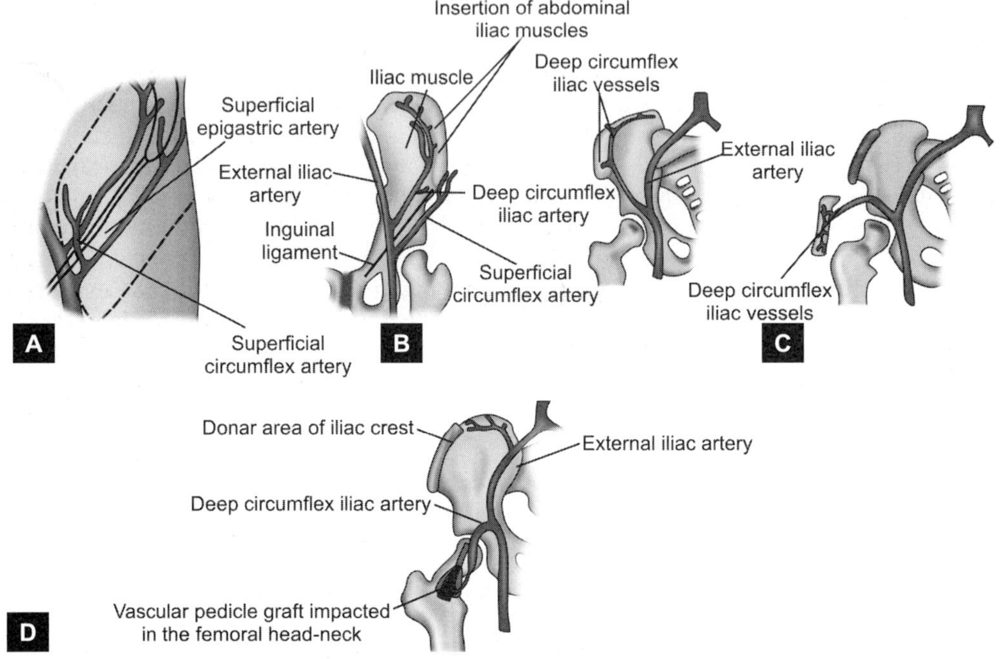

Figs 15.1A to D Line diagram (LD) showing anatomical landmarks and diagrammatic representation of the vascular pedicle of deep circumflex iliac artery in the vicinity of hip joint and iliac bone (A and B); Diagrammatic representation of isolation of deep circumflex iliac vascular pedicle along with part of iliac bone in the region of the hip (C); Diagrammatic representation showing implantation of vascular pedicle graft of deep circumflex iliac artery with part of iliac crest into the head and neck of femur (D)

the femoal head is exposed and the necrotic lesion is confirmed under an image intensifier. Now a window is made at the junction of the femoral head and neck by drilling initially by 4.5 mm extending upwards through the ischemic area. Now the entire core decompression procedure has to be done under image control. The size of drilling is increased gradually and the entire ischemic sectoral involvement is drilled, usually up to 12 to 14 mm, then the created core tract, cavity and ischemic segment of the femoral head is curetted. If there is depressed subchondral bone, it is raised up by using impactor under image control and the collapsed part of the femoral head is raised up, and the subchondral area and part of the cavity is filled with a few pieces of cancellous bone removed from the iliac crest procured during harvesting the vascular pedicle. The

trough and cavity is now ready for receiving the vascular iliac crest graft (Figs 15.1C and D). Now the graft is tunneled through the intermuscular plane between the rectus femoris and pectineus muscle and is swung in to the trochanteric region, and is introduced into the trough created in the femoral head and confirmed under the image intensifier (Fig. 15.1D). The graft is secured by taking the stitch through the hole prepared by drilling in the neck and graft.

Postoperative Protocol

Postoperatively the limb is kept in 20-degree abduction and 30-degree flexion and 10-degree of internal rotation to avoid tension on the vascular pedicle. The patient is mobilized by allowing free movements of flexion-extension and adduction-abduction after 15 days in bed and after four to six weeks patient is mobilized out of bed on nonweight-bearing crutch walking with encouragement to perform all movements. The patient is allowed partial weight-bearing after 10 weeks and full weight-bearing after 14 to 16 weeks depending upon the incorporation of the graft. Digital substraction arteriography was performed in nine patients only at the end of 12 weeks, which showed the patency of the deep circumflex artery in all the cases. Similarly bone scan was performed at 12 weeks in six other patients, showed high uptake in the grafted area of all the femoral heads. This investigation to confirm patency of the vascular pedicle and viability of the graft was not routinely done subsequently after these 15 patients, which were conclusive about the viability of the graft.

Results

Of the 31 femoral heads, almost all patients had relief of pain with the improvement in the range of movements at the end of 10 to 12 weeks. Six patients of stage III had residual low-intensity pain for a period of 24 weeks. Eight patients had painless limp for a period of 16 to 18 weeks. Four patients of stage III had restriction of flexion beyond 100 to 110 degrees till the last follow-up at five years. Only one hip from stage III progressed to further collapse and got deformed, but without any progression to arthrosis and surgery of total hip was advised at six years of follow-up. Another one patient had superficial infection at the operative site, and the wound responded nicely to dressing and short course of antibiotics within 15 days of surgery. No other complications occurred in any other patient. Nine patients of stage II improved completely without any further deterioration with complete relief of pain. The postoperative bone scan and digital substraction arteriogram performed after 12 weeks, showed hundred percent patency of the vascular pedicle and viability of the graft. The clinical and radiological results were available for all these patients.

The mean ± SD improvement in Harris Hip Score at five to eight years follow-up was 28.6 ± 6.4. The difference in the preoperative and postoperative score across the whole sample was significant ($p < 0.05$). When analyzed separately for patients with stage II and stage III disease, there was no significant difference in the Harris Hip Score suggesting that at least in the present sample, the stage of the disease had no effect on the improvement seen after surgery. Seventy percent of patients had improvement of > 25 points in the Harris Hip Score while, 48 percent had improvement of more than > 28 points in the score.

Observation

Osteonecrosis was commonly seen in the young male patients between the age of 31 to 40 years with mean age of 32 years. Loss of internal rotation and positive axis deviation test are cardinal clinical signs to suspect osteonecrosis. Whenever there is sectoral involvement of the femoral head, axis deviation test is positive. Normally if the hip is flexed more than 90 degree with flexed knee, the knee and patella faces towards the opposite shoulder, where as if it faces to the same axilla or shoulder it should be considered as positive axis deviation test. The test was positive in all patients with loss of internal rotation and bone scan, and MRI confirmed the diagnosis. The disease was commonly seen in association with alcohol abuse and corticosteroid consumption. There were 22 patients in stage III and 9 patients in stage II of ARCO's classification. Out of 31 patients who were operated, 9 patients of stage II recovered completely and no collapse occurred till the last follow-up of more than 7 to 8 years. Out of 22 patients of stage III, 12 patients had excellent results and had no symptoms of pain or restricted movements and all of them returned to their respective jobs (Figs 15.2A to H).

Out of the remaining ten patients, six patients had residual pain for about six months, but these patients also had complete relief from pain and returned to their

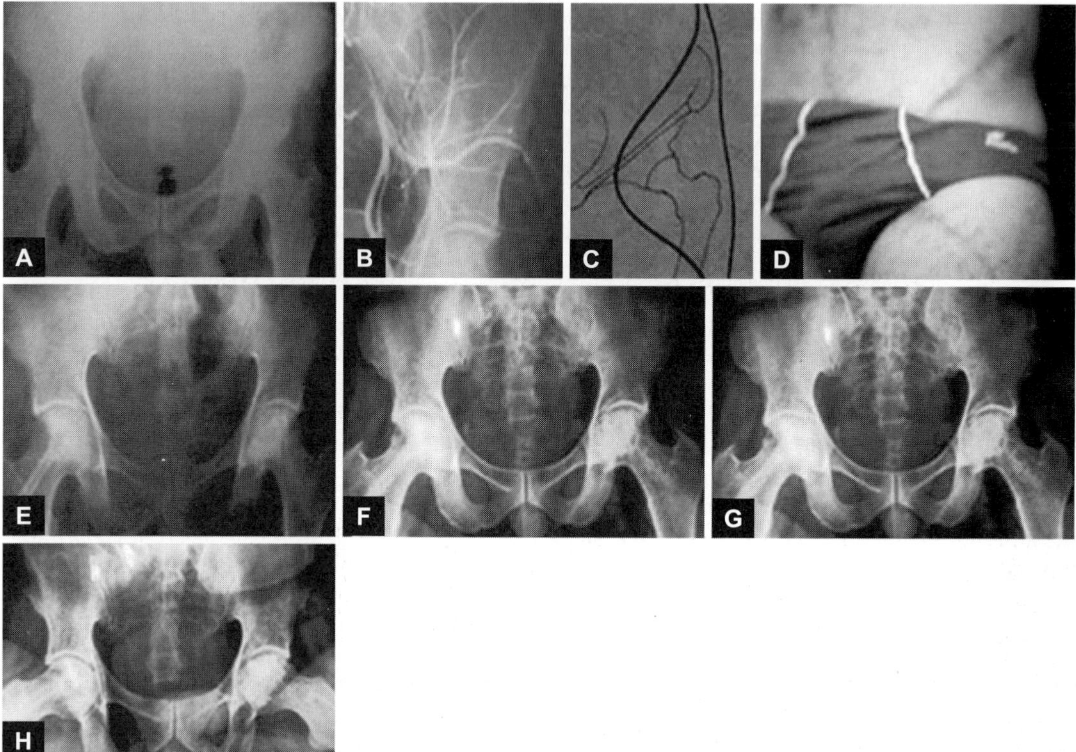

Figs 15.2A to H A young male 9 (LK) 35 years showing bilateral osteonecrosis femoral head? drug induced osteonecrosis (Preoperative X-ray A); Preoperative angiography showing presence of deep circumflex iliac pedicle (B); Line diagram of proposed surgical incision for exploration of vascular pedicle graft and its implantation into the head and neck femur (C); Clinical photograph showing operative scar (D); Postoperative X-rays at three years showing good revascularization on both sides with preservation of joint space (E and F); Postoperative X-rays at ten years showing good revascularization, maintained joint space, no arthritic changes and no deformation (G and H)

employment (Figs 15.3 and 15.4). Amongst the remaining four patients, in one patient the head progressively collapsed and developed deformity causing disturbing pain, and the surgery of total hip replacement was advised, the other three patients accepted the limitation of flexion. The sphericity of the femoral head was maintained in all the patients at five years follow-up, except that slight flattening and dome depression occurred in two patients. The postoperative bone scans and digital substraction arteriogram showed conclusive favorable results. The clinical and radiological results were available for all these patients.

Certainly with this surgery, most of the patient got the pain relief and improvement in the function of the hip, though rarely in some circumstances the progressive collapse may occur but the need for joint replacement can be prolonged and postponed by seven to eight years more in a few selected patients of this stage III, as in one of our patients.

Discussion

Need to treat ischemia of the femoral head is becoming more common since many cases are detected in the early stages in young

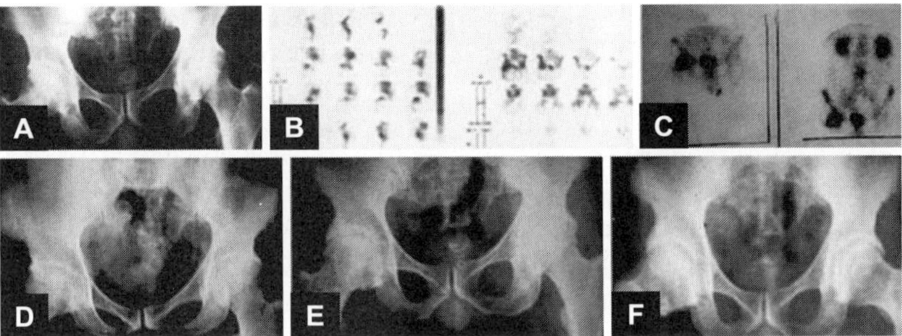

Figs 15.3A to F A young male 38 (SK) years preoperative X-ray with osteonecrosis right femoral head (A); Preoperative radionuclide bone scan with osteonecrosis right femoral head (B and C); Postoperative X-ray at 14 months with good revascularization of right femoral head (D); Postoperative X-rays at 15 years with good revascularization of right femoral head without any collapse nor arthritic changes (E and F)

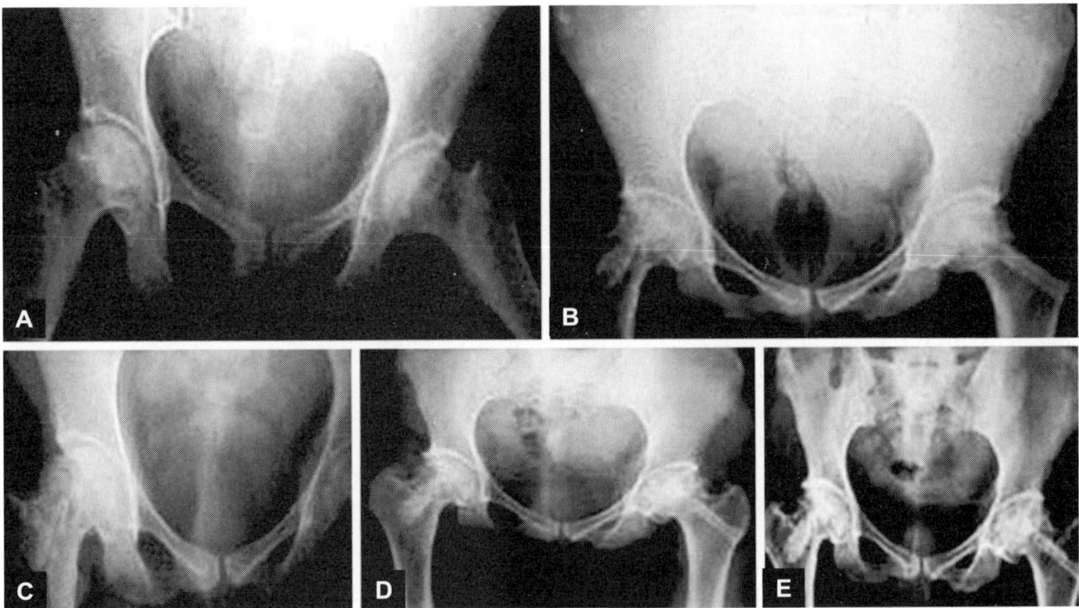

Figs 15.4A to E Young lady (PC) with osteonecrosis both femoral heads preoperative X-rays (A); Postoperative X-rays at 2 years with vascular pedicle graft from the deep circumflex iliac artery right side and fibular bone graft left side (B and C); Postoperative X-ray at 5 years showing good vascularization right femoral head (D); Postoperative X-ray at 10 years showing with good revascularization of femoral head without any collapse or arthritic changes (E)

patients. One must consider the possibility of osteonecrosis if individual has pain in the vicinity of the hip with history of chronic alcoholism, corticosteroid consumption, associated disease like sickle cell, Gaucher's, Gout, etc.[8,31,32] Early diagnosis prior to the appearance of radiological changes is crucial in the treatment of ischemic necrosis. Its diagnosis is based on clinical examination and confirmation by bone scan, CT, MRI, as osteonecrosis is the response to the vascular impairment of the bone marrow circulation. X-ray examination is of limited value in early diagnosis but has importance in staging since it helps in planning the treatment and the prognosis. The X-rays become positive late in the condition after the process of repair has started. Osteonecrosis is a disease characterized by ischemic death of bony and marrow tissues. Different imaging modalities provide different information on the mineralized and nonmineralized component of the bone. The advent of MRI has dramatically improved the diagnosis of osteonecrosis, though bone scan is also important, since in about 30 to 70 percent cases of the femoral head osteonecrosis, the other hip is affected in due course of time. Hence, it is necessary to exclude early involvement of the contralateral hip, which is asymptomatic, by either bone scan or MRI. MRI is the most accurate imaging modality for the diagnosis of osteonecrosis of the femoral head, especially in the early stages when there are only bone marrow changes. Characteristic MRI signal alterations in the anterosuperior portion of the femoral head surrounded by a band of low signal intensity on T1 and T2-weighted images represent the diagnostic criteria of osteonecrosis on MRI.[18] The occurrence of a double-line sign on the T2-weighted image represents a pathognomonic sign, but its absence does not eliminate the diagnosis of osteonecrosis.[33]

There are a number of staging systems for osteonecrosis, but with inherent problems of poor reliability.

Neel Marcus et al. 1973[34]	Florida system
Steinberg et al. 1984[13,35]	Philadelphia/Pensylavania system (Table 15.1)
Ficat and Arlet 1985[36-38]	French system
ARCO's Classification 1993	Gardeniers (Table 15.2)[15]

The Steinberg staging (Table 15.1) is widely accepted and is used in planning the treatment by many workers. The Association Research Circulation Osseous (ARCO) has proposed a new international classification system including radiographs, CT, bone scans, and MRI (Table 15.2).

This classification system incorporates the Pennsylvania system based on lesion size and the Japanese system based on lesion location. Quantitation (% area involvement of the femoral head, length of crescent sign, % surface collapse, and dome depression) and location of the lesion (medial, central or lateral) represent important prognostic factors. This ARCO's classification has been proposed as the preferred system for the future.[15] Core decompression offers the opportunity to study histological changes of early bone ischemia. It also achieves reduction in the symptoms of the pre-collapse stage of ischemic necrosis because of reduction of pressure in the compartment.

Barring exceptional circumstances there is hardly any role of conservative treatment of osteonecrosis of the femoral head and

Table 15.1 Steinberg staging of osteonecrosis of the femoral head

Stage	X-ray findings	MRI	CT
0	Normal roentgenogram, normal bone scan	+	+/-
I	Normal roentgenogram, abnormal bone scan	+	+/-
II	Sclerosis or cyst formation in the femoral head	+	+
III	Subchondral collapse (crescent sign) without flattening	+	+
IV	Flattening of head with joint narrowing or acetabular involvement	+	+
V	Flattening of head with joint narrowing and acetabular involvement	+	+
VI	Advanced degenerative changes in the hip joint	+	+

Table 15.2 ARCO's classification

Stage	0	1	2	3	4
Findings	All present techniques normal or non-diagnostic	X-ray and CT are normal. At least one of the below is positive	No crescent sign: X-ray abnormal: Sclerosis, lysis, focal porosis	Crescent sign on the X-ray and/or flattening of articular surface of femoral head	Osteoarthritis joint space narrowing, acetabular changes, joint destruction
Techniques	X-ray CT Scintigraph MRI	Scintigraph MRI * Quantitate on MRI	X-ray, CT Scintigraph MRI *Quantitate MRI and X-ray	X-ray, CT only Quantitate on X-ray	X-ray only
Sub-classification	No	Medial	Central	Lateral	No
Quantitation	No	% Area Involvement Minimal A<15% Moderate B 15-30% Extensive C>30%	Quantitation Length of crescent A<15% B 15-30% C >30%	% surface collapse dome depression A < 2 mm B 2-4 mm C > 4 mm	No

surgery is inevitable. Steinberg et al.[13] reported that progression occurred in 92 percent of 48 hips that had undergone nonoperative management. While observing the patients with protected weight-bearing, more than 85 percent patients had collapse of the femoral head at two years when symptomatic hips with stages I and II were left untreated.[17,20] More studies have shown that nonoperative treatment yields poor results. The only condition for which the protected weight-bearing might be effective is a Type A lesion to involvement of medial aspect of the femoral head. No drugs have been useful and specific in the treatment of osteonecrosis though recently the use of alendronate has been advised.

Once diagnosed it is desirable to subject the patient to early surgical intervention. The rationale for the treatment of osteonecrosis of the femoral head requires a lot of consideration.[5,20] Of prime importance in this is the age of the patient, whether both the hips are affected, etiology of the associated diseases, and demands and requirement of the patients, and the stage of the disease when the patient presents for treatment is equally important. Only core decompression may relieve the pain[21] but is not useful for revascularization of the femoral head, hence, core decompression should always be supplemented by one of the procedures of bone grafting. Core decompression is the effective treatment in the preradiological and precollapse stage of the avascular necrosis of the femoral head,[8,36-38] especially if coupled with bone grafting. Core decompression may be effective in symptomatic relief, but is of no greater value than conservative management in preventing collapse in early osteonecrosis of the femoral head.[20,21] Jones (1994)[39] analyzed nine studies and showed that in 218 of 369 patients where, 59 percent core decompression performed in the precollapse stage the prevention of progressive collapse failed. Steinberg et al. (1984)[13] concluded that the core decompression provided more predictable pain relief and changed the indications for arthroplasty more consistently than conservative management. However, only core decompression should be avoided and it must be coupled with bone grafting in the tract of the core to avoid iatrogenic fractures.[40] Despite many reports on salvage procedures no method has clearly demonstrated the arrest of disease before subchondral fracture or slowed down the progression of collapse of the femoral head and arthrosis.[6]

Certainly early diagnosis is the key to the success of head preserving operations. In the patients where changes are evident radiologically before the collapse (stage II and III), core decompression and various bone grafting procedures are advised.[22,24] The use of a nonvascularized bone graft, as originally described by Phemister, has had variable success in the treatment of osteonecrosis. Marcus et al.[34] reported satisfactory clinical results in seven of eleven hips at the time of short-term follow-up (range, 2 to 4 years). The other workers concluded the Phemister bone-grafting technique is not effective once collapse has occurred. Boettcher et al.[24] reported success in 27 (71%) of 38 hips six years after nonvascularized tibial strut grafting. However, in a longer term evaluation (performed at a mean of 14 years postoperatively) that included the original thirty-eight hips in the study by Boettcher et al. found that only 16 (29%) of 56 hips still had a good result.[41] The study by Plakseychuk AY et al.[27,28] on free vascular fibular grafting showed better clinical results and prevention of radiographic signs of progression and collapse of the femoral head more frequently than does nonvascularized fibular grafting. A marked difference with regard to signs of radiographic progression and collapse was noted between the A and B subgroups in the precollapse groups (stages I and II). To achieve early vascularization[25,26] vascular pedicle grafting using deep circumflex iliac vessel with the iliac crest is a very useful (Figs 15.1 to 15.4). This procedure though easy, is technically demanding and time consuming. Preoperative femoral angiography is necessary to confirm the presence of the deep circumflex iliac artery pedicle (Fig. 15.2B). Vascularized grafting provided a significant benefit for the hips in stages IB, IIA, and IIB.[27]

Once the crescent sign appears without collapse it is desirable to couple the bone grafting procedure with the core decompression preferably vascular or muscle pedicle grafting, to achieve early revascularization. Vascularized pedicle graft by using part of the iliac crest with the deep circumflex iliac vessels is more advantageous since a high percentage of marrow and osteogenic cells survive within a living graft, which helps for early vascularization.[25-29] However, muscle pedicle graft using tensor fascia lata graft is very easy and is commonly performed whenever both hips need simultaneous surgery. Muscle pedicle graft using quadratus femoris (Meyer's procedure)[23] was also propagated in the treatment of osteonecrosis, but it did not achieve satisfactory early revascularization and fell into disrepute since the results were not encouraging, though Meyer's[23] reported a success rate of 57 percent and Baksi[30] reported 93 percent good results. Use of tensor fascia lata graft (Baksi DP)[30] is commonly advocated when bilateral hips are involved and surgery is performed in a single sitting, as discussed in previous chapter.

The rationale of this procedure of vascularized pedicle bone grafting is based on the following three points:

1. Decompression of the femoral head, which act as compartment syndrome following increased intraosseous pressure, and interrupting the circulation that is thought to contribute to the disease.

2. Excision of the necrotic tissue which inhibits revascularization of the head.

3. Filling of the defect that is created after core with vascular pedicle is a osteo-inductive cancellous graft, which is a viable and it support the subchondral bone and articular surface and enhances the revascularization process.

The procedure has the advantages, any orthopedic surgeon can perform it, it does not require advanced training of microsurgical technique, nor any special equipment are required. Morbidity of the donor site is minimal and operative time required is comparable to a total hip arthroplasty. The potential disadvantages of vascularized fibular grafting include—it requires a longer operation time, microvascular technique, leaves a longer operative scar, and is associated with more donor site morbidity such as ankle instability, toe-clawing, subtrochanteric fracture, and heterotopic ossification, which are avoided by this technique.[41]

Head-preserving operation of core decompression and vascular pedicle grafting certainly gives excellent results in stage II, III. The prognosis of stage II and III is fairly good whereas in stage IV it is satisfactory, since about one-third of the stage IV group are likely to progress further and may require total hip joint replacement (THR) or resurfacing operations.[42,43] Prosthetic replacement is frequently an unappealing option for patients who have osteonecrosis because many are young and the etiological factors associated with the disease are also associated with complications after total hip arthroplasty, hemiarthroplasty, and surface replacement.[6] Though at our institute many patients of sickle cell disease with osteonecrosis are studied and treated, this procedure of vascular pedicle grafting was not performed on any patient, because of the possibility and high prevalence of thromboembolism in the vascular tree in this disease. Out of 103 patients treated by Urbanaiak et al.[6] free vascular fibular grafting, total hip replacement was performed in 34 percent cases in stage II and III within five years. There was survival and the probability of conversion within five years to THR rate of 11 percent in stage II and 23 percent survival for stage III. In the study by Shin Yoon Kim[41] the rate of conversion to THR was 13 percent (three of twenty-three hips) in the vascularized graft group and 22 percent (five of twenty-three hips) in the nonvascularized graft group, as compared to this study requiring THR in one patient out of 31 patients of vascular pedicle grafting at the end of six years. The hips treated with vascular pedicle grafting seemed to have less dome depression of the femoral head, and the retention of sphericity, probably because of more rapid revascularization and increased osteoinductive potential of the vascularized graft. It has been observed that there is an early failure of THR in osteonecrosis than in age-matched patients with other diagnoses because of abnormal remodeling of bones, and subsidence of prosthesis because of

Table 15.3 Stage of osteonecrosis, age and sex

Stage of osteonecrosis	No. of patient	No. of patient and sex	Age of patient			
			16–20	21–30	31–40	41 and Above
II	9 patients	7 Males	-	3	1	3
		2 Female	1	1	-	-
III	22 patients	19 Males	2	3	11	3
		3 Females	-	1	2	-
Total	31 patients	26 Males	3	8	14	6
		5 Females				

poor quality of proximal femoral bone.[40] Other contributory factors for failure are—on going systemic disease, defects in mineral metabolism, use of steroids, high level of activity in young patients and increased body weight. Hence, we prefer to delay or eliminate the need for hip replacement by performing head preserving surgeries, of which core decompression and vascular pedicle grafting is the surgery of choice.[40]

CONCLUSION

Basically osteonecrosis of the femoral head is a multifactorial, heterogeneous group of disorder that leads to final common pathology of mechanical failure of the femoral head. In this study more than 50 percent patients had osteonecrosis because of alcohol abuse, 40 percent secondary to steroid consumption and in 10 percent cases exact cause could not ascertained. It is common in the young age group where a conservative surgical approach is chosen, rather than a radical approach of reconstructive surgery. If diagnosed early head-preserving operation of core decompression and vascular pedicle bone grafting yields good to excellent results. Essentially, the result depends on the preoperative condition of the joint, the site of necrotic focus and the associated disease, which may be the cause of osteonecrosis. With the experience, if the ischemic necrosis of the femoral head is diagnosed early in stage II and III core decompression and vascular pedicle grafting gives very good results. In stage III even if there is slight collapse with deformation, the depressed segment can be elevated and deformity corrected after elevation and bone grafting. However, in a few patients the osteonecrotic segment can still deteriorate and may collapse in due course, wherein one may succeed in prolonging the need of joint replacement for seven to eight years by this surgery. Out of 31 patients only one patient progressed to collapse and surgery of joint replacement was advised. The long standing effects of surgery were excellent with great improvement in the Harris Hip Score, achieving improvement between 70 and 80 points in about 65 percent of patients at the final follow-up period.

REFERENCES

1. Glimcher MJ, Kenzora JE. The biology of osteonecrosis of the human femoral head and its clinical implications: Part III. Discussion of the etiology and genesis of the pathological sequelae; comments on treatment. Clin Orthop. 1979;140:273-312.
2. Herndon JH, Aufranc OE. Avascular necrosis of the femoral head in the adult. A review of its incidence in variety of conditions. Clin Orthop. 1972;86:43-62.
3. Glimcher MJ, Kenzora JE. The biology of osteonecrosis of the human femoral head and its clinical implications: Part II. The pathological changes in the femoral head as an organ and in the hip joint. Clin Orthop. 1979;139:283-312.
4. Mankin HJ. Nontraumatic necrosis of bone (osteonecrosis). N Eng J Med. 1992;326:1473-9.
5. Mont MA, Hungerford DS. Non-traumatic avascular necrosis of the femoral head. J Bone Joint Surg. 1995;77A:459-74.
6. Urbaniak JR, Coogan PG, Gunneson EB, et al. Treatment of osteonecrosis of the femoral head with free vascularised fibular grafting: A long term follow-up study of one hundred and three hips. J Bone Joint Surg. 1995;77A:681-94.
7. Bradway JK, Morrey BF. The natural history of the silent hip in bilateral atraumatic osteonecrosis. J Arthroplasty. 1993;8:383-7.
8. Hungerford DS, Jones LC. Diagnosis of osteonecrosis of the femoral head. In: Schoutens A, Arlet J, Gardeniers JWM, et al (Eds). Bone Circulation and Vascularisation in Normal and Pathological Conditions. New York, NY, Plenum Press; 1993.pp.265-75.
9. Kozinn SC, Wilson PD Jr. Adult hip disease and total hip replacement. Clin Symp. 1989;39:1-32.
10. Shimizu K, Moriya H, Akita T, et al. Prediction of collapse with magnetic resonance imaging of avascular necrosis of the femoral head. J Bone Joint Surg. 1994;76A:215-23.
11. Beltran J, Knight CT, Zuelzer WA, et al. Core decompression for avascular necrosis of the femoral head: Correlation between long-term results and preoperative MR staging. Radiology. 1990;175:533-6.

12. Steinberg ME, Brighton CT, Hayken GD, et al. Electrical stimulation in the treatment of Osteonecrosis of the femoral head—a 1 year follow-up. Orthop. Clin North Am. 1985;16:747-56.

13. Steinberg ME, Hayken GD, Steinberg DR. The conservative management of avascular necrosis of the femoral head. In Bone Circulation. Edited by Arlet A, Ficat RP, Hungerford DS. Baltimore; Williams and Wilkins; 1984.pp.334-7.

14. Stulberg BN, Davis AW, Bauer TW, et al: Osteonecrosis of the femoral head: A prospective randomised treatment protocol. Clin Orthop. 1991;268:140-51.

15. Gardeniers JWM. ARCO international classification of osteonecrosis. ARCO News. 1993;5:79-82.

16. Kenzora JE, Glimcher MJ. Pathogenesis of idiopathic osteonecrosis: The ubiquitous crescent sign. Orthop Clin North Am. 1985; 16:681-96.

17. Norman A, Bullough P. The radiolucent crescent line: An early diagnostic sign of avascular necrosis of the femoral head. Bull Hosp Joint Dis. 1963;24:99-104.

18. Mitchell DG, Steinberg ME, Dalinka MK, et al. Magnetic resonance imaging of the ischaemic hip: Alterations within the osteonecrotic, viable, and reactive zone. Clin Orthop. 1989;244:60-77.

19. Harris WH. Traumatic arthritis of the hip. J Bone Joint Surg Am. 1969;51A:738-43.

20. Kerboul M, Thomine J, Postel M, et al. The conservative surgical treatment of idiopathic aseptic necrosis of the femoral head. J Bone Joint Surg. 1974;56B:291-6.

21. Robinson HJ Jr. Success of core decompression in the management of early stages of avascular necrosis: A four-year prospective study. Proceedings of the American Academy of Orthopaedic Surgeons 59th Annual Meeting, Washington DC, Park Ridge, IL, American Academy of Orthopaedic Surgeons; 1992.p.177.

22. Saito S, Ohzono K, Ono K. Joint preserving operations for idiopathic avascular necrosis of the femoral head: Results of core decompression, grafting and osteotomy. J Bone Joint Surg. 1988;70B:78-84.

23. Meyers MH. The treatment of osteonecrosis of the hip with fresh osteochondral allografts and with the muscle-pedicle graft technique. Clini Orthop. 1978;130:202-9.

24. Boettcher WG, Bonfigilo M, Smith K. Non-traumatic necrosis of the femoral head: II. Experiences in treatment. J Bone Joint Surg. 1970;52A:322-9.

25. Leung PC, Chow YY. Reconstruction of proximal femoral defects with a vascular-pedicle graft. J Bone Joint Surg Br. 1984;66B:32-7.

26. Leung PC. Vascular bone grafts from iliac crest Microsurgical Technique in Orthopaedics Pho Robert WH (Ed), Butterworths; pp.135-144.

27. Plakseychuk AY, Bogov AA, Plakseychuk YA. vascularised Iliac crest Graft in the treatment of aseptic necrosis of femoral head; Reconstructive Microsurgery Current Trends Proceedings 12th Symposium International Society of Reconstructive Microsurgery, Singapore; 1996.pp.85-7.

28. Plakseychuk AY, Kim SY, Park BC, Varitimidis SE, Rubash HE, Sotereanos DG. Vascularised compared with nonvascularised fibular bone grafting for the treatment of osteonecrosis of the femoral head. J Bone Joint Surg Am. 2003; 85:589-96.

29. Iwata H, Torii S, Hasegawa Y, Itoh H, et al. Indications and results of vascularised pedical iliac bone graft in avascular necrosis of femoral head. Clin Orthop. 1993;295:281.

30. Baksi DP. Treatment of osteonecrosis of the femoral head by drilling and muscle-pedicle bone grafting. J Bone Joint Surg Br. 1991;73B:241-5.

31. Jones JP Jr. Intravascular coagulation and osteonecrosis. Clin Orthop. 1992;277:41-53.

32. Jones JP Jr. Fat embolism, intravascular coagulation, and osteonecrosis. Clin Orthop. 1993;292:294-308.

33. Kramer J, Hofmann S, Imhof H. The non-traumatic femur head necrosis in the adult: II. Radiologic diagnosis and staging. Radiologe. 1994;34:11-20.

34. Marcus ND, Enneking WF, Massam RA. The silent hip in idiopathic aseptic necrosis: treatment by bone grafting. J Bone Joint Surg Am. 1973;55A:1351-66.

35. Steinberg ME, Hayken GD, Steinberg DR. A quantitative system for staging avascular necrosis. J Bone Joint Surg. 1995;77B:34-41.

36. Arlet J, Ficat P. Forage-biopsie de la tete femorale dans l'osteonecrose primitive. Observations histo-pathologiques portant sur huit forgaes. Rev Rhumat. 1964;31:257-64.

37. Ficat P, Arlet J, Hungerford DS (Eds). Ischaemia and Necrosis of Bone. Baltimore, MD, Williams and Wilkins, 1980.

38. Ficat RP. Idiopathic bone necrosis of the femoral head: Early diagnosis and treatment. J Bone Joint Surg Br. 1985;67B:3-9.

39. Jones JP Jr. Concepts of etiology and early pathogenesis of osteonecrosis. In Schafer M (Ed):

Instructional Course Lectures 43. Rosemont, IL, American Academy of Orthopaedic Surgeons; 1994.pp.499-512.

40. Babhulkar SS. Osteonecrosis of the femoral head (in young individuals). Indian Journal of Orthopaedics. 2003;37(2):77-86.

41. Shin Yoon, Young Goo, Poong Taek Kim, Joo Chul Ihn, Byung Chae Cho, Kyung Hoi Koo. Vascularized Compared with Nonvascularized Fibular Grafts for Large Osteonecrotic Lesions of the Femoral Head. J Bone and Joint Surg. 2005;87A:2012-8.

42. Koo KH, Kim R. Quantifying the extent of osteonecrosis of the femoral head: A new method using MRI. J Bone Joint Surg Br. 1995; 77B:875-80.

43. Dutton RO, Amstuz HC, Thomas BJ, Hedley AK. Tharies surface replacement for osteonecrosis of femoral head. J Bone Joint Surgery Am. 1982; 64:1225-37.

16 PLACE OF OSTEOTOMY IN OSTEONECROSIS

Intertrochanteric osteotomy has been recommended as a way to unload the necrotic segment of the femoral head, allowing it to heal in the early stages of the disease, and as palliative treatment after collapse of the head and osteoarthrosis of the joint.[1] However, most of the results of that procedure have been inconsistent and have deteriorated rapidly with time. The most successful experience with intertrochanteric osteotomy was reported by Scher and Jakim,[2] in a prospective study of for 43 hips in a young and highly selected population. A valgus extension osteotomy combined with curettage and bone-grafting of necrotic lesions after subchondral collapse resulted in an 87 percent rate of success according to a survivorship analysis at five years, and these results remained relatively good even after longer follow-up. Sugioka et al.[3,4] reported excellent results with their technique of rotational osteotomy, however, efforts to duplicate their rate of success have been disappointing. Core decompression, when performed before subchondral collapse, has been advocated as a technique capable of interrupting the disease process and allowing the femoral head to heal. Conflicting clinical results continue to be reported, however, the variable and poorly defined natural history of the early stages of osteonecrosis of the femoral head make these studies particularly difficult to interpret.

It is believed that once the crescent sign appears and there is a collapse of necrotic bone segment, even if it is a minimal on X-ray, further collapse is inevitable and the hip joint is likely to degenerate.[5] Once the collapse of the ischemic segment occurs all the procedures of core decompression and bone grafting are not expected to do any more good, and at this stage osteotomies amongst head preserving operative groups are indicated.[2-12] In such a situation, one must analyze the possible future development in osteonecrosis, so that failed osteotomies do not affect or worsen the situation for performing total hip joint replacement. However, this does not reduce the importance of the effectiveness of osteotomies. Since at this stage, this is the only group of operations in which relatively young patients do not undergo joint replacement and a benefit of 10 to 15 years can be easily drawn. Different types of intertrochanteric osteotomies, which preserve the joint are an important and efficient method to treat the cases of ischemic necrosis of the femoral head, which usually threatens the younger patients by its rampant destruction of joint, which may result in severe disability. There are various types of osteotomy performed depending upon the site and location of the necrotic segment, which has collapsed.[2-24]

TYPES OF OSTEOTOMY

- Ventral rotation osteotomy
- Flexion osteotomy
- Valgus/varus osteotomy
- McMurray's osteotomy.

Intertrochanteric osteotomy has been recommended as a way to unload the necrotic segment of the femoral head, allowing it to heal in the early stages of the disease, and as palliative treatment after collapse of the head and osteoarthrosis of the joint. However, most of the results of that procedure have been inconsistent and have deteriorated rapidly with time. The most successful experience with intertrochanteric osteotomy was reported by Scher and Jakim,[1] in a prospective study of 43 hips in a young and highly selected population. A valgus extension osteotomy combined with curettage and bone-grafting of necrotic lesions after subchondral collapse resulted in an 87 percent rate of success according to a survivorship analysis at five years, and these results remained relatively good even after longer follow-up. Sugioka et al.[2,4,12,13] reported excellent results with their technique of rotational osteotomy: however, efforts to duplicate their rate of success have been disappointing.

Transtrochanteric ventral rotational osteotomies[3,4,7,12-18] in stage IV are done primarily in cases with collapse of femoral head without any degenerative changes (Figs 16.1 and 16.2). At times instead of ventral rotation, flexion osteotomies are done (Figs 16.3A to C).[6,8] Basically, in both these osteotomies the weight bearing superolateral segment is rotated anteromedially in the nonweight-bearing region. Angular valgus/varus osteotomy is also advised depending upon the situation of the collapsed femoral head segment, for proper containment of the undamaged femoral head underneath the acetabulum for weight-bearing (Figs 16.4 and 16.5).[18-22] McMurray's osteotomy frequently done in earlier days, is presently not considered as a suitable operation for osteonecrosis of the femoral head. In all these operated patients, early mobilization is done but nonweight bearing is maintained for four to five months.

OSTEOTOMY

The purpose of an osteotomy for the treatment of avascular necrosis of the femoral head is

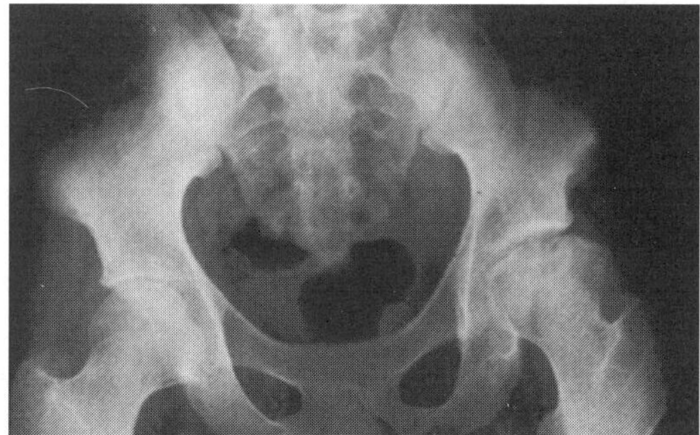

Fig. 16.1 Preoperative X-ray: Young patient of osteonecrosis with segmental collapse of the femoral head

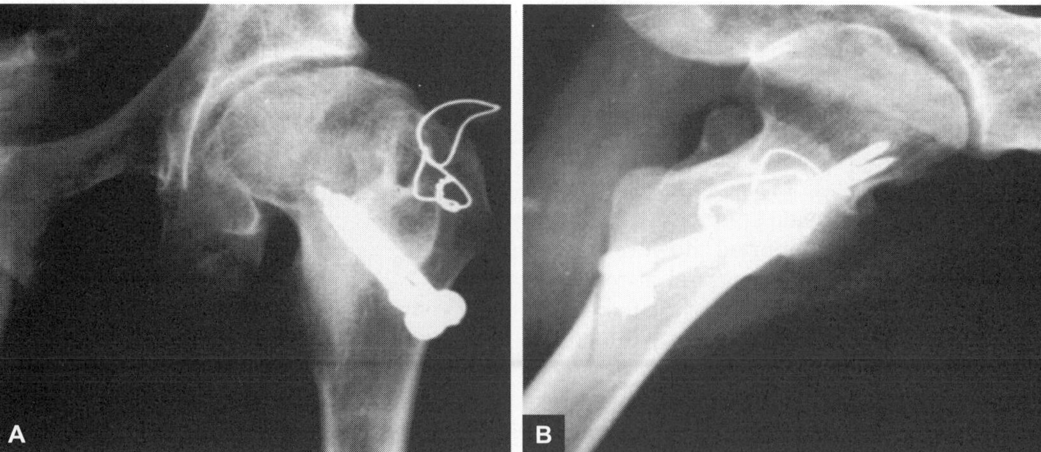

Figs 16.2A and B Postoperative X-ray of the same patient treated by ventral rotation osteotomy showing good vascularization and restoration of articular surface of femoral head at the end of one year

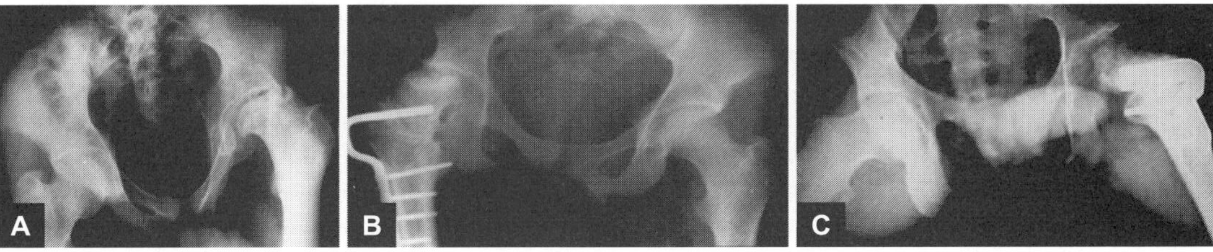

Figs 16.3A to C X-ray of a young 18 years male with sickle cell disease showing marked collapse of the femoral head, two years after flexion osteotomy of the hip at intertrochanteric region. At this young age with collapse, surgery of THR was not considered

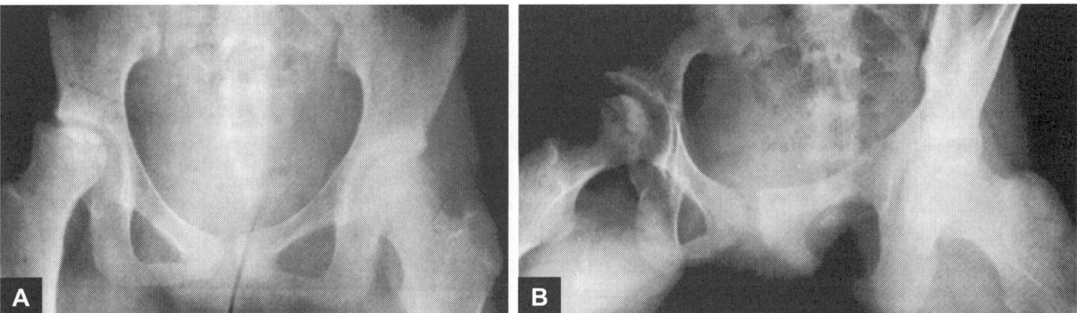

Figs 16.4A and B X-ray of young female 20-year-old with sickle cell disease showing segmental collapse affecting superolateral segment of the femoral head, properly seen in AP and Dunn's view

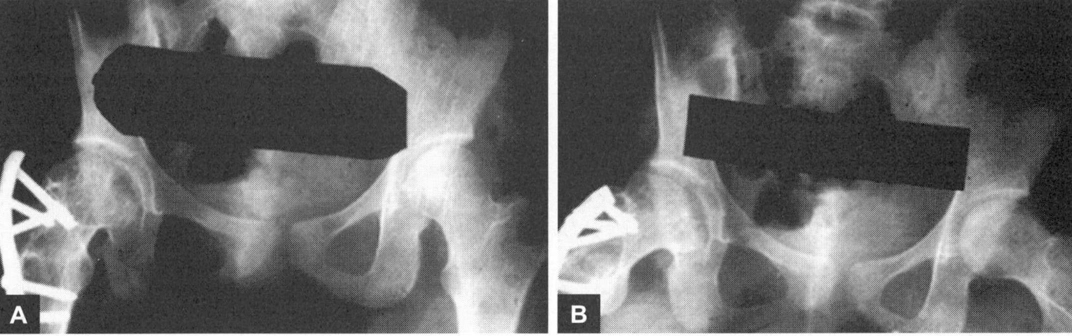

Figs 16.5A and B X-ray of the same patient Figure 16.4 six months after varus osteotomy showing complete revascularization of the femoral head with good containment hip, within the acetabulum

to move the necrotic segment away from the major load-transmitting area of the acetabulum and to redistribute the weight-bearing forces to articular cartilage that is supported by healthy bone. There are many reports in the European and Japanese literature concerning the use of osteotomies for salvage of hips with stages II and III disease. All of these osteotomies require a period of restricted weight-bearing lasting from three months to one year and usually until there is a radiographic evidence of healing of the osteotomy.[5,8] One of the more well-known osteotomies is the transtrochantenic procedure described by Sugioka et al.[3,4,12] It is technically demanding and its reported success has been variable.[14,15] Masuda et al.[16] reported a satisfactory result in 36 (69%) of 52 hips that had been followed for an average of five years (range, one to ten years). Sugano et al.[17] in 1992 reported a similar rate of success in 23 (56%) of 41 hips at six years. However, other surgeons,[14,15] have reported less favorable results than those reported in these series.[14,15]

In the study by M Mont and Hungerford[18] in 1995, varus intertrochanteric osteotomy resulted in the preservation of 23 (74%) of 31 hips with stage III disease at an average of 11 years. When only the patients who did not have corticosteroid-associated disease are considered, 15 of 18 hips survived. When the combined necrotic angle was less than 200 degrees, 13 of 15 hips survived. In another recent report, Scher and Jakim[1] found that valgus osteotomy combined with bone-grafting was successful in 36 (80%) of 45 patients who were not taking corticosteroids. Other reported rates of failure of varus and valgus osteotomies have ranged from 23 to 40 percent after approximately five years.[5,19-21] One possible problem with the use of an osteotomy is that it may make it more difficult to obtain a good clinical result if the hip ever needs to be converted to an arthroplasty.[25] In a study of 105 arthroplasties performed in 93 patients, who had had a previous osteotomy,[25] the surgeons encountered intraoperative problems, such as difficulty with removal of a plate or screw as well as with reaming of the femur. However, the clinical outcomes were good. It appears that these difficulties are acceptable as long as the surgeon can manage them intraoperatively.

Presently the opinion regarding osteotomy for osteonecrosis of the femoral head is with proper selection of the patient, angular or rotational osteotomies are useful for the treatment of this condition. The ideal candidate has stage III disease, a small lesion (a combined necrotic angle of less than 200 degrees, and no ongoing causes for avascular necrosis, such as the use of high doses of corticosteroids.[18] Several kinds of femoral osteotomies may also be effective in some hips with advanced stages of osteonecrosis. The principal concept of femoral osteotomies in the treatment of femoral head osteonecrosis is that the necrotic femoral head focus is moved away from the major weight-bearing portion underneath the acetabulum and weight-bearing forces are transmitted to living areas of the femoral head. The main purpose of the anterior femoral rotational osteotomy described by Sugioka is for the remaining posterior noncollapsed living femoral head bone to be transferred to the loaded portion opposite to the acetabular roof.[3,4,12,13] Postoperatively, results of that procedure have been linked to the extent of the intact articular surface of the affected lateral portion of the femoral head that can be seen on the anteroposterior radiographs. According to Sugioka et al. a success rate of 93 percent was achieved with anterior femoral rotational osteotomy if the postoperative living lateral portion of the femoral head articular surface exceeded 36 percent on anteroposterior radiographs.[25] However, the rate of good results decreased in stage III hips with collapse. In the present study, further collapse was prevented when an adequate amount of living femoral head bone had been placed under the acetabular roof as seen on conventional anteroposterior and 45 degree flexion anteroposterior radiographs. Sugioka et al. originally proposed an anterior rotational osteotomy if the necrotic area of the femoral head was localized anteriorly and if it involved less than two-thirds of the head.[3,4,12,13] It is found that many young patients have extensive lesions with advanced collapse that would not be candidates for the procedure of Sugioka et al.[25,26]

Sugioka et al.[3,4,12,13] have reported on a transtrochanteric anterior femoral rotational osteotomy to treat osteonecrosis of the femoral head and have described excellent results. According to Sugioka, the absolute indication for this operation is a necrotic focus that includes less than the posterior one-third of the entire femoral head, as seen on lateral radiographs, so that this area can be rotated and placed under the loaded portion of the acetabulum. Sugioka has mentioned indications for posterior rotational osteotomies to be used for femoral heads with anterior living bone but has not reported on this procedure in detail.[25]

Atsumi et al. have previously reported on the use of a modified approach to posterior rotational osteotomy for the treatment of femoral head osteonecrosis with extensive lesions.[25,26] One possible advantage of the posterior femoral rotational osteotomy is that the posterior column artery branch from the medial femoral circumflex artery is shifted medially and is not put under tension with posterior rotation. This benefit has been confirmed by angiographic studies.[27,28] Thus, a large amount of posterior rotation can be performed even when the patient has an extensive femoral head lesion that is beyond the scope of traditional anterior rotational osteotomy according to the indications suggested by Sugioka. Another advantage of the posterior osteotomy is that the necrotic femoral head lesion is transferred to the posteromedial nonweight-bearing portion of the joint and the areas of living bone of the femoral head are moved to the lateral loaded portion below the acetabular roof with hip flexion. After posterior rotation, articular surface congruency can be expected when the hip is flexed. Atsumi et al.[25-29] reviewed their patients and expressed the effectiveness of joint preservation by means of this posterior femoral neck rotational osteotomy for extensively collapsed lesions due to osteonecrosis of the femoral head in young patients.

■ REFERENCES

1. Merle d' Aubigue R Vaillant JM. Correction simultanee des angles d' inclinations et de torsion du col femoral part I osteotomies plane oblique. Rev Chir Orthop. 1961;47:94-103.
2. Scher MA, and Jakim I. Intertrochanteric osteotomy and autogenous bone grafting for avascular necrosis of the femoral head. J Bone Joint Surg Am. 1993;75A:1119-33.
3. Sugioka Y. Transtrochanteric anterior rotational osteotomy of the femoral head in the treatment of osteonecrosis affecting the hip in a new osteotomy operation, Clin Orthop. 1978; 130:191-201.
4. Sugoika Y, Hotokebuchi T, Tsutsui H. Transtrochanteric anterior rotational Osteotomy for idiopathic and steroid induced necrosis of the femoral head; indications and long-term results. Clin Orthop. 1992;277:111-20.
5. Kerboul M, Thomine J, Postel M, Merle d' aubigne R. The conservative surgical treatment of idiopathic aseptic necrosis of the femoral head. J Bone Joint Surg Br. 1974;56B:291-6.
6. Simonnet JH, Aubaniac JM. The results of intertrochanteric flexion osteotomy in idiopathic avascular necrosis of femoral head - 52 cases. Rev Chir Ortho. 1984;70:219-29.
7. Kempt I, Karger C, associates. Post rotational osteotomy of femoral head in avascular necrosis. Rev Chir Ortho. 1984;70:271-82.
8. Willert HG, Buchhom G, Zichner L. Results of flexion osteotomy on segmental femoral head necrosis in adults. In: Weil UH (Ed). Segmental idiopathic necrosis of the femoral head. Progress Orthop Surg. 1981;5:63-80.
9. Wagner H, Zeiler G. Idiopathic necrosis of the femoral head. Results of intertrochanteric osteotomy and joint resurfacing. In: Weil UH, (Ed). Segmental Idiopathic necrosis of the femoral head. Progress Orthop Surg. 1981;5:87-116.
10. Saito S, Ohzono K, Ono K. Joint preserving operations for idiopathic avascular necrosis of the femoral head. J Bone Joint Surg Br. 1988; 70B:78-84.
11. Giunti A, Vicenzi G, Toni A, et al. Intertrochanteric osteotomy in the treatment of idiopathic osteonecrosis of the head of the femur in adults: A study of 76 cases with a follow up of 3-16 years. Ital J Orthop Traumatol. 1984; 10:31-7.
12. Sugioka Y. Transtrochanteric rotational osteotomy in the treatment of idiopathic and steroid induced femoral head necrosis, Perthes disease, slipped capital femoral epiphysis, and osteoarthritis of the hip. Indications and results. Clin Orthop. 1984;184:12.
13. Sugioka Y, Kotsuki I, Hotokebuchi T. Transtrochanteric anterior rotational Osteotomy of the femoral head for the treatment of osteonecrosis. Follow-up statistics. Clin Orthop. 1982;169: 115-26.

14. Dean MT, Cabanela ME. Transtrochanteric anterior rotational osteotomy for avascular necrosis of the femoral head. Long term results. J Bone Joint Surg Br. 1993;75-B:597-601.

15. Tooke SMT, Amstutz HC, Hedley AK. Results of transtrochanteric rotational osteotomy for the femoral head osteonecrosis. Clin Orthop. 1987;224:150-7.

16. Masuda T, Matsuno T, Hasegawa, et al. Results of transtrochnateric rotational osteotomy for non-traumatic osteonecrosis of the femoral head. Clin Orthop. 1988;228:69-74.

17. Sugano N, Takaoka K, Ohzono K, Matsui M, Saito M, Saito S. Rotational osteotomy for non-traumatic avascular necrosis of the femoral head. J Bone Joint Surg Br. 1992;74B:734-9.

18. Mont MA, Hungerford DS. Non-traumatic avascular necrosis of the femoral head. J Bone Joint Surg Am. 1995;77A:459-74.

19. Ganz R, Buchler U. Overview of attempts to revascularise the dead head in aseptic necrosis of the femoral head osteotomy and revascularization. Hip. 1983;296-305.

20. Gottschalk F. Indication and results of intertrochanteric osteotomy in osteonecrosis of femoral head. Clin Orthop. 1989;249:219-22.

21. Maistrelli G, Fusco U, Avai A, Bombelli R. Osteonecrosis of the hip treated by intertrochanteric osteotomy. A 4 to 15 years follow up. J Bone and Joint Surg Br. 1988;70B:761-6.

22. Jacobs MA, Hungerford Ds, Krackow KA. Intertrochanteric osteotomy for avascular necrosis of the femoral head. J Bone joint Surg Br. 1989;71B:200-4.

23. Sugano N, Takaoka K, Ohzono, et al. Rotational osteotomy for non-traumatic avascular necrosis of the femoral head with large lesion. Clinc Orthop. 1997;334:98-10.

24. Kenzora JE, Glimcher MJ. Pathogenesis of idiopathic osteonecrosis: The ubiquitous crescent sign. Orthop Clin North Am. 1985; 16:681-96.

25. Benke GJ, Baker AS, Dounis E. Total hip replacement after upper femoral osteotomy. A clinical review. J Bone joint Surg Br. 1982;64B:570-1.

26. Atsumi T, Kuroki Y. Modified Sugioka's osteotomy more than 130 degrees posterior rotation for osteonecrosis of the femoral head with large lesion. Clin Orthop. 1997;334:98-107.

27. Atsumi T, Kajiwara T, Hiranuma Y, Tamaoki S, Asakura Y. Posterior rotational osteotomy for nontraumatic osteonecrosis with extensive collaped lesions in young patients. J Bone Joint Surg Am. 2006;88A (Supplement 3):42-7.

28. Atsumi T, Yamano K. Role of impairment of blood supply of the femoral head in the pathogenesis of idiopathic osteonecrosis. Clin Orthop. 1992;277:22-30.

29. Atsumi T, Yamano K. Superselective angiography in osteonecrosis of the femoral head. In: Urbaniak JR, Jones JP (Eds). Osteonecrosis: Etiology, diagnosis and treatment. Rosemont, IL: American Academy of Orthopaedic Surgeons. 1997.pp.247-52.

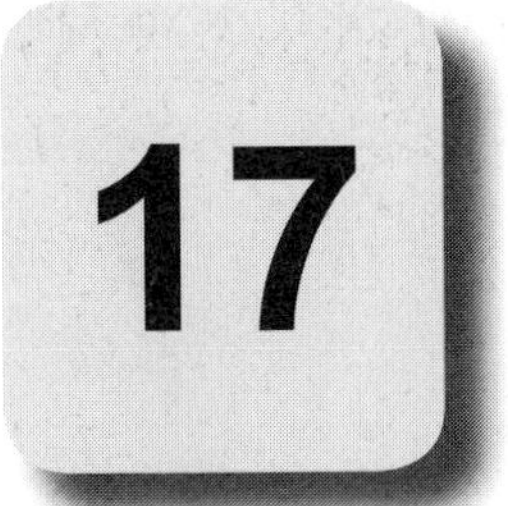

OSTEONECROSIS AND JOINT REPLACEMENT ARTHROPLASTY

Prosthetic replacement is frequently an unappealing option for patients who have osteonecrosis because many are young and the etiological factors associated with the disease are also associated with complications after total hip arthroplasty, hemiarthroplasty, and surface-replacement arthroplasty. Proponents of replacement arthroplasty have stated that the results have improved and that the life expectancy frequently shorter than normal in patients who are at risk for osteonecrosis of the femoral head justifies prosthetic replacement in some. Enthusiasm for arthrodesis of the hip has been diminished by the realization that in more than 50 percent of patients who have nontraumatic osteonecrosis of the femoral head, the condition is bilateral. Similarly, obtaining fusion of a necrotic head might be more difficult.

Osteonecrosis of the femoral head is a common debilitating cause of hip pain, particularly among patients in their third to sixth decades of life. It is a frequent disease of the young, where collapse of the femoral head is inevitable on many occasions, causing secondary arthritis. Femoral head osteonecrosis occurs in young patients with a mean age of younger than 50 years and treating these young patients remains a major therapeutic challenge. The prognosis of osteonecrosis depends heavily on the size of the necrotic lesion; involvement greater than 30 percent involvement of the femoral head leads to progressive femoral head collapse and further joint deterioration. There are many different underlying etiologies and factors which predispose to the development of osteonecrosis, the more common of which are steroid use, alcoholism, sickle cell disease, idiopathic and trauma. Treatment of osteonecrosis of the femoral head remains difficult and controversial, and is based on multiple factors, such as patient age, stage of disease, and degree of involvement. Prior to significant head collapse, treatment generally consists of head-preserving procedures such as core decompression, bone grafting, or osteotomy. When debilitating pain is associated with significant collapse and joint degeneration, total hip replacement is indicated. A large osteonecrotic lesion of the femoral head collapse, resulting in pain and deformity, frequently requires a major reconstructive procedure for symptom control. Replacement arthroplasty offers good functional and symptomatic outcome; however, long life expectancy and increased physical activity in young patients puts them at increased risk of multiple revisions resulting from implant failure.

Traditionally, osteonecrosis of the femoral head as the reason for total hip arthroplasty has had outcomes inferior to the hips with osteoarthritis as the cause of the operation. Specifically, the osteonecrotic hips have had more loosening of components. Many previous reports suggest that total hip arthroplasty performs suboptimally in young patients with osteonecrosis. Total hip replacement is considered as the treatment of choice in advanced osteonecrosis of the femoral head with significant collapse of the head and

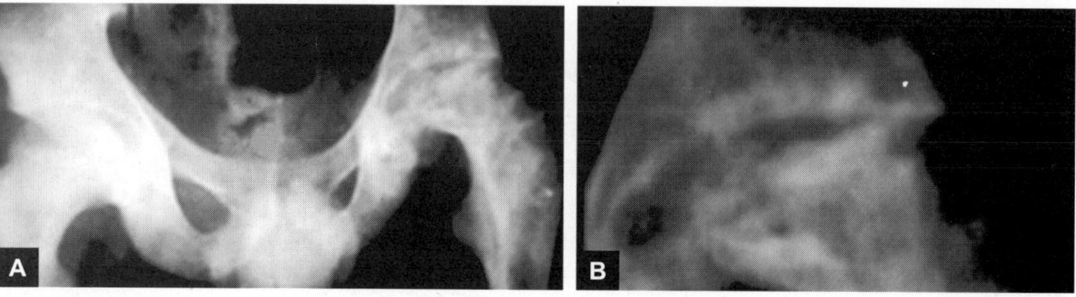

Figs 17.1A and B X-ray of a 45 years young sickle-cell disease patient with complete collapse of the femoral head and arthritic changes—Stage IV-V

joint degeneration. The most experience has been with cemented total hip replacement, and although no previous minimum ten-year follow-up results have been reported for patients with osteonecrosis of the femoral head, the medium-term results have generally been inferior to those in other patient populations (Figs 17.1 and 17.2). Failure with cemented components was frequently noticed in many young patients of osteonecrosis and may be related to changes in cancellous bone structure and remodeling with osteonecrosis. Defective cancellous bone might not support the interdigitation of cement and the increased load placed on it. The framework of cancellous bone in osteonecrosis is apparently weak. Calder et al.[1] described extensive osteocyte death and an abnormal remodeling capacity in the proximal femur in osteonecrosis, and proposed that premature loosening of implants in patients with osteonecrosis may be related to this presence of abnormal cancellous bone at the implant-bone and cement-bone interfaces. Some of the explanations given for poor results of cemented total hip replacement in patients with osteonecrosis of the femoral head include the relatively young population of patients affected by osteonecrosis and the associated systemic illness and metabolic bone disease which may underlie osteonecrosis. Cornell et al.[2] reported an overall failure rate of 37 percent in 28 hips which underwent cemented total hip replacement for osteonecrosis of the femoral head with five to ten year follow-up.

Thirty-two percent of the hips were revised for aseptic loosening. Saito et al.[3] reported on 29 cemented total hip replacements in patients with osteonecrosis of the femoral head with five to eleven year follow-up: 48 percent developed aseptic loosening and 28 percent required revision. These results were significantly worse than in their patients with osteoarthritis. Stauffer's[4] ten year follow-up of cemented total hip replacement included ten hips with osteonecrosis of the femoral head and five of these had loosening of the femoral component, a loosening rate which was higher than in the rest of the series. Salvati and Cornell[5] reviewed a series of 28 hips in 24 patients treated by cemented total hip replacement, and reported a rate of failure of 37 percent at a mean of eight years after implantation, with 100 percent failure in those under 30 years of age. Acetabular loosening was responsible in five patients, three had a fracture of the femoral stem, two a deep infection and in one the femoral component was loose. Saito et al.[3] reported the results of cemented THA in 23 patients with 29 hips diagnosed as nontraumatic AVN. The rate of revision was 28 percent (eight hips) with a mean follow-up of seven years. Overall, the results were unsatisfactory in 48 percent of patients.

Chandler et al.[6] reviewed the results of 33 total hip arthroplasties undertaken in patients under the age of 30 years, of whom 11 were known to have avascular necrosis. Complications were reported in over 50 percent and

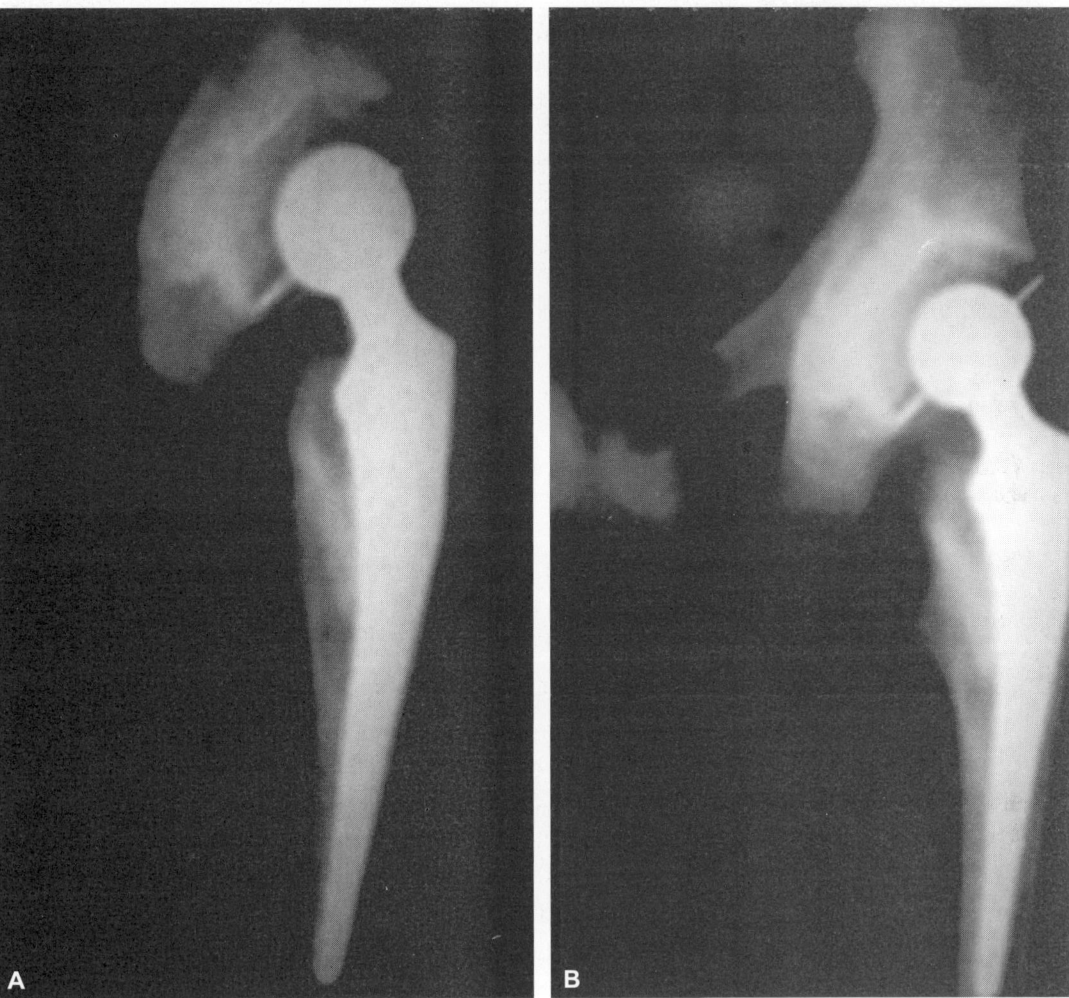

Figs 17.2A and B Postoperative X-ray of same patient (Fig. 17.1) one year after surgery, hip was treated with cemented total hip replacement

the revision rate at five years was 21 percent, with a further 33 percent showing either migration of the component or progressive radiolucent lines. The poor results appeared primarily in the younger age patient at the time of total hip replacement. Aseptic loosening of cemented acetabular components has been a problem. Contemporary cement techniques did not improve results. Modern cementing techniques have improved the results of total hip arthroplasty. Kantor et al.[7] using second-generation cementing techniques, reported an overall rate of revision of 12.5 percent at a mean follow-up of 7.5 years in 28 hips of 20 patients with nontraumatic osteonecrosis.

In view of the high rate of failure and revision in this group of patients, a few authors—Lieberman JR et al.[8] and Hungerford MW et al.[9] have advocated the use of uncemented implants. Cementless total hip arthroplasty was developed to obtain biologic fixation and increase the longevity of the implant (Figs 17.3A

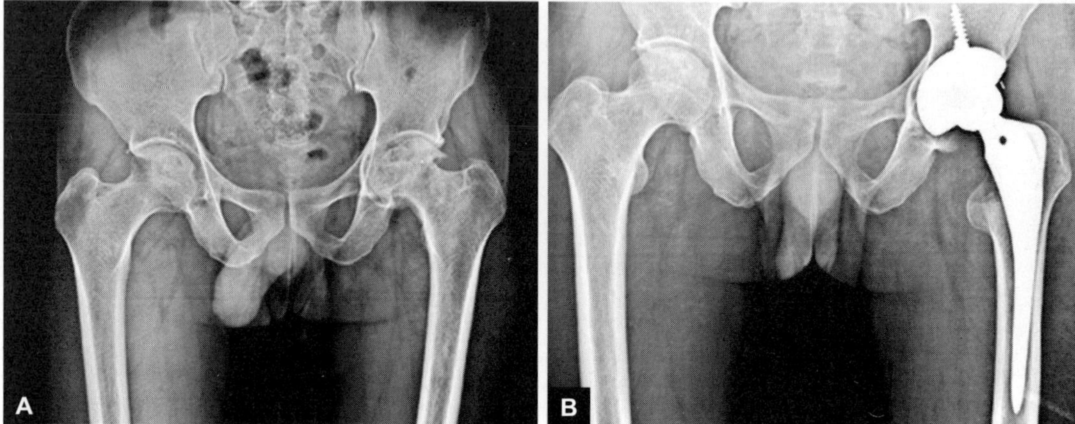

Figs 17.3A and B X-ray showing osteonecrosis left hip with arthritic changes stage IV in a 52 years alcoholic male treated by uncemented total hip replacement

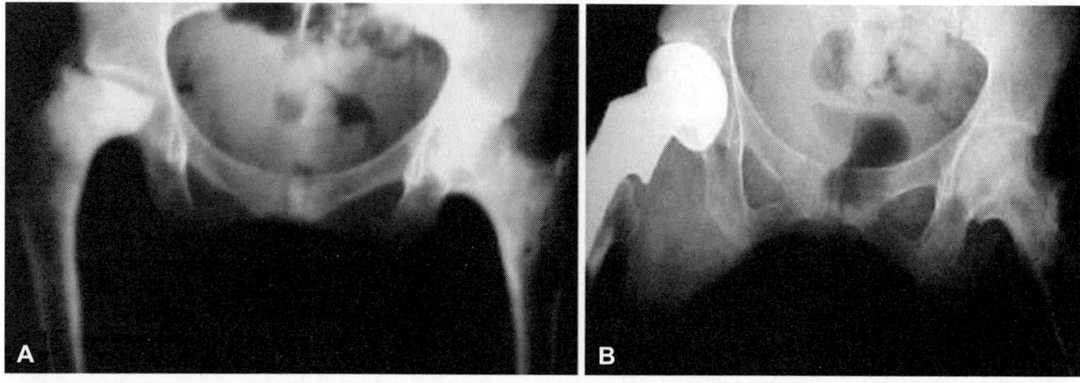

Figs 17.4A and B X-ray of a young lady of 32 years with sickle-cell disease, had multiple joint involvement. Her both hips had osteonecrosis: left hip showed a big osteonecrotic segmenetal involvement with spared hip joint and was treated by core decompression and free fibular graft on left side, within 8 months right hip was very painful and was treated with bipolar hip replacement

and B, 17.7 to 17.12). Short-term results of various types of cementless total hip arthroplasty were encouraging. However, arthroplasty using the first-generation straight femoral stems was associated with high rates of failure as a result of thigh pain, subsidence of the femoral stem, aseptic loosening, proximal loss of bone attributable to stress shielding, and polyethylene particle-induced osteolysis. Anatomic stems were designed to maximize the proximal fit in both the coronal and the sagittal planes and hopefully enhance implant survival compared to that of the first-generation stems. Implant survival would, of course, be particularly important for the younger patients with osteonecrosis. However, the effectiveness of the anatomic stem remains controversial and it is not known whether the design criteria solved the problems with the first generation straight stems.

The survival of cementless, porous-coated acetabular components implanted by a press-fit technique, with or without multiple

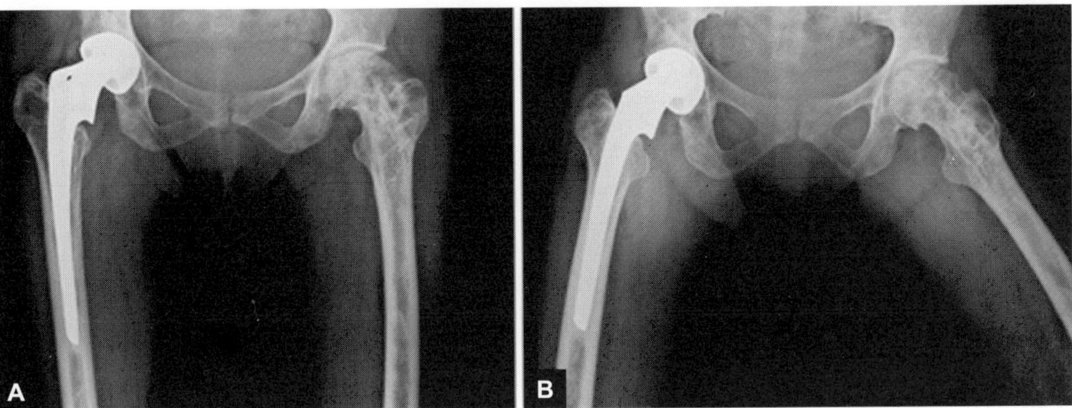

Figs 17.5A and B Postoperative X-ray of the same patient (Fig. 17.4), after 5 years of surgery showing good vascularization of left hip and good function with bipolar on right side

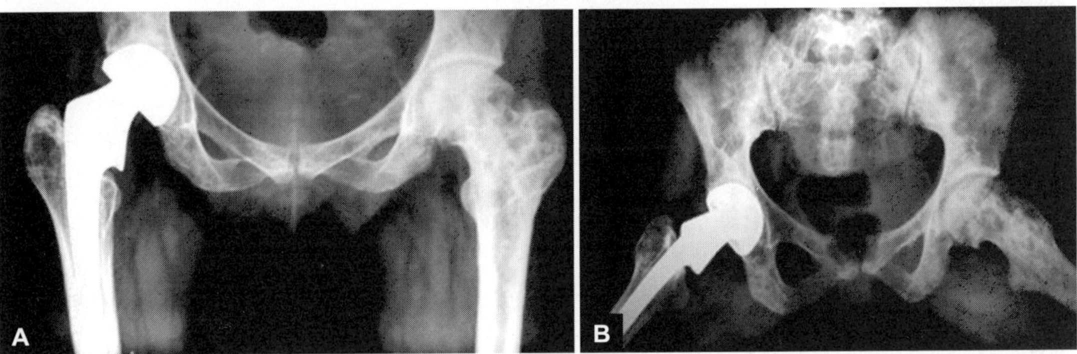

Figs 17.6A and B Postoperative X-ray of the same patient (Fig. 17.4), after 20 years of surgery showing good vascularization of left hip and well functioning bipolar on right side without any symptoms

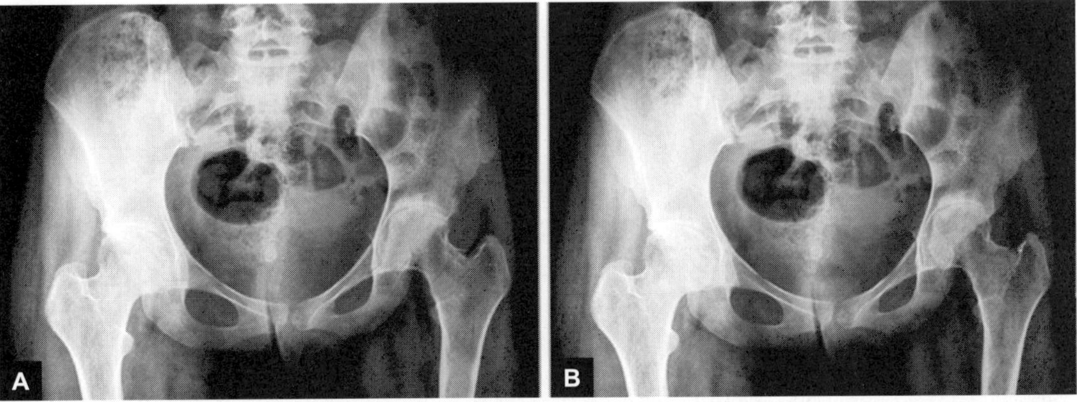

Figs 17.7A and B X-ray of a young lady of lupus eryhromatosis on corticosteroid has advanced osteonecrosis both sides. Had painful hips with restricted walking ability

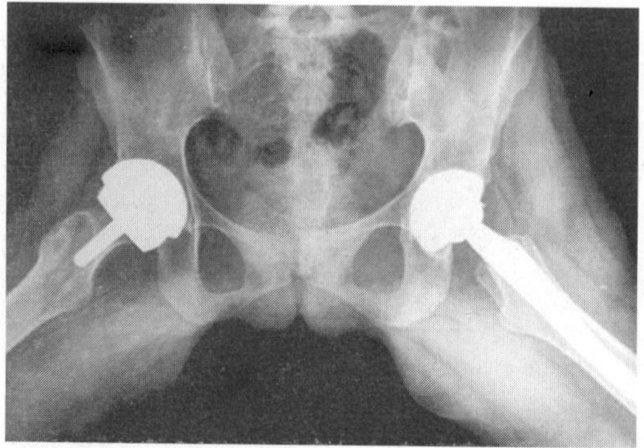

Fig. 17.8 Postoperative X-ray of the same patient (Fig. 17.7) which was treated by surface replacement on right side and uncemented hip replacement on left side

screws, has been excellent although wear of polyethylene and periprosthetic osteolysis have still been major problems.

Brinker et al.[10] described 81 uncemented arthroplasties in 64 patients with osteonecrosis of differing etiologies. In a follow-up period of four to eight years, the rate of revision was 10 percent. Piston et al.[11] in a series of 35 uncemented arthroplasties in 30 patients with osteonecrosis, found a rate of revision of 6 percent at a mean of 7.5 years metal-on-metal articulations in younger active patients have a low rate of wear and osteolysis. Low wear has been the most important factor in long-term performance of metal-on-metal articulations.

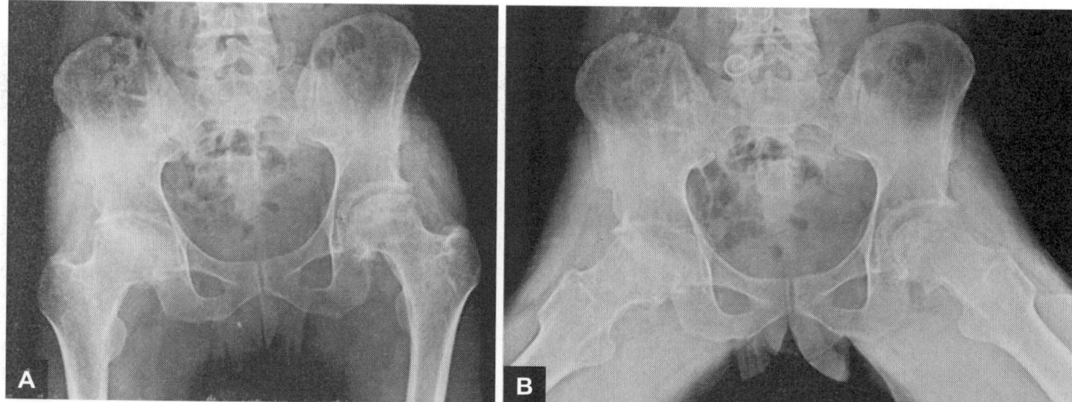

Figs 17.9A and B X-ray of a young male on corticosteroid for one year for dermatological problem, has advanced osteonecrosis both sides. Had painful hips with restricted walking ability

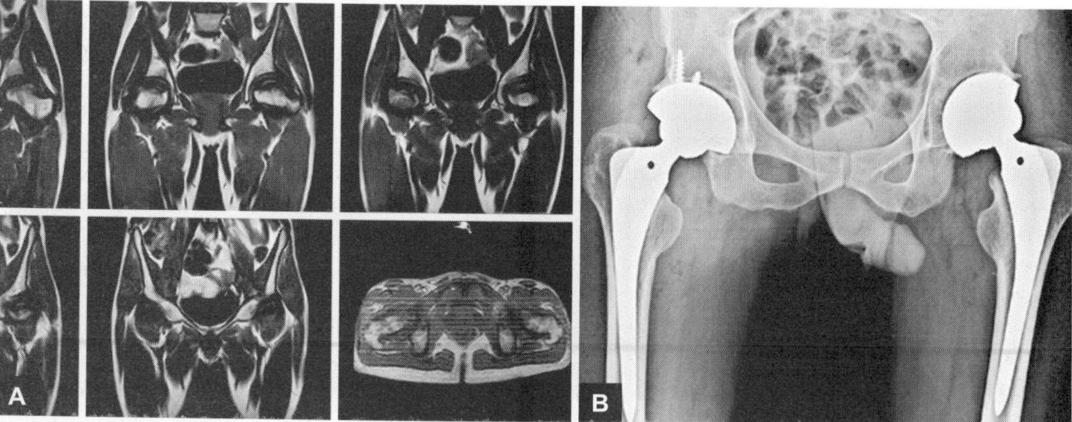

Figs 17.10A and B MRI of the same patient as Figures 17.9 to 17.10A showing bilateral osteonecrosis. (Fig. 17.10B) Postoperative X-ray of the same patient which was treated by uncemented total hip replacement

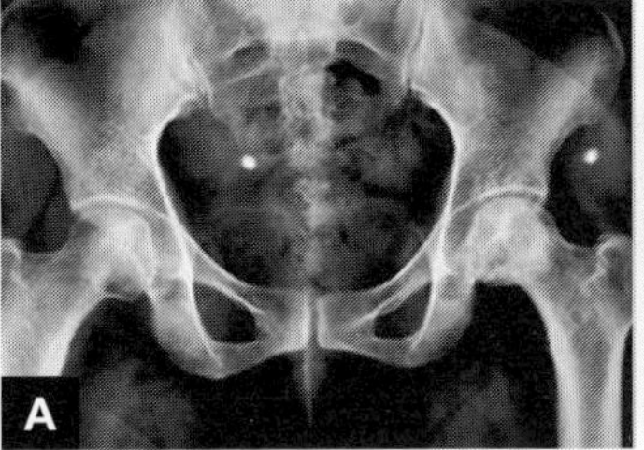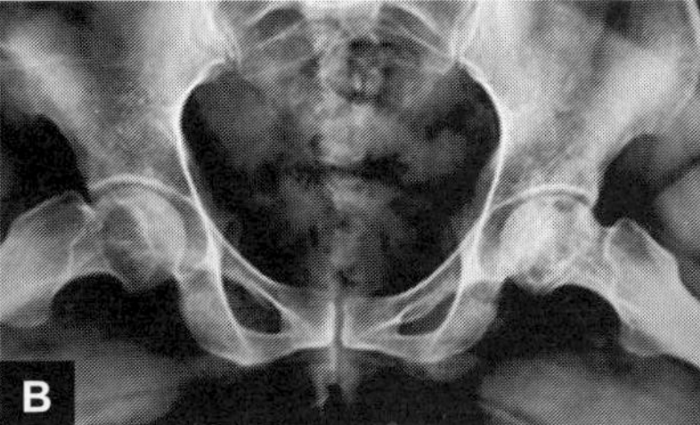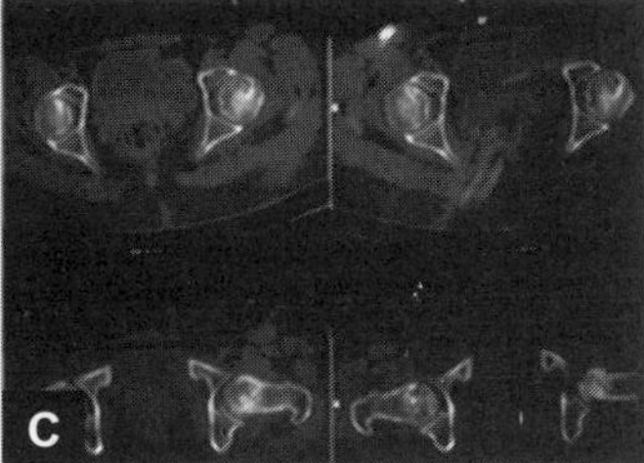

Figs 17.11A to C X-ray of a young lady of 45 years with osteonecrosis steroid induced: plain X-ray showing segmental involvement of left femoral head, stage II/III. CT scan (Fig. 17.11C) confirms the lesion

Revisions and rerevisions are associated with subsequent lower quality of life and patient satisfaction, higher failure rates (26-57 percent at 10 years) and more early (readmission, infection, hip dislocation) and late (nonunion of the trochanter, thigh pain, heterotopic bone formation, rerevision, recurrent dislocation) complications than primary total hip arthroplasty. Because of these considerations, bone-conserving procedures such as resurfacing provide a possible alternative for young patients with advanced osteonecrosis. Resurfacing hemiarthroplasty preserves the acetabulum and proximal femur and does not violate the femoral medullary canal. The utility of the resurfacing procedure as treatment of osteonecrosis is a subject of disagreement. The results of femoral head resurfacing are unpredictable, with an overall failure rate of 64 percent at 33 months follow-up.[12] Others offer this procedure as a treatment option for osteonecrosis, based on satisfactory results in 62.5 percent of patients at three years follow-up (Figs 17.7, 17.8, 17.13 to 17.15).[13]

Bose and Baruah[14] in 2010 has emphasized that the utility of resurfacing hemiarthroplasty probably lies in delaying total hip arthroplasty in a young patient with osteonecrosis who otherwise would have received a total hip arthroplasty.[14] The important questions are, how long a delay is meaningful and are there any factors that could extend this period?

Preliminary results by Evguenia J et al.[15] showed that resurfacing hemiarthroplasty may delay the need for THR by three years in the majority of patients and by seven to eight years in select patients. Another theoretical advantage of resurfacing hemiarthroplasty is the potential to perform a total resurfacing in the future should acetabular wear occur. Hypothetically, the femoral component can be left in place and the acetabulum can be resurfaced.

Uncemented prostheses are not without problems; Kim, Oh and Oh[16, 17] reviewed a series of 78 uncemented total hip arthroplasties in 61 patients with a rate of femoral revision of 5.1 percent, of the acetabulum of 6.4 percent and an overall failure of 20.5 percent. Callaghan, Dysart and Savory[18] in their series of porous-coated anatomic uncemented prostheses, had a 16 percent incidence of thigh pain. Katz et al.[19] in their series of 34 total hip arthroplasties (31 patients), of which 14 had uncemented components, described a 29 percent incidence of severe thigh pain. Lins et al.[20] in a series of 37 hips in 33 patients had an 25 percent incidence of thigh pain with nine patients (20%) requiring the aid of a stick. Several studies have shown a variable outcome depending on the etiology; patients with traumatic or idiopathic osteonecrosis were better than those whose osteonecrosis was associated with steroids or alcohol.[21,22]

Those hips which are grossly disorganized after the collapse of the femoral head might require one of the following procedures depending upon its merit, the need and demand of the patient and the etiology of the osteonecrosis.

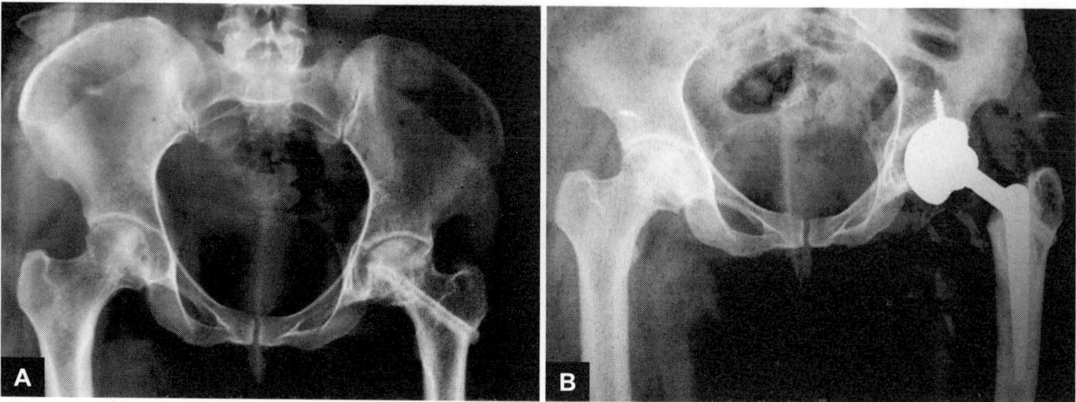

Figs 17.12A and B X-ray of the same patient as Figure 17.11A, a young lady of 45 years with osteonecrosis steroid induced: treated initially by core decompression and free fibular graft. She had no benefit from surgery and continued to have painful hip with restricted movements. She was operated and uncemented total hip was performed (Fig. 17.11B)

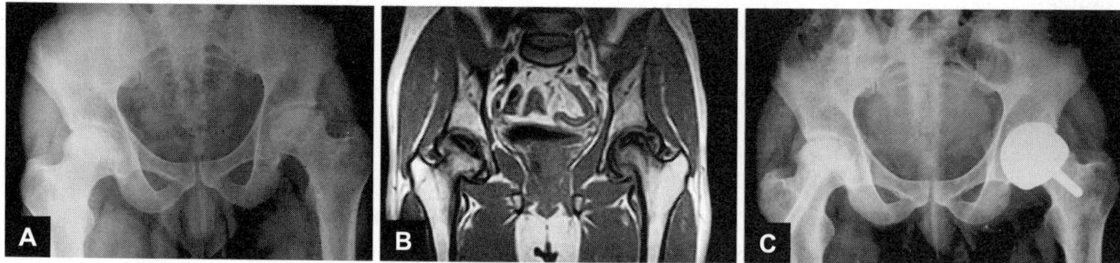

Figs 17.13A to C X-ray of a young patient of 40 years with bilateral steroid induced osteonecrosis (A) and MRI confirming both hip involvement (B). Changes were advanced on left side and was treated by surface replacement on left and stage II on right was treated with core decompression and free fibular graft on right side (C)

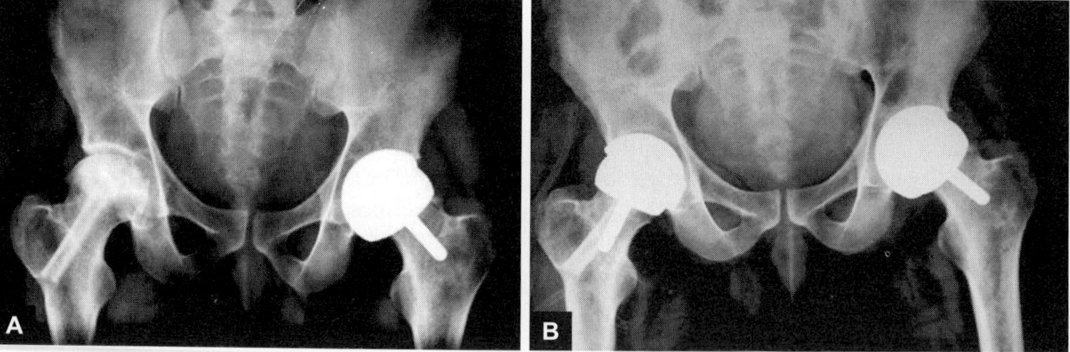

Figs 17.14A and B X-ray of the same patient (Fig. 17.8), treated initially with core decompression and free fibular grafting on right side (Fig. 17.14A). After surgery on both hips, right hip became painful and had to be treated with replacement arthroplasty. Surface replacement was performed on right side one year after core decompression and bone grafting

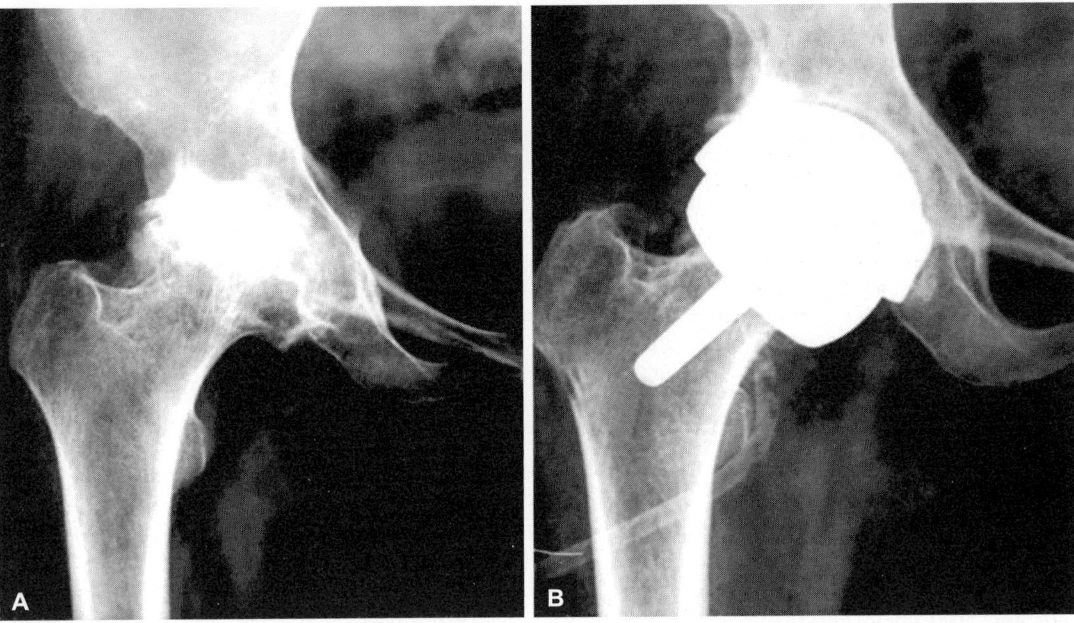

Figs 17.15A and B X-ray of a lady with steroid induced advanced osteonecrosis right hip with arthritic changes treated by surface replacement arthroplasty

Arthroplasty and arthrodesis:
1. Hemiarthroplasty
2. Bipolar hip replacement (Figs 17.4 to 17.6)
3. Surface replacement
4. Total hip replacement
5. Arthrodesis
6. Excision head neck femur (Girdlestone operation).

▉ REFERENCES

1. Calder JD, Pearse MF, Revell PA. The extent of osteocyte death in the proximal femur of patients with osteonecrosis of the femoral head. J Bone Joint Surg Br. 2001;83:419-22.
2. Cornell CN, Salvati EA, Pellicci PM. Long-term follow-up of total hip replacement in patients with osteonecrosis. Orthop Clin North Am. 1985;16:757-69.
3. Saito S, Saito M, Nishina T, et al. Long-term results of total hip arthroplasty for osteonecrosis of the femoral head: a comparison with osteo-arthritis. Clin Orthop. 1989;244:198-207.
4. Stauffer RN. Ten-year follow-up study of total hip replacement. J Bone Joint Surg Am. 1982; 64:983-90.
5. Salvati EA, Cornell CN. Long-term follow-up of total hip replacements in patients with avascular necrosis. In: AAOS Instructional Course Lectures. St Louis, CV Mosby. 1988; 37:67-73.
6. Chandler HP, Reineck FT, Winson RL, McCarthy JC. Total hip replacement in patients younger than thirty years old: a five-year follow-up study. J Bone Joint Surg Am. 1981;63A: 1426-34.
7. Kantor SG, Huo MH, Huk OL, Salvati EA. Cemented total hip arthroplasty in patients with osteonecrosis: a 6-year minimum follow-up study of second-generation cement techniques. J Arthroplasty. 1996;11:267-71.
8. Lieberman JR, Berry DJ, Mont MA, et al. Oteonecrosis of the hip: management in the 21st century. Instr Course Lect. 2003;52:337-55.
9. Hungerford MW, Hungerford DS, Jones LC. Outcome of uncemented primary femoral stems for treatment of femoral head osteonecrosis. Orthop Clin North Am. 2009;40(2):283-9.
10. Brinker MR, Rosenbury AG, Kull L, Galante JO. Primary total hip arthroplasty in patients with osteonecrosis of the femoral head. J Arthroplasty. 1994;9:457-68.

11. Piston RW, Engh CA, De Carvalho PI, Suthers K. Osteonecrosis of the femoral head treated with total hip arthroplasty without cement. J Bone Joint Surg Am. 1994;76A:202-14.

12. Squire M, Fehring TK, Odum S, Griffin WL, Bohannon MJ. Failure of femoral surface replacement for femoral head avascular necrosis. J Arthroplasty. 2005;20(7 suppl 3):108-14.

13. Adili A, Trousdale RT. Femoral head resurfacing for the treatment of osteonecrosis in the young patient. Clin Orthop. 2003;417:93-101.

14. Bose VC, Baruah BD. Resurfacing arthroplasty of the hip for avascular necrosis of the femoral head: a minimum follow-up of four years. J Bone Joint Surg Br. 2010;92(7):922.

15. Evguenia J, Karimova MD, Shesh N Rai, et al. Femoral Resurfacing in Young Patients with Hematologic Cancer and Osteonecrosis. Clin Orthop. 2008;466:3044-50)

16. Kim YH, Oh JH, Oh SH. Cementless total hip arthroplasty in patients with osteonecrosis of the femoral head. Clin Orthop. 1995;320:73-84.

17. Kim YH, Choi Y, Kim JS. Cementless total hip arthroplasty with ceramic-on-ceramic bearing in patients younger than 45 years withfemoral-head osteonecrosis. Int Orthop. 2010;34(8):1123-7.

18. Callaghan JJ, Dysart SH, Savory CG. The uncemented porous-coated anatomic total hip prosthesis: two-year results of a prospective consecutive series. J Bone Joint Surg Am. 1981;63A:1426.

19. Katz RL, Bourne RB, Rorabeck CH, McGee G. Total hip arthroplasty in patients with avascular necrosis of the hip. Clin Orthop. 1992;281:145-51.

20. Lins RE, Barnes BC, Callaghan JJ, Mair SD, McCollum DE. Evaluation of uncemented total hip arthroplasty in patients with avascular necrosis of the femoral head. Clin Orthop. 1993;297:168-73.

21. Alpert B, Waddell JP, Morton J, Bear RA. Cementless total hip arthroplasty in renal transplant patients. Clin Orthop. 1992;284:164-9.

22. Dorr LD, Luckett M, Conaty JP. Total hip arthroplasties in patients younger than 45 years: a nine to ten year follow-up study. Clin Orthop. 1990;260:15-219.

OSTEONECROSIS OF THE HUMERAL HEAD

Osteonecrosis of the humeral head is fairly common and the larger studies are infrequently reported. The most common cause of osteonecrosis of the humeral head in my region is sickle cell hemoglobinopathy, which results in various complications affecting the musculoskeletal system. In central India the multisystem disease of sickle cell disease may manifest in various forms. Skeletal changes are seen in a large number of patients and may be the first manifestation of the disease. Osteonecrosis of the bone is one of the skeletal manifestations of sickle cell hemoglobinopathy. The sites commonly involved are the femoral head, the humeral head and rarely the lunate, talus, tarsal navicular and the vertebral end plates. Osteonecrosis of the humeral head though rare, was commonly observed in this series. Changes of osteonecrosis of the humeral head are also seen in association with other disorders. We have seen such changes in two patients of Gaucher's disease, six patients of corticosteroid consumption and five cases of alcohol abuse. In spite of the fact that most of the patients are asymptomatic in the early stages of the disease and the condition may not be detected; a large number of patients were detected and followed in this study.

EPIDEMIOLOGY

Osteonecrosis of the humeral head was seen in 191 patients affecting 276 humeral head (Table 18.1).

In contrast to the femoral head osteonecrosis, there is little information in the literature about the rate of progression of humeral head osteonecrosis or about the risk factors for progression of the osteonecrosis in symptomatic shoulders in adults. Chung and Ralston[1] provided initial descriptions of humeral head osteonecrosis and Milner et al.[2] reported the frequency of the condition in patients with sickle cell disease, but no report has described the natural evolution of symptomatic shoulder osteonecrosis in patients with sickle cell disease.

Table 18.1 Epidemiology of osteonecrosis of the humeral head

Associated disease	No. of patients	Unilateral	Bilateral	Total no. of humeral heads
Sickle cell hemoglobinopathy	178	98	80	258
Gaucher's disease	2	2	-	2
Corticosteroid consumption	6	4	2	8
Alcohol abuse	5	2	3	8
Total	191	106	85	276

Changes of osteonecrosis were seen and observed in 258 humeral heads in 178 patients of sickle cell hemoglobinopathy, as per our data compiled in the year 1996. Eighty patients had bilateral affection of the shoulder joints. There were 13 patients of other disorder affecting 18 humeral heads. Pain on movement was the usual complaint, and in general rest pain and night pain were not prominent. Late in the course of the disease crepitus and an audible click on movement was often heard in the shoulder; the click was always painful. The active range of movement gradually decreased, mainly because of pain. On the other hand, passive movement was nearly always free until late in the course of the disease.

It is a common belief that the humeral head has abundant blood supply compared to the femoral head (Figs 18.1A and B). Our observation on dissecting 50 cadaveric shoulders in the Anatomy Department was different.

The observations were consistent in over 70 percent of shoulders dissected. About 80 percent of the size of the humeral head has vascular supply from the ascending branch of the anterior circumflex humeral artery. This relatively large vessel supplies the supero-medial, superolateral and inferomedial quadrants. The inferolateral quadrant is supplied by a branch from the posterior circumflex humeral artery which pierces the humerus after traversing the quadrangular space along with the articular branch of the axillary nerve (Figs 18.2 to 18.4). It has been observed that in patients with sickle cell hemoglobinopathy the vaso-occlusive changes of osteonecrosis of the humeral head mainly involve the quadrants supplied by anterior

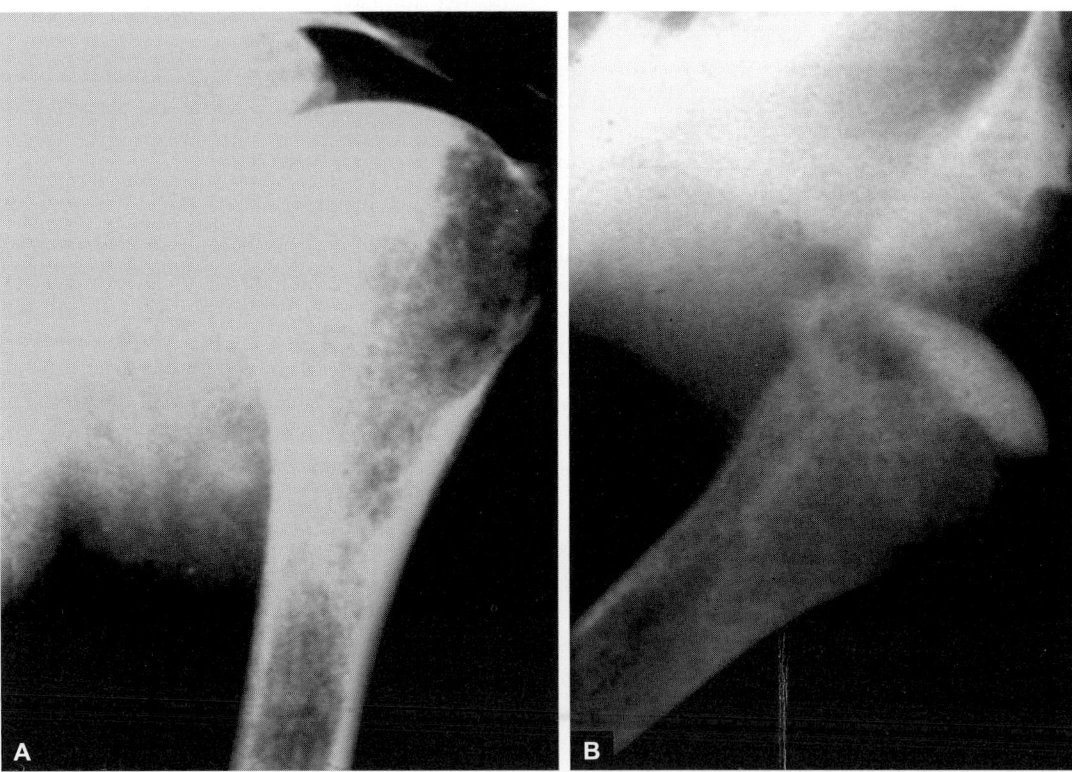

Figs 18.1A and B Osteonecrosis of the humeral head. Segmental sclerosis is seen involving about 90 percent of the articular surface with relative porosis in the metaphysis

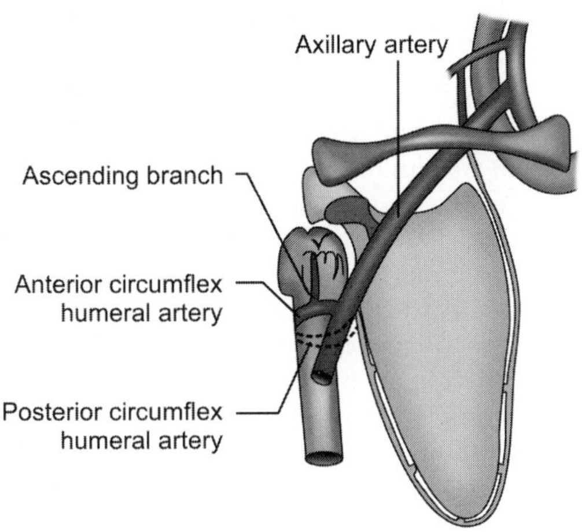

Fig. 18.2 Diagrammatic representation of anterior view of shoulder showing consistent presence of ascending branch of anterior circumflex humeral artery (vascular supply of the humeral head)

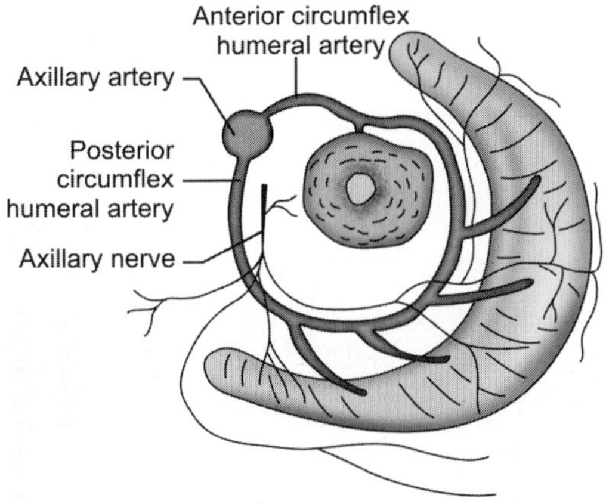

Fig. 18.3 Cross-section at upper end of the humerus showing vascular supply of proximal humerus

circumflex humeral artery and the inferolateral quadrant is usually spared. Another explanation for peculiar affection is the longer course of this artery and the susceptibility for impingement underneath the subscapularis during abduction and rotation of shoulders as against the lax posterior circumflex artery which lies mainly posteroinferiorly. These findings appear similar to the changes of osteonecrosis of the femoral head secondary

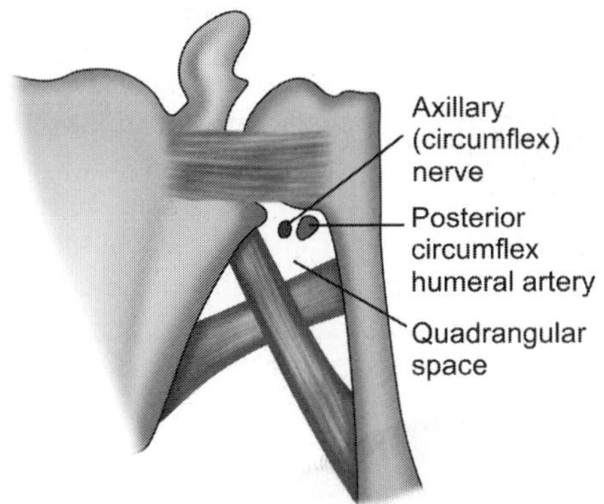

Fig. 18.4 Posterior view of shoulder showing quadrangular space with a branch from posterior circumflex humeral artery traversing to the humeral head along with the articular branch of the axillary nerve

to vaso-occlusive changes in the ascending branch of the lateral femoral circumflex artery seen frequently in sickle cell disease.

Review of Literature

Osteonecrosis is an important chronic complication of sickle cell disease in developed countries. The first case of avascular necrosis was described by Bauer and Fischer in 1943 (Taylor 1985[3]). The prevalence of osteonecrosis of the femoral head in sickle cell disease (SCD) is well described.[2,4-13] Involvement of the humeral head is well recognized though very few studies have been done in details.[1,2,5-7,11,14-17] Hernigou et al. (1991)[18] recorded a 32.5 percent incidence of femoral head involvement in 160 patients with either homozygous or heterozygous SCD. Of these 80 percent had pain and impaired function, with secondary osteoarthritis in 30 percent; 16 percent had undergone surgery. SCD was the most common cause of hip deformity in black children. Involvement of the humeral head is well recognized[5-7,11,14,15] (Ehrenpreis and Schwinger, 1952; Smith and Conley, 1954; Tanaka, Clifford and Axelrod, 1956; Cockshott, 1958; Golding, MacIver and Went, 1959; Reynolds, 1965), but little has been reported about the clinical and functional problems of such patients.

Pathophysiology in Sickle Cell Disease

Blood containing long, multipointed, curved and rigid sickle cells are more viscid and flows less readily through terminal vessels. Utilization of oxygen by living blood cells and by endothelial and tissue cells favors an exaggeration of sickling. Chronic stasis of blood in capillaries and defective oxygenation leads to infarction in various tissues. Sickle cells are mechanically more fragile, are phagocytosed more readily and are subject to hemolysis in the circulating blood. The imbalance between blood destruction and formation leads to chronic hemolytic anemia, the degree of anemia depending on the type of disease.

Radiographic Changes

Routine radiography is used for assessment of these patients. Advanced investigations like CT and MRI scan were not used routinely, due to cost restraints and nonavailability in many sickle cell centers in earlier days. A new classification is proposed according to the changes seen in the humeral head in this study. The MRC classification of McCallum et al.[19] does not give details of pathological stages in the progression of osteonecrosis even in type A (Table 18.2). The type B lesions are essentially different stages of infarcts and osteomyelitic changes rather than changes of osteonecrosis of the humeral head.

The changes of osteonecrosis of the humeral head usually occur in the supero-medial quadrant where maximum pressure occurs with shoulder in abduction. The radiographic findings were staged according to the initial assessment. In a few patients progression of the disease was observed at follow-up. A large number of patients had regression of the changes.

■ CLASSIFICATION

Though there are several staging and classification systems of osteonecrosis of the humeral head, as described by McCallum and Walder in 1966,[19] Cruess in 1976 (Table 18.3)[20]

and Ficat and Arlet in 1980 (Table 18.4).[21] I described my own classification depending upon the radiological picture at the time of first presentation and routinely the MRI findings were not considered, as this facility did not exist at this center in the early period of the study (Table 18.5, Figs 18.6 to 18.12).[22,23] The majority of the patients (55%) were detected in stage I and II before the development of crescent sign. Sickle cell disease with SS pattern had a great risk factor for an increase in the size of the lesion, rapid progression of the disease, and collapse, though the patients of sickle cell trait were more in this study. The size of the lesion increased in more than 40 percent patients with the SS pattern of sickle cell disease. The time between symptoms and collapse was less than six months in most of the shoulders. The duration of survival before collapse for shoulders that presented with stage I or stage II was significantly shorter for the shoulders with the SS pattern than for the shoulders with sickle cell trait with AS pattern.

Medical Research Council Decompression Panel (McCallum and Walder 1966)[19] in which type A or juxta-articular lesions, are distinguished from type B lesions of the head, neck and shaft (Table 18.2).

Table 18.2 Medical Research Council Decompression Panel classification of avascular necrosis of the upper humerus (McCallum and Walder, 1966)

A	Juxta-articular lesions
	Dense areas with intact articular cortex
	• Spherical segmental opacities
	• Linear opacity
	• Structural failure
	• Translucent subcortical band
	• Collapse of articular cortex
	• Sequestration of cortex
	• Osteoarthrosis
B	Head, neck and shaft lesions
	Dense areas
	Irregular calcified areas
	Translucent areas and cysts

Table 18.3 Cruess 1976[20] method of grading osteonecrosis of the humeral head

Criteria for staging		No. of shoulders	
		At initial visit	At final follow-up
Stage I	Abnormal MRI, normal radiograph	38	0
Stage II	Abnormal radiograph with sclerotic or cystic changes in the humeral head, but no crescent line	42	15
Stage III	Abnormal radiograph showing a crescent sign with humeral head flattening of <1 mm	5	0
Stage IV	Collapse of the humeral head of >1 mm without joint space narrowing	19	14
Stage V	Joint space narrowing	0	46
Stage VI	Advanced degenerative changes	0	29

Table 18.4 Radiographic classification of avascular necrosis of the shoulder according to Ficat and Arlet (1980)[21]

Stage	Joint space	Head contour	Trabecular pattern
I	Normal	Normal	Osteoporosis, mottled areas
II	Normal	Normal	Wedge sclerosis
III	Normal or slightly decreased	Subchondral collapse	Sequestrum appearance
IV	Decreased	Collapse	Extensive destruction

Table 18.5 Author's radiological staging[22,23] and number of patients

Stage	Features	No.	Figs no.
I	Area of spotty irregularities and densities in the subchondral region	92	18.6A and B
II	Rim like area of increased density in juxta-articular portion of the humeral head. At times larger dense shadows in the humeral head without any separation	40	18.7A and B 18.8A and B
III	Crescent sign with increased density as in stage II with clear cleavage	15	18.9A and B
IV	Increased density with fragmentation without change in the contour of the humeral head	47	18.10A and B
V	Mild collapse of humeral head with reduction of vertical height and width with irregularity of articular surface	53	18.11
VI	Severe collapse of humeral head with hypertrophic arthritic changes	11	18.12A and B

Table 18.6 Age and sex distribution

Age (Years)	Total	Male	Female
0–5	1	1	0
6–10	9	8	1
11–15	12	7	5
16–20	62	38	24
21–25	57	31	26
26–30	29	13	16
Over 30	8	6	2
Total	178	104	74

Table 18.9 Radiological staging at first presentation of sickle cell patients

Stage	Number of humeral heads
I	92
II	40
III	15
IV	47
V	53
VI	11
Total	258

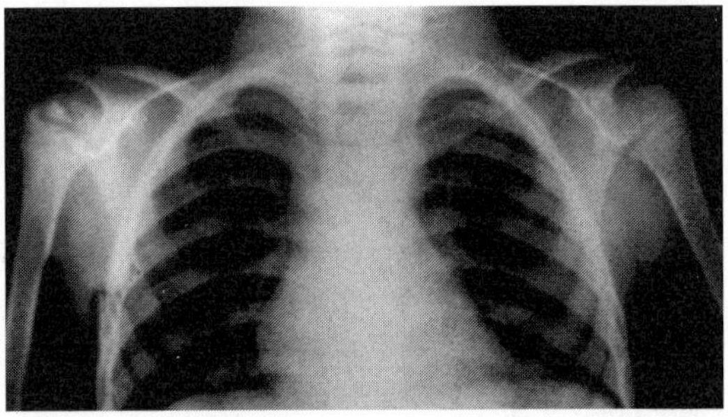

Table 18.7 Stage wise clinical features

Stage	No. of shoulders	No. of symptomatic
I	92	10
II	40	19
III	15	-
IV	47	22
V	53	27
VI	11	10

Fig. 18.5 Radiograph of a four-year-old child showing classical changes of osteonecrosis of the humeral head with fragmentation

Table 18.8 Electrophoresis pattern

Pattern	Total	Males	Age (Years)
AS	106	67	39
SS	43	22	21
ASF	29	15	14
Total	178	104	74

To know the severity of affection of the humeral head, we have classified osteonecrosis of the humeral head in different stages. One of the important observations of this study was predominant involvement of three-fourths of the humeral head and the sparing of inferolateral quadrant in osteonecrosis. The patients were classified into various stages according to the radiological changes observed at the first presentation. Significant number of patients had progression of the disease on follow-up. This gives us clear picture at a glance for better assessment (Table 18.5).

OBSERVATIONS

Age and sex distribution: There were 104 males and 74 females. The maximum numbers of patients were between 15 to 25 years of age. There were 4 patients under the age of 10 years and one of this presented at 4 years of age (Table 18.6 and Fig. 18.5).

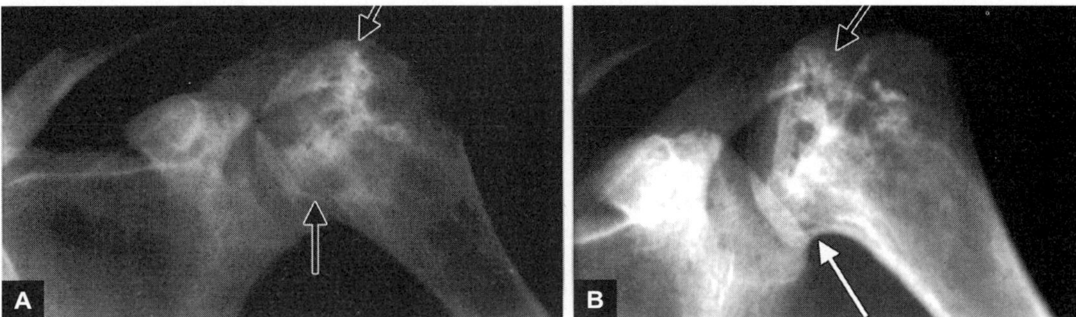

Figs 18.6A and B 'Stage I'—radiograph showing multiple dense sclerotic spots in the humeral head, at places fused to each other, delineating the possible segmental involvement in osteonecrosis

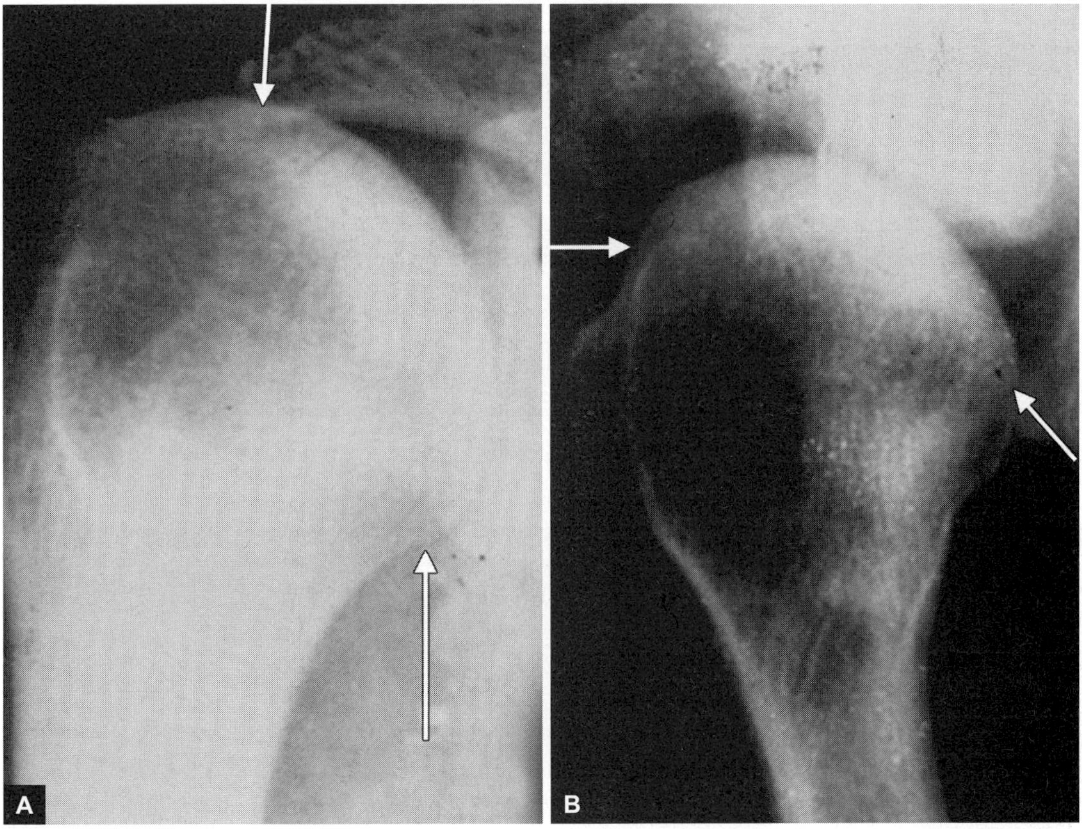

Figs 18.7A and B 'Stage II'—radiograph showing the juxta-articular dense of sclerosis seen in AP and lateral views. There is no cleavage or separation

Table 18.10 Age and sex-wise bilateral affection of sickle cell patients

Age (Years)	Total	Male	Female
0–5	0	0	0
6–10	1	1	0
11–15	11	7	4
16–20	13	7	6
21–25	32	21	11
26–30	14	10	4
Over 30	9	6	3
Total	80	52	28

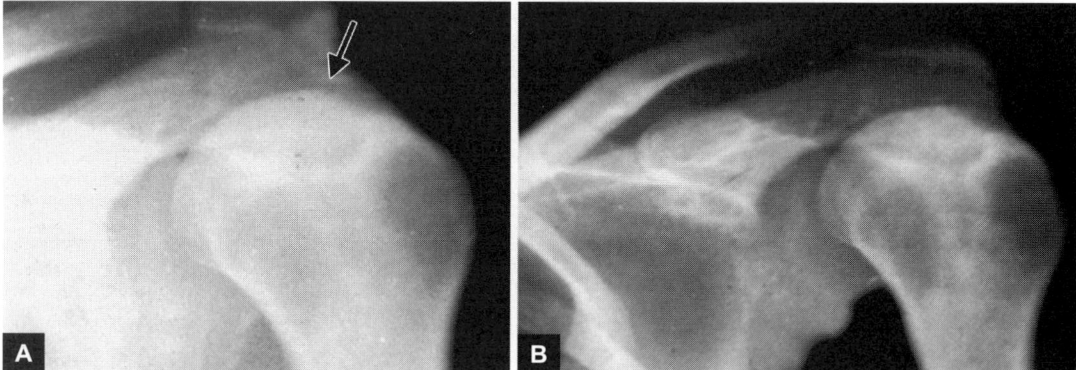

Figs 18.8A and B 'Stage II'—radiograph showing segmental involvement of the humeral head in osteonecrosis without separation, with relative osteoporosis

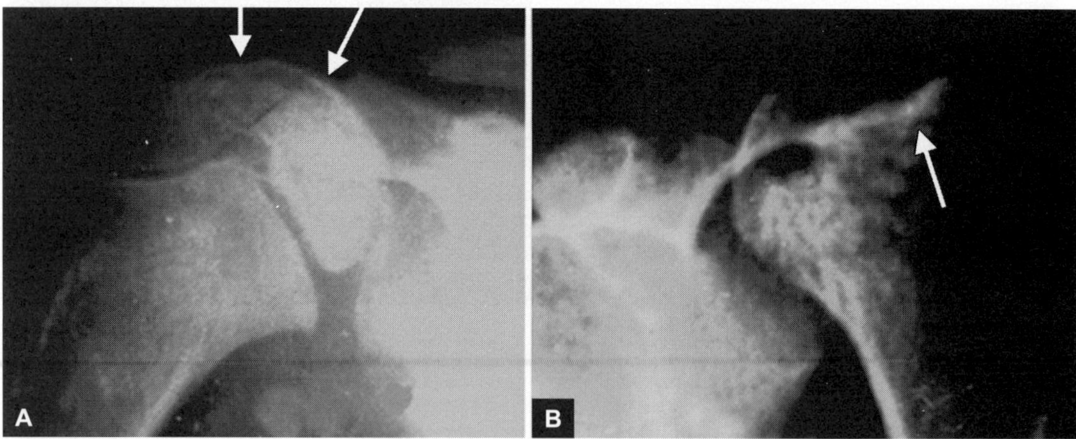

Figs 18.9A and B 'Stage III'—radiograph of shoulder showing clear separation of subchondral segment without deformation of the humeral head

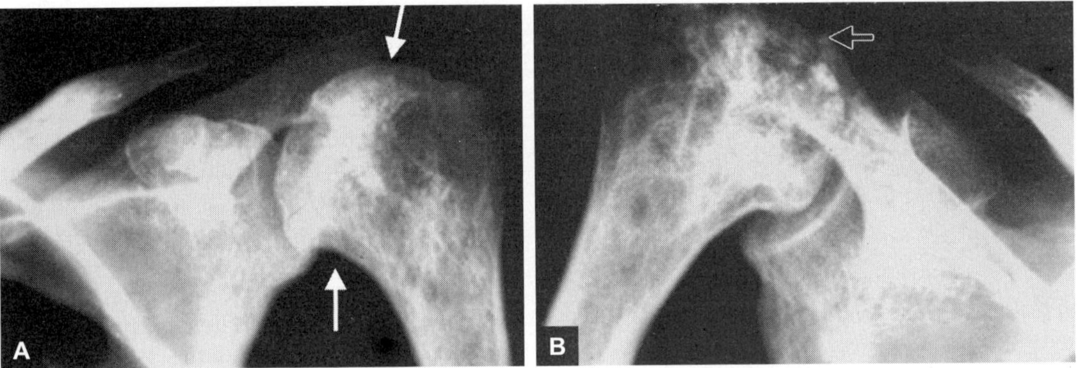

Figs 18.10A and B 'Stage IV'—radiograph of shoulder showing multiple dense areas with fragmentation of the humeral head without change in the contour

Hematology

The test for sickling was positive in all the cases as per the criterion of Daland and Castle.[24] The electrophoretic pattern observed is as follows:

The radiographic findings were staged according to the initial assessment. In a few patients progression of the disease was observed at follow-up. A large number of patients had regression of the changes. The findings are presented as seen in 258 humeral heads (Tables 18.7 to 18.9).

Bilateral Affection

Of the 178 sickle cell patients 80 had bilateral involvement and maximum number of patients were between the age of 20 to 25 years (Table 18.10).

Management

It is difficult to predict early in the course of the lesion the degree of deformity that will occur in the humeral head, and equally difficult to assess how much disability will arise. For these reasons the early management in these cases has been conservative. All patients were instructed as to how to try to maintain the range of movement of the shoulder joint with pendulum exercises, but were discouraged from active abduction or heavy work with their arms. The rationale was, of course, to diminish the stresses across the joint in the hope of minimizing collapse and avoiding serious degenerative changes when revascularization occurred. Because these patients suffered from serious systemic illness, some difficulties were encountered with the program. In particular, when painful hip lesions occurred simultaneously the patients had to use crutches.

A few patients had more severe deformity of the humeral head with limitation of active movement and inability to use the arm above the shoulder. However, their daily living did not require extensive use of the arm and of the shoulder. Most of the patients with osteonecrosis of the humeral head were managed by conservative treatment. During the painful episode, the shoulder was rested in a sling till the pain subsided. Patients presenting during sickle cell crisis were managed by similar means in addition to the specific treatment for crisis. Treatment has usually been by exercises and the avoidance of strenuous use and overhead movements of the shoulder (Cruess[20]). When these measures failed to relieve disability, hemiarthroplasty or total shoulder replacement was used (Cruess[20]). Core decompression for the treatment of avascular necrosis of the humeral head has been advised for intractable pain in the shoulder, affecting the normal daily

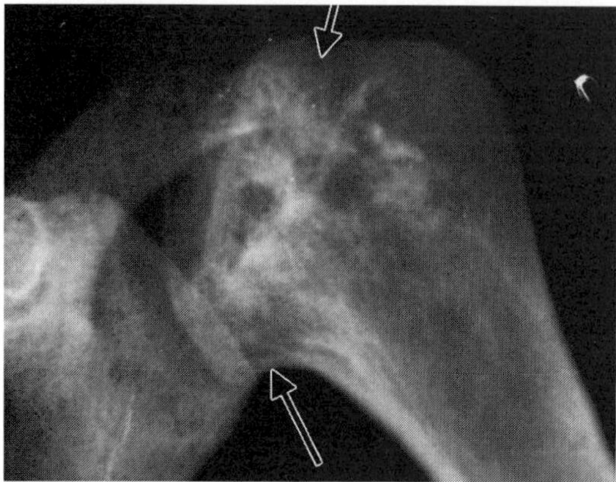

Fig. 18.11 'Stage V'—advanced changes of osteo-necrosis with partial collapse of the humeral head causing deformation and reduction in the vertical height of the humeral head

activities.[25,26] As with avascular necrosis of the hip, the results were better if decompression was done early, before the humeral head had collapsed. Although the anatomy of the humeral head is in some ways similar to that of the femoral head, the glenoid is much shallower and less conforming than the acetabulum and the shoulder does not sustain the body-weight. For these reasons the shoulder may continue to function satisfactorily despite considerable deformity, and shoulder decompression may be more efficacious in later stages of the disease, stage III, than it is in the hip. Since the only other effective treatment for pain in the shoulder from avascular necrosis is arthroplasty, the minimally invasive procedure of core decompression would seem to be the procedure of choice.

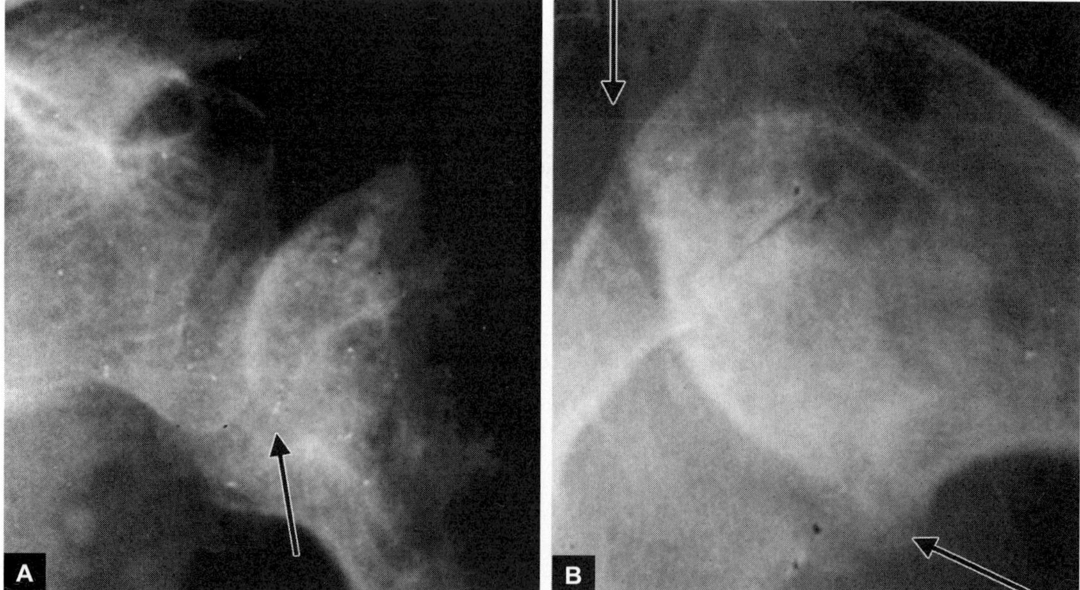

Figs 18.12A and B 'Stage VI'—residual changes of osteonecrosis with collapse of the humeral head causing irregularity of the articular surface and secondary hypertrophic arthritic changes

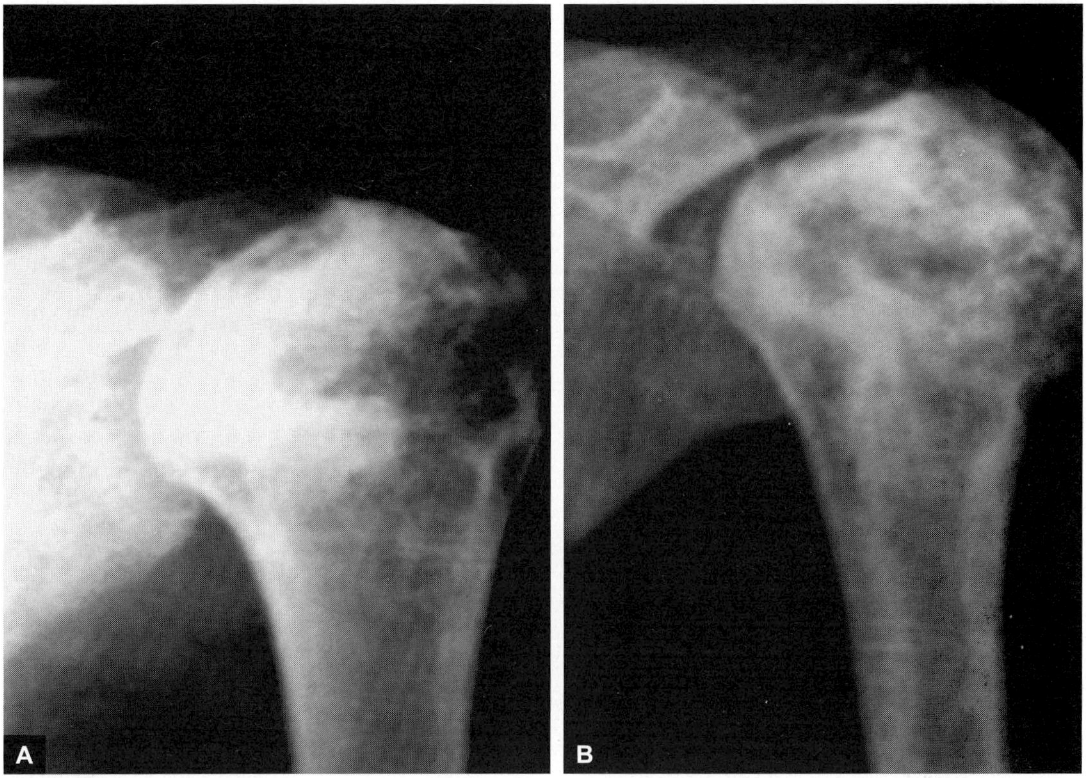

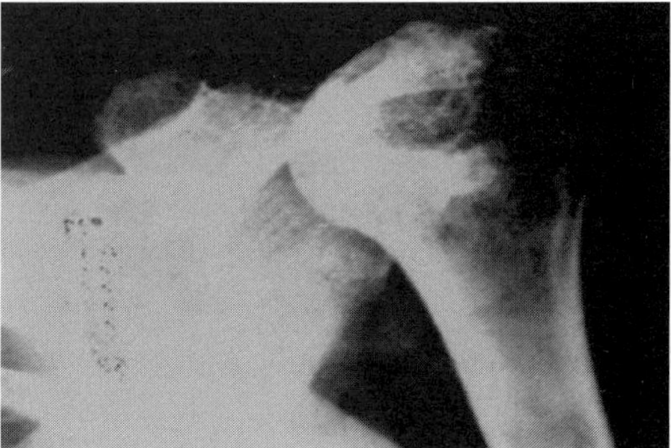

Figs 18.13A and B X-ray showing stage III-IV type of osteonecrosis of humeral head treated by core decompression

Core decompression was done in 12 humeral heads without bone grafting. Core decompression and free iliac bone grafting (Figs 18.13 to 18.15) was done twice. Arthroplasty was indicated in only six patients but not done due to the morbid condition of the patient.

Evaluation and Results

Clinical evaluation was done by the UCLA Shoulder Rating System.[27] Ten points were assigned in each of the three categories, pain, function and active movements (Table 18.11). The maximum score possible was 30 points.

Fig. 18.14 X-ray of same patient (Fig. 18.13B) 1 year postoperatively after core decompression showing good attempt towards revascularization

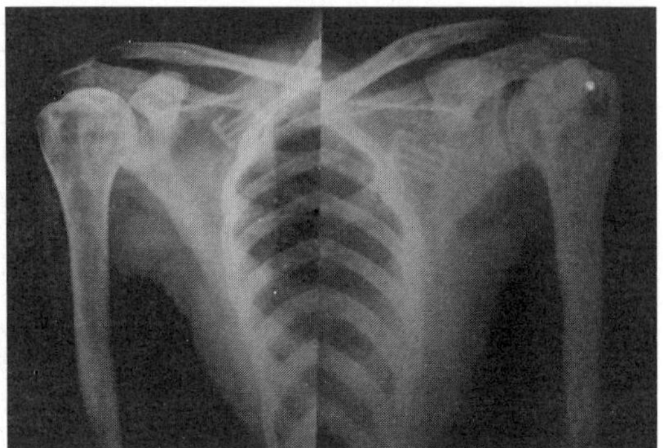

Fig. 18.15 X-ray of same patient (Fig. 18.13A) 20 years after core decompression showing good attempt towards revascularization

An excellent result scored 27 points or more, a good result 24 to 26, a fair result 21 to 23 and a poor result scored less than 21.

A total of 10 patients in whom core decompression was performed in stage I or II had excellent to good result. Four patients had fair results (Figs 18.13 to 18.15). Humeral heads with changes of stage V and VI had consistently poor result. Twenty patients had progress of lesion during the follow-up and the result was fair at the end of two years of follow-up (Table 18.12).

Discussion

Chung and Ralston[1,28] were the first to review the literature and describe the orthopedic

Table 18.11 UCLA shoulder rating[27]		
Criterion	Score	Findings
Pain	1	Constant, unbearable, strong medications frequently
	2	Constant but bearable, strong medications occasionally
	4	None or little at rest, occurs with light activity, salicylates frequently
	5	With heavy or particular activities only salicylates occasionally
	8	Occasional and slight
	10	No pain
Function	1	Unable to use arm
	2	Very light activities only
	4	Light house work or most daily living activities
	5	Most house work, washing hair, putting on brassiere, shopping, driving
	8	Slight restriction only, able to work above shoulder level
	10	Normal activities
Muscle power and motion	1	Ankylosis with deformity
	2	Ankylosis with good functional position
	4	Muscle power poor to fair, elevation less than 60°, internal rotation less than 45°
	5	Muscle power fair to good, elevation 90° internal rotation 90°
	8	Muscle power good or normal, elevation 140°, external rotation 20°
	10	Normal muscle power, motion near normal

Table 18.12 Results of osteonecrosis

Result	No. of shoulders
Excellent	125
Good	46
Fair	53
Poor	34

implications of osteonecrosis of the humeral head in sickle cell disease. There are a very few reports on the osteonecrosis of the humeral head.

The incidence of osteonecrosis of humeral head in sickle cell disease in this study was 3.5 percent. The reported incidence of humeral head involvement ranges from 0 percent (Becker, 1962[9]) to 31.5 percent (Golding et al. 1959[15]). Milner et al.[2] (1993) reported an incidence of 5.6 percent and David et al.[17] (1993) found humeral head involvement in 28.3 percent patients (Table 18.13).

Early reports from Smith and Conley[6] (1954) suggested that only patients with sickle cell trait were affected by osteonecrosis. It has now been shown that it occurs in all types of sickle cell hemoglobinopathy with the same frequency, giving a distribution proportional to that of the types of hemoglobin electrophoretic pattern in any given population or geographical area.[7,15,22,23,27-31]

As reported earlier, we found a higher incidence of osteonecrosis of the humeral head in patients with heterozygous SC disease than in those with homozygous SS disease.[6,7,14,17,28-33] Milner et al.[2] (1993) found a higher incidence in patients with SS pattern. Osteonecrosis of the humeral head has not been reported in a child below five years of age.[17] There was no patient under the age of ten years in their study. Milner et al.[2] reported six patients under the age of ten years. In this study, there were four cases under the age of ten years and one of them had radiological changes at the age of four years (Fig. 18.5). The age distribution otherwise is comparable to other studies.[2,17] There were 80 patients (45%) with bilateral involvement in this study. Chung and Ralston[1] reported six cases with bilateral involvement out of ten. The reported incidence of bilateral disease in the study of Milner et al.[2] and David et al.[17] was 67.2 percent and 28 percent respectively.

It is generally agreed that the patients with osteonecrosis of the humeral head are not as disabled as those with involvement of the femoral head.[1] In the study of Milner et al.[2] 79 percent patients were asymptomatic at the

Table 18.13 Review of literature

Author	Hb	No. of patients	Humeral head no.	AVN %
Ehrenpreis and Schwinger (1952)	-	72	1	1.4
Smith and Conley (1954)	SC	16	1	6.2
Tanaka et al. (1956)	SS	38	1	2.6
Cockshott (1958)	SC	20	3	15.0
Golding et al. (1959)	SS	51	5	9.8
	SC	19	6	31.5
Barton and Cockshott (1962)	SC	117	4	3.4
Becker (1962)	SC	12	0	0
Reynolds (1965)	SS	63	10	15.9
	SC	34	7	20.6
Chung and Ralston (1971)	SS	40	2	5

time of diagnosis. Only 22 percent patients reported pain and limitation of movement. In the present study, 34 percent patients were symptomatic at the initial assessment. In contrast to the above reports, Haddad[34] (1967) found significant pain and disability in a similar group of patients.

Diggs[12] (1967) opined that since the humerus does not bear weight, the cartilage is usually spared, hypertrophic changes are minimal and the glenoid fossa is normal. Only in rare instances, deformity and secondary hypertrophic arthritic changes are seen.

Changes of osteonecrosis of the humeral head have also been reported by many workers.[33-44] Changes of osteonecrosis of the humeral head are also seen with other disorders.[33-39] Changes of osteonecrosis of the humeral head were seen in two patients of Gaucher's disease, six patients of corticosteroid consumption and five cases of alcohol abuse. We did not observe similar changes of osteonecrosis of the humeral head in any other disease known to cause osteonecrosis like hyperuricemia, alkaptonuria or following renal transplantation.

Various classifications have been proposed for the osteonecrosis of the humeral head,[19-22] David et al.[17] have used the Medical Research Council Decompression Panel Classification proposed by McCallum and Walder[19](1966). A conservative treatment comprising heat, massage, range of motion exercises and protection from undue stresses has been recommended in the early stages of the disease.[1,27] A large number of patients in this study were satisfactorily managed by conservative means.

Chung and Ralston[1] and other workers[24,25] reported decompression and bone grafting for patients of osteonecrosis of the humeral head who did not respond to conservative treatment with good results. In this study a similar procedure without grafting was done in 12 shoulders and twice with bone grafting. In 10, the results were good to excellent and 4 patients had fair results. It was, thus, possible to arrest the progression of the disease. The results of this procedure are comparable to those obtained by Mont et al.[25] (1993) in patients with osteonecrosis of the humeral head due to causes other than sickle cell disease. In this series no patient was treated with arthroscopic assisted surgery as reported by Hayes et al.[45]

Replacement arthroplasty using Neer's prosthesis has been advocated in patients with intractable pain and secondary osteoarthritic changes.[1,2,17,46,47] Infection and prosthetic loosening are common following this procedure in sicklers.[17] No patient in this study was subjected to replacement arthroplasty though it was indicated in six cases.

SUMMARY

Osteonecrosis of the humeral head is more common than is usually recognized since a large number of patients are asymptomatic. It is less common than osteonecrosis of the femoral head. Pain and disability in these cases is mild and the progression of the disease is slow and most of them are managed conservatively with good results. Patients with sickle cell disease and trait are equally affected with osteonecrosis of the humeral head. Early detection is important to prevent progression of the disease, as the results of replacement arthroplasty are not satisfactory. Core decompression with or without grafting yields good results and helps in arresting the progress of the disease.

REFERENCES

1. Chung SKM, Ralston EL. Necrosis of the humeral head associated with Sickle cell anaemia and its genetic variants. Clin. Orthop. 1971;80:105-17.
2. Milner PF, Kraus AP, Sebes JI, et al. Osteonecrosis of the humeral head in Sickle Cell Disease. Clin Orthop. 1993;289:136-43.
3. Taylor L. Sickle cell disease in Britain: A review. Jacksonian Prize Essay, 1985.
4. Diggs LW, Pulliam HN, King JC. The bone changes in Sickle cell anaemia. Southern Med Jr. 1937;30:249-59.

5. Ehrenpreis B, Schwinger HN. Sickle Cell Anaemia. Am J Roentgenol. 1952;68:28-36.

6. Smith EW, Conley Cl. Clinical features of the genetic variants of Sickle cell disease. Bull John Hopkins Hosp. 1954;94:289-318.

7. Tanaka KR, Clifford GO, Axelrod AR. Sickle cell anaemia (homozygous S) with aseptic necrosis of the femoral head. Blood. 1956;11:988-1008.

8. Barton CJ, Cockshott WP. Bone changes in Haemoglobin SC Disease. Am J Roentgenol. 1962;88:523-32.

9. Becker JA. Haemoglobin SC Disease. Am J Roentgenol. 1962;88:503-11.

10. Moseley JE. Bone changes in haematologic disorders. New, Grune and Stratton, 1963.

11. Reynolds J. The roentgenological features of Sickle cell disease and related haemoglobinopathies. Springfield, Ill: Charles C. Thomas, 1965.

12. Diggs LW. The bone and joint leisons in Sickle cell disease: Clin Orthop. 1967.p.119.

13. Lee REJ, Golding JSR, Sergeant GR. The radiological features of avascular necrosis of the femoral head in homozygous Sickle cell disease. Clin Radiol. 1981;32:205.

14. Cockshott WP. Haemoglobin SC Disease. J Fac Radiologists. 1958;9:211-6.

15. Golding JSR, MacIver JE, Went LH. The bone changes in Sickle cell anaemia and its genetic variants. J Bone Joint Surg Br. 1959;41B:71-8.

16. Theis JC, Owen R. Skeletal Complications in Sickle cell disease in the UK JR Coll Surg Edinb. 1988;33:306-10.

17. David HG, Bridgman SC, Davies SC, Hine AL, Emery RJH. The Shoulder in Sickle cell disease. J Bone Joint Surg Br. 1993;75B:538-45.

18. Hernigou P, Galacteros F, Bachir D, Goutaliier D. Deformities of the hip in adults who have Sickle cell disease and had avascular necrosis in childhood: a natural history of fifty-two patients. J Bone Joint Surg Am. 1991;73A:81-92.

19. McCallum RI, Walder DN. Bone lesions in compressed air workers with special reference to men who worked on the Clyde tunnels 1958 to 1963. J Bone & Joint Surg Br. 1966:48B;207-35.

20. Cruess RL. Steroid-induced avascular necrosis of the head of the humerus. Natural history and management. J Bone Joint Surg Br. 1976; 58:313-7.

21. Ficat P, Arlet J, Hungerford DS (Eds). Ischaemia and Necrosis of Bone. Baltimore, MD, Williams & Wilkins, 1980.

22. Babhulkar Sudhir. Orthopaedic manifestations and bone changes in sickle cell haemoglobinopathy. Monogram by CBS Publishers. 1997. pp.78-93.

23. Babhulkar Sudhir, Babhulkar Sushrut. Sickle cell haemoglobinopathy. Osteonecrosis etiology, Diagnosis and treatment. In: Urbaniak JR, Jones JP, (Eds). Osteonecrosis: Etiology,diagnosis, and treatment. Rosemont, IL: American Academy of Orthopaedic Surgeons. 1997.pp.131-133 (Monogram by AAOS 1997).

24. Daland GA, Castle WB. A simple and Rapid method of demonstrating sickling of red blood cells, the use of reducing agents. J Lab Clin Med. 1948;33:1082.

25. Mont MA, Marr DC, Urquhart MW, Lennox D, Hungerford DS. Avascular necrosis of the humeral head treated by core decompression. J. Bone Joint Surg Br. 1993;75B;785-8.

26. LaPorte DM, Mont MA, Mohan V, et al. Osteonecrosis of the humeral head treated by core decompression. Clin Orthop. 1998;355: 254-60

27. Kay SP, Amstutz HC. Shoulder Hemiarthroplasty at UCLA. Clin Orthop. 1988;288:42-8.

28. Chung SKM, Ralston EL. Necrosis of the femoral head asociated with Sickle cell anaemia and its genetic variants. J Bone Joint Surg Am. 1969; 51A:33-58.

29. Nachamie BA, Dorfman HD. Ischaemic necrosis of bone in Sickle cell trait. Mt Sinai J Med NY. 1974;41:527-36.

30. Nixon JE. Avascular necrosis of bone: A review. J of the Royal Soc Med. 1983;76:681-92.

31. Ebong WW. Avascular necrosis of the femoral head associated with haemoglobinopathy. Tropical & Geographical Medicine. 1977;29: 19-23.

32. L'Insalata JC, Pagnani MJ, Warren RF, Dines DM. Humeral head osteonecrosis: clinical course and radiographic predictors of outcome. J Shoulder Elbow Surg. 1996;5:355-61.

33. Hattrup SJ, Cofield RH. Osteonecrosis of the humeral head: relationship of disease stage, extent, and cause to natural history. J Shoulder Elbow Surg. 1999;8:559-64.

34. Haddad RJ Jr. Sickle cell disease involvement of the hip and its surgical treatment. Clin Orthop. 1967;55:135-49.

35. Jones JP Jr, Engleman EP, Steinbach HL, et al. Fat embolization as a possible mechanism

producing avascular necrosis. Arthritis Rheum. 1965;8:449.

36. Jones JIP, Jamenson RM, Engelman EP. Alcoholism, Fat embolism and avascular necrosis of femoral head. J Bone and Joint Surgery Am. 1968;50A:1065.

37. Hunder GG, Worthington JW, Bickel WH. Avascular necrosis of femoral head in a patient with Gout. JAMA. 1968;203(1):47-9.

38. Fischer DE, Bickel WH. Corticosteroid induced avascular necrosis. A clinical study of seventy seven patients. J Bone Joint Surg Am. 1971;53A: 859-73.

39. Solomon L. Idiopathic necrosis of the femoral head: Pathogenesis and treatment. Can J Surg. 1981;24:573.

40. Hungerford DS. Pathogenic considerations in ischemic necrosis of bone. J Bone and Joint Surgery, Orthopaedic Transactions. 1983;7:215.

41. Hernigou P, Bachir D, Galacteros F. The natural history of symptomatic osteonecrosis in adults with sickle-cell disease. J Bone Joint Surg Am. 2003;85:500-4.

42. Hernigou P, Galacteros F, Bachir D, Goutallier D. [164 epiphyseal necroses (hips,

shoulders, knees) in 55 patients with sickle cell anemia. Characteristics, epidemiologic and etiopathogenic aspects]. Rev Rhum Mal Osteoartic. 1989;56:869-75. French.

43. Hernigou P, Flouzat-Lachaniette CH, Roussignol X, Poignard A. The natural progression of shoulder osteonecrosis related to corticosteroid treatment. Clin Orthop. 2010; 468:1809-16.

44. Poignard A, Lachaniette CH, Amzallag J, et al. The Natural Progression of Symptomatic Humeral Head Osteonecrosis in Adults with Sickle Cell Disease. J Bone Joint Surg Am. 2012; 49A:156-62.

45. Hayes JM. Arthroscopic treatment of steroid-induced osteonecrosis of the humeral head. Arthroscopy. 1989;5:218-21.

46. Lau MW, Blinder MA, Williams K, Galatz LM. Shoulder arthroplasty in sickle cell patients with humeral head avascular necrosis. J Shoulder Elbow Surg. 2007;16:129-34-37.

47. Naranja RJ Jr, Iannotti JP. Surgical options in the treatment of arthritis of the shoulder: alternatives to prosthetic arthroplasty. Semin Arthroplasty. 1995;6:204-13.

19 OSTEONECROSIS OF VERTEBRAL END PLATES

Osteonecrosis of vertebral end plates is a rare presentation following a vaso-occlusive phenomenon commonly seen in patients of sickle cell hemoglobinopathy. A stage-wise radiological interpretation is evaluated in detail. Hypothesis for the etiopathology of this peculiar pathognomonic feature following vascular insult and ischemia in patients of sickle cell hemoglobinopathy is explained.[1-3]

Commonly the patients are in the age group of young adolescents and adults between the ages of 12 to 32 years with equal incidence in both the sexes.

CLINICAL FEATURES

Patients report backache and deformity of spine. The onset of pain might be sudden without any relation to any stress, weight lifting or trauma. At times the clinical changes are detected during regular periodical check up at a sickle cell center. The changes of osteonecrosis were frequently observed in adolescents and young adults, in the group of sickle cell disease (SS) patients and are infrequently seen in sickle cell trait (AS) patients. The epiphyseal vertebral end plate changes were not noticed in any children and were not seen in patients less than 12 years of age. All patients were investigated by sickling test (Daland and Castle 1948[4]) and hemoglobin electrophoresis in addition to routine blood investigations.

RADIOGRAPHIC FEATURES

In all patients radiographic changes were peculiar and identical. The changes were fre-quently noticed in the thoracic and lumbar region especially in the adjoining disk surface of the vertebral body. The normal rectangular shape of the vertebrae was changed and a peculiar shape of vertebral body was noticed. The changes were very obvious in the center of the vertebral end plates close to intervertebral disc spaces. The changes were mirror image changes on the disc surface of the vertebral body changing the vertebral configuration, which showed central depression with an abrupt transition to the more normal shape of the vertebral body in the periphery (Figs 19.1 to 19.4). There was no collapse of the vertebral body but simply a failure of growth in the central portion of the growth plate. The probable sequence of changes is bone infarct in the center of the metaphyseal region of the vertebral body, which becomes sclerosed and fragmented (Figs 19.5 to 19.8). Subsequently there is growth arrest and localized central collapse of the vertebral end plate giving rise to "step off" deformity. There was reactive sclerosis parallel to the end plates in some vertebral bodies as a straight zone of condensation 1 to 2 mm below the vertebral end plate in the center of the involved centrum. This zone of condensation resembles a short growth arrest line observed commonly in the distal femur. This zone of condensation of the vertebral end plates causes squaring of the vertebral body and at times gives the appearance of 'bone within bone' (Fig. 19.9). This central cup depression called as 'step off' or H vertebrae, might look like a dome, might be asymmetrically irregular or flattened at the

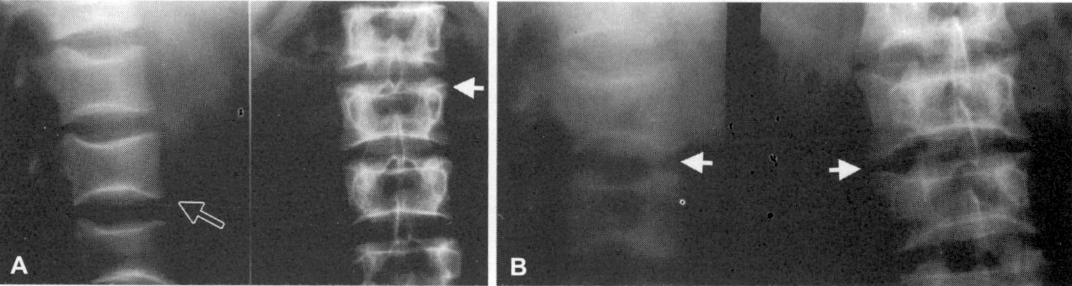

Figs 19.1A and B X-ray of lumbar spine anteroposterior and lateral view showing osteoporosis with ballooning of disk spaces and changes like cod fish vertebra with deformation of vertebral body

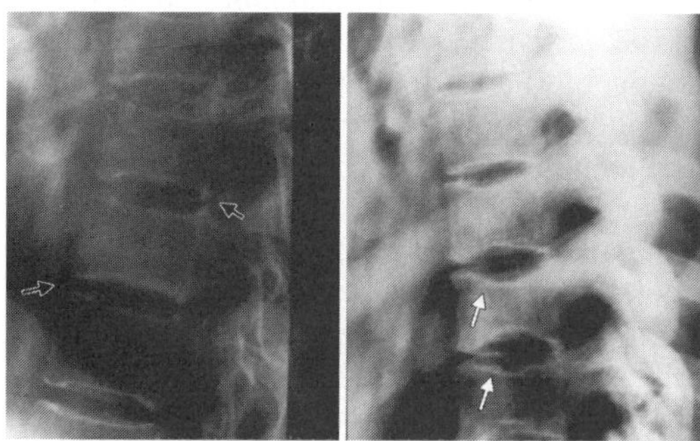

Fig. 19.2 X-ray of thoracic spine showing typical "step off" deformity in the vertebral body with normal appearance at the periphery (early changes)

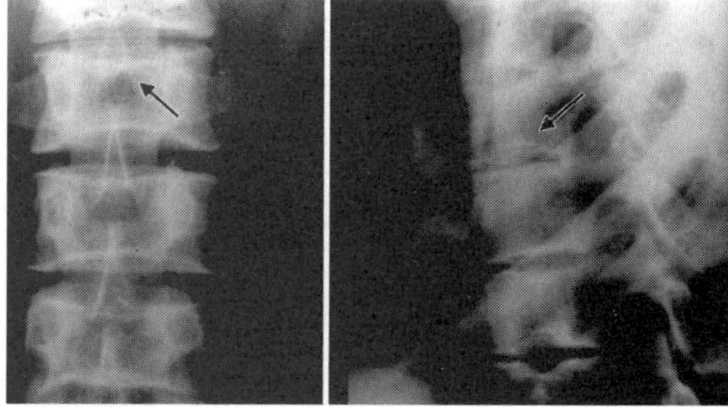

Fig. 19.4 X-ray lumbar spine anteroposterior and lateral view showing development of step off deformity—Early changes close to the arrow and advanced central cupping in the next disk space

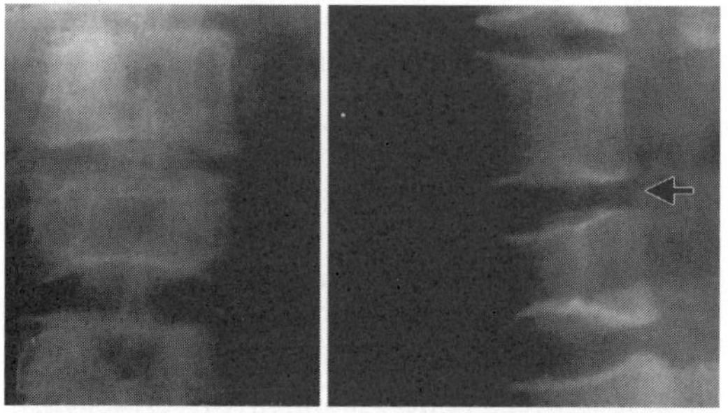

Fig. 19.3 X-ray of another patient showing advanced central cupping (step off deformity) showing mirror image central depression, fragmentation, and collapse of vertebral end plates with normal periphery

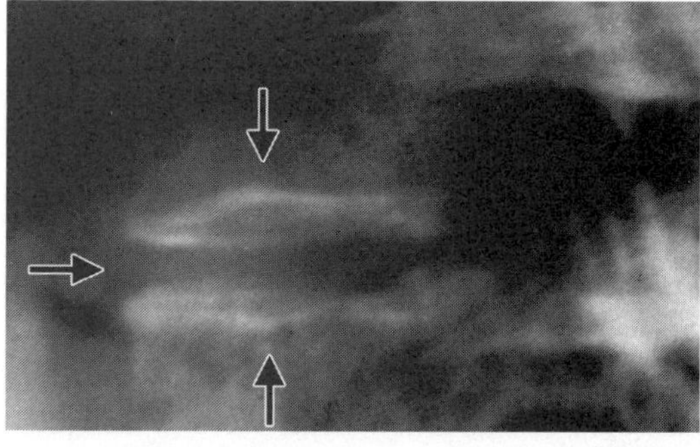

Fig. 19.5 X-ray Lumbar spine lateral view showing infarcts in the center close to arrow

top giving the profile of a truncated triangle.[1,2] These changes are different from fish mouth vertebrae in which a smooth biconcave depression of end plates extends from corner to corner of the vertebral body, usually secondary to osteoporosis. Associated tuberculous infection is infrequently seen. There is typical destruction of adjoining disk surfaces of the vertebral body with loss of intervertebral space giving a typical appearance of Pott's spine (Fig. 19.10).[5]

ETIOPATHOLOGY OF OSTEONECROSIS

Though these changes were attributed as ischemic changes secondary to vaso-occlusion following increased viscosity, thrombosis and infarction they could also be because of vascular compression from overactive marrow (hyperplasia). As per observation of these patients, it was felt that these are classical changes of osteonecrosis of the vertebral end plates akin to the changes seen in long bones and osteonecrosis of the femoral head and humeral head. The major portion of the blood supply of vertebral body to the extent of 75%

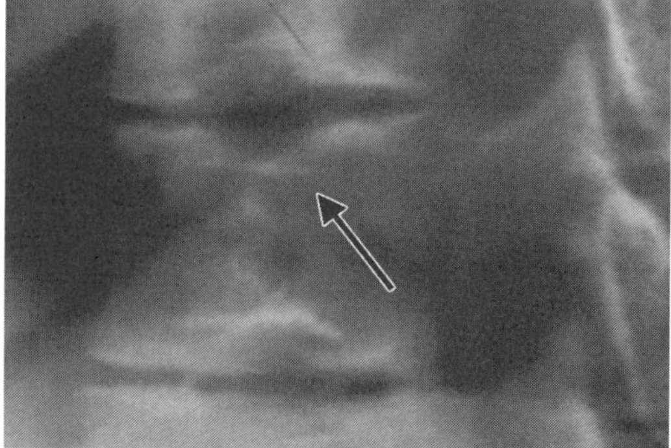

Fig. 19.6 X-ray thoracic spine lateral view, lower arrow showing bone infarct in the center of vertebral end plate with fragmentation and collapse. These are early changes before developing step off deformity

Fig. 19.8 Localized lateral view of spine showing straight zone of condensation 1–3 mm away from the vertebral end plate of involved vertabrae—en early presentation before developing step off deformity

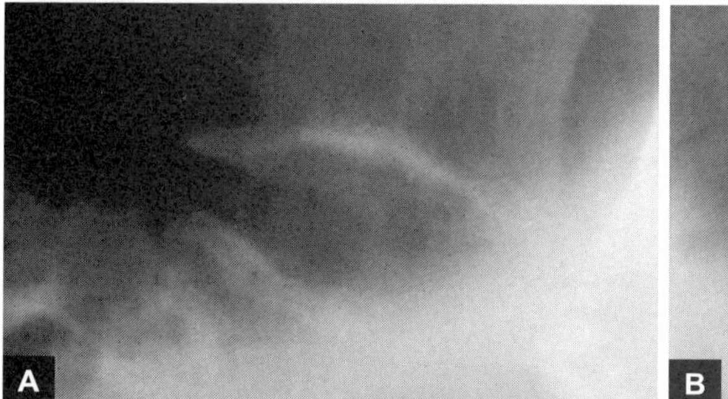

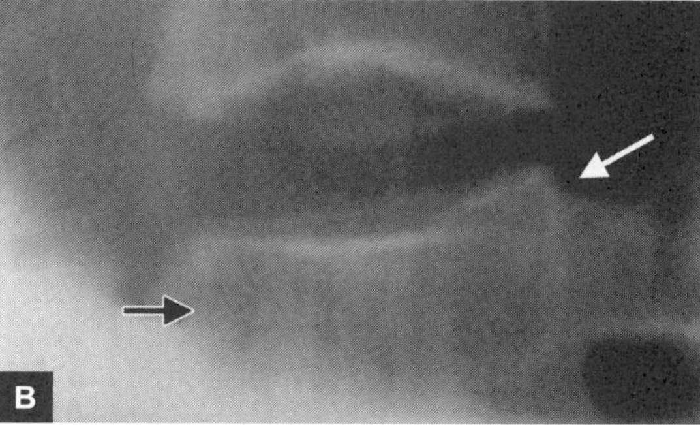

Figs 19.7A and B Localized view of intervertebral disk space showing early changes of vertebral end plates

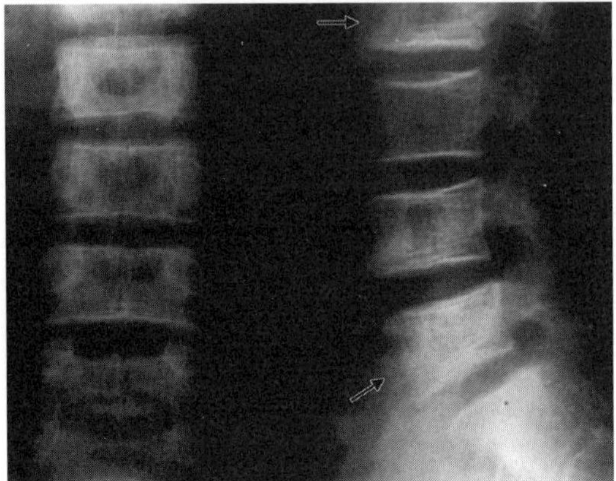

Fig. 19.9 X-ray showing marked porosis with sclerotic zone of subchondral bone from vertebral end plate nicely seen in L4 and L5 vertebrae (Growth arrest lines) and lateral view showing the typical appearance of "bone within the bone"

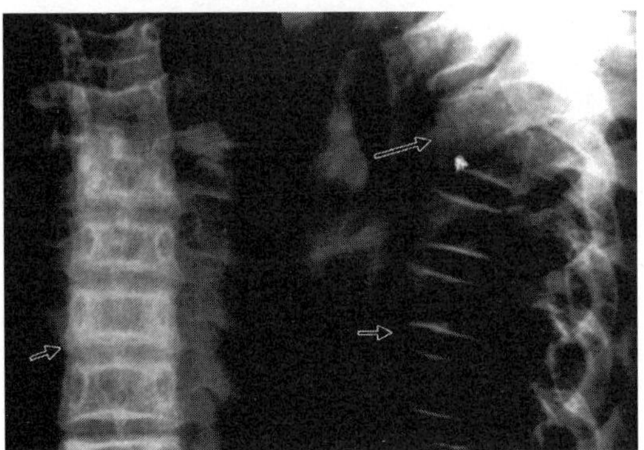

Fig. 19.10 Typical Pott's spine appearance of destruction with loss of disk space in the upper portion with typical changes of step off deformity in the vertebrae

(which mainly involve the central core) comes from the nutrient vessels which is a branch from ventral tributary of spinal branch, which itself is a dorsal branch of a segmental artery. The remaining 25% of blood supply belonging to the peripheral zone comes from periosteal vessels, which are the branches of the segmental artery and are small and multiple (Hollinshead et al. 1985[6]). The ischemia is produced because of vaso-occlusion of major

nutrient artery of the vertebral body, which affects the central part of the growth plate of vertebra since the periphery continues to grow at a normal rate because of supplementary periosteal blood supply (Fig. 19.11). Various stages in the development of typical step off deformity in these patients of sickle cell disease may be seen in one of the skiagram at one time (Fig. 19.12). In sickle cell disease blood containing long, multipointed, curved and rigid sickled cells is more viscid and flows less readily through terminal vessels. Utilization of oxygen by living blood cells and by endothelial tissue cells favors an exaggeration of sickling which increases viscosity and sludging of RBCs.

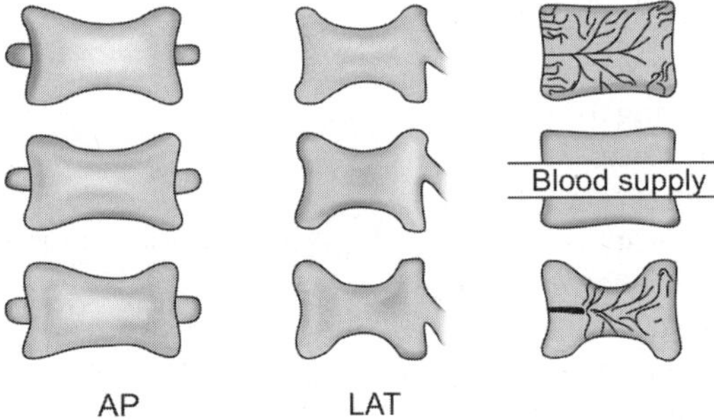

Fig. 19.11 Diagrammatic representation of the hypothesis for step off deformity and diagrammatic picture showing the vascular supply of vertebral body

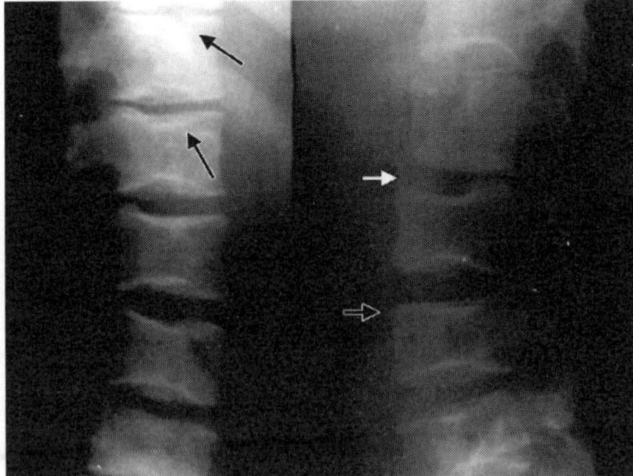

Fig. 19.12 X-ray lumbar spine showing various stages in the development of typical step off deformity in the same skiagram—lower vertebrae showing early changes and upper vertebrae showing typical established deformity

Chronic stasis of blood in capillaries and defective oxygenation leads to thrombosis, infarction in various tissues. Sickle cells, which are mechanically more fragile, are phagocytosed more readily and are subjected to hemolysis in the circulating blood. This ischemia is produced because of sludging of RBC's and increased vascular compression resulting from marrow hyperplasia causing classical changes of osteonecrosis like in the femoral head and humeral head (Fig. 19.13). There might be bone infarct, followed by classical changes of osteonecrosis in the form of spotty irregularities, increased densities, subsequent fragmentation and collapse of end plates. Since the symptoms are few the fragmentation of vertebral epiphysis is not properly seen as the X-rays are usually done late during the stage of revascularization and repair process. However in case the patients of sickle cell disease are followed roentgenographically, a proper sequence of radiological changes can be observed and many times at different vertebral levels on the same skiagram. Weight transmission through these vertebral bodies might also play a significant role in flattening the vertebral end plates and in its repair process. Basically all the changes of epiphyseal growth arrest are following ischemia, which results in osteonecrosis.

Management

These patients require follow-up and a general line of treatment for sickle cell disease. No specific treatment is required for changes of osteonecrosis. Supportive treatment for porosis in the form of vitamin D, calcium, anabolics and in grossly porotic bones with compression spinal support may be necessary. Systemic treatment by soda bicarbonate, zinc, folic acid and correction of fluid imbalance is required.

In the cases where there was associated secondary TB infection, treatment on the lines of Pott's disease—anti-tubercular treatment, rest and spinal support, is necessary. Rarely surgical decompression may be necessary if there is associated neurodeficit which is not responding to conservative treatment.

Discussion

Reynolds[7] in 1966 hypothesized that essentially stasis and ischemia retard the growth in the central portion of the vertebral cartilaginous growth plate in sickle cell disease. The periphery of the growth plate with a different blood supply continues to grow at a normal rate whereas there is slow growth in the centre of vertebral body because of compromised vascular supply to the major nutrient-feeding artery of the vertebral body. The periphery of the vertebral body receives a supplementary blood supply from periosteal feeding vessels whereas the center depends on the major nutrient artery. In a stage of vaso-occlusion as by sludging in patients of sickle cell disease peripheral growth continues whereas the centre would have ischemic retardation of the vertebral growth plate. This results in the classical 'step off' sign and these central end plate depressions or cupping are due to growth arrest. Reynolds (1973, 1977)[8,9] compared this cartilaginous growth plate of the vertebral body to the epiphyseal plate of long bones which when injured in toto resulted in odd shaped epiphysis and cupped metaphysis with greater growth peripherally. It is clear from these radiological pictures that the changes are because of vascular insult, which results in osteonecrosis of vertebral end plates. Though Reynolds (1978)[10] thought this to be ischemic he never postulated these as

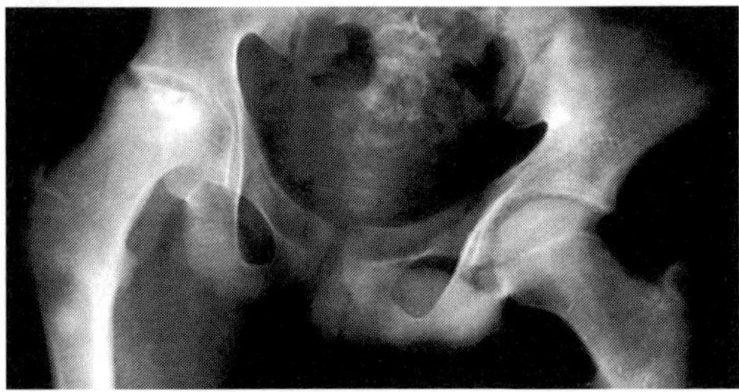

Fig. 19.13 X-ray showing typical changes of osteonecrosis of the femoral head with central collapse

changes of osteonecrosis. I feel that changes of osteonecrosis (avascular necrosis) which are commonly seen in the femoral head and humeral head are identical to these changes of osteonecrosis of vertebral end plates as observed by me with probably the same etiopathological process. This 'step off' sign was also observed in Gaucher's disease.[11-13] It was also seen in patients of thalassemia major and hereditary spherocytosis.[9,14]

In the presentation of the 'step off' sign the vascular supply of the end plate an important role since it is simply a failure of growth. The squared appearance of the vertebral body is due to a straight zone of condensation, which resembles short growth arrest lines seen in long bones. This type of epiphyseal growth disturbance was reported by Currarino and Erlandson (1964)[15] in thalassemia major showing premature closure of a portion of the epiphyseal plate with progressive deformity in the proximal humeral epiphysis and distal femoral epiphysis of adolescent patients. The changes were seen in adolescents and young adults and not in children in our series possibly because blood supply to the epiphysis is best during the growth.

Cupping or dome-like changes in the cartilaginous plate resemble those seen in tubular bones of the hand which is due to central infarcts with arrest of growth in sclerotic area and more rapid growth in the marginal bone which has better blood supply (Diggs LW, 1967).[16] These epiphyseal infarcts give a classical appearance of a combination of sclerotic and lucent changes in long bones (Bohrer SP 1974),[17] femoral head, humeral head and tubular bones of hand and foot (Babhulkar SS et al. 1995).[3]

The etiology of these osteonecrotic changes is ischemic and the vascular insult in these patients of sickle cell disease is not clearly understood. The accepted explanation is that hypoxia induces sickling which leads to sludging of RBCs and vascular stasis, which may cause thrombosis and infarction. Ischemia could be partly because of hyperplasia of the bone marrow causing vascular compression. Bone infarcts have no roentgenographic changes unless the infarct is revascularized. Re-ossification is accompanied by deposition of new bone on the framework of the dead bone. These re-ossified bones may not be strong and usually collapses and it looses its growth potential.

REFERENCES

1. Babhulkar Sudhir. Orthopaedic manifestations and bone changes in sickle cell haemoglobinopathy. Monogram by CBS Publishers;1997.pp.78-93.
2. Babhulkar Sudhir, Babhulkar Sushrut. Sickle cell haemoglobinopathy. Osteonecrosis etiology, Diagnosis and treatment; In Urbaniak JR, Jones JP, Editors; Osteonecrosis: Etiology,diagnosis, and treatment. Rosemont, IL: American Academy of Orthopaedic Surgeons: 1997, P 131-3 (Monogram by AAOS 1997)
3. Babhulkar SS, Pande KC, Babhulkar S. Hand foot syndrome in Sickle cell hemoglobinopathy. J Bone Joint Surg Br. 1995;77B:310-2.
4. Daland GA, Castle WB. A simple and Rapid method of demonstrating sickling of red blood cells, the use of reducing agents. J Lab Clin Med. 1948;33:1082.
5. Babhulkar Sudhir, Pande Sonali. Unusual manifestations of osteoarticular tuberculosis. Clin Orthop. 2002;398:114-20.
6. Hollinshead WH, Rosse Cornelius. Textbook of Anatomy, 4th edn. Harper and Row Publishers Inc. Philadelphia; 1985.pp.298-9.
7. Reynolds J. A re-evaluation of the "fish vertebra" sign in Sickle cell hemoglobinopathy. AJR. 1966; 97:693-707.
8. Reynolds J, Pritchard JA, Ludders D, Mason RA. Roentgenographic and clinical appraisal of Sickle cell beta- thalassemia disease. AJR. 1973; 118:378-400.
9. Reynolds J. Radiologic manifestations of sickle cell haemoglobinopathy. JAMA. 1977;238:247-50.
10. Reynolds J, Jack AP, Darrell Ludders, Ruble A M. Roentgenographic and clinical appraisal of sickle cell beta-thalassemia disease. Radiology. 1978;118:378-97.
11. Moseley JE. Skeletal changes in the anemias, Semin Roentgenol. 1974;9:169-84.

12. Hansen GC, Gold RH. Central depression of multiple vertebral end plates: A pathognomonic sign of Sickle hemoglobinopathy in Gaucher's disease. AJR. 1977;129:343-4.

13. Schwartz Alan M, Marc J, Homer and Roy GK, McCauley. "Step-off" vertebral body: Gaucher's disease versus Sickle cell haemoglobinopathy. AJR. 1979;132:81-5.

14. Cassady JR, Berdon WE, Baker DH. The "typical" spine changes in Sickle cell anemia in a patient with thalassemia major (Cooley's anemia). Radiology. 1967;89:1065-8.

15. Currarino & Erlandson. Premature fusion of epiphysis in Cooley's anemia. Radiology. 1964; 83:655-64.

16. Diggs LW. Bone and joint lesions in sickle cell disease. Clin Orth; 1967.pp.119-43.

17. Bohrer SP. Growth disturbances of the distal femur following Sickle cell bone infarcts and/or osteomyelitis. Clinical radiology. 1974;25: 221-35.

OSTEONECROSIS OF THE KNEE

Osteonecrosis is a disease characterized by a derangement of osseous circulation that leads to necrosis of osseous tissue of the distal femur. Ahlbäck et al[1] first described osteonecrosis of the knee in the year 1968. In osteonecrosis, the lesion can extend to the subchondral plate and result in collapse of the necrotic segment. This can lead to disruption of the joint line, resulting in painful secondary arthritis. The condition was initially described as having a spontaneous presentation that typically involved the medial femoral condyle. The true incidence of the disease is unknown, but osteonecrosis of the knee is believed to account for approximately 10 percent of cases of osteonecrosis. Early reports noted a greater prevalence in women aged more than 60 years, often following minor trauma or increased activity. Later studies identified patients whose characteristics and symptoms did not match these initial descriptions, which led to the recognition of three unique entities:[2]

1. Secondary osteonecrosis
2. Spontaneous osteonecrosis of the knee (SPONK)
3. Postarthroscopic osteonecrosis.

However, the etiology, associated risk factors, diagnostic evaluation, prognosis, and management approach may differ for each type.

SECONDARY OSTEONECROSIS

Epidemiology

The incidence of secondary osteonecrosis of the knee has been estimated to be 10 percent that of hip osteonecrosis.

Although the etiology of secondary osteonecrosis is unknown, several risk factors are associated with the disease. Corticosteroid consumption is the most significant risk factor; other risk factors include alcohol abuse, sickle cell disease, systemic lupus erythematosus, Caisson's disease, Gaucher's disease, patients with organ transplantation, and so on. The two risk factors most commonly associated with secondary knee osteonecrosis are use of corticosteroid and alcohol abuse amounting to approximately 90 percent.[3] The pathogenesis of this condition is poorly understood, although the mechanism may be similar, the specific pathogenesis remains unclear. Some authors have implicated elevated intraosseous pressure resulting from adipocyte hyperproliferation.[2,4] Alternatively, fat emboli may occlude vessels in the subchondral bone. In persons who abuse alcohol, these emboli are likely to originate from a fatty liver. One possible mechanism is microvascular disruption in the subchondral bone that causes infarction. This circulatory compromise leads to bone marrow edema, with resultant ischemia and necrosis.

The mechanism by which corticosteroids contribute to osteonecrosis is also unclear. One hypothesis is that an increase in the size of the marrow fat cells decreases circulation and leads to ischemia. Other possible contributors to the etiopathogenesis are coagulopathies, fat emboli, and thrombus formation. There are anecdotal reports of osteonecrosis occurring after the administration of low-dose corticosteroids or intra-articular injections; however, there is no sufficient evidence to suggest a cause-and-effect relationship. Conditions such as sickle cell disease, Caisson's disease, Gaucher's disease, and myeloproliferative disorders are considered to be direct causes of knee osteonecrosis. The pathomechanism in sickle cell and Caisson's disease is similar, with direct occlusion of blood vessels. Gaucher's disease, leukemia, and myeloproliferative disorders are thought to increase intraosseous pressure by displacing marrow. Osteonecrosis of the knee is also more prevalent in certain patients, such as those who have undergone organ transplantation.

The knee is the fourth most common site of osteonecrosis, the most common being the femoral head, humeral head and vertebral end plates as seen in our study. Secondary osteonecrosis, spontaneous osteonecrosis of the knee, and postarthroscopic osteonecrosis are distinct pathologic entities, but they share some similarity in their presentation. Secondary osteonecrosis often involves both femoral condyles and presents with multiple lesions. The epiphysis, metaphysis, and diaphysis may be affected. The femur is affected in ≤90 percent of cases, and >80 percent of patients have bilateral disease.

Controversy exists regarding whether spontaneous osteonecrosis of the knee represents insufficiency fracture or part of the progression of osteoarthritis. Postarthroscopic osteonecrosis is associated with subchondral collapse and may be associated with altered knee mechanics. MRI is the most sensitive and specific diagnostic tool for all three entities. Disease progression is monitored on standard radiographs.

Nonsurgical management with analgesics and protected weight-bearing is recommended for early-stage spontaneous osteonecrosis of the knee and postarthroscopic osteonecrosis, but it may not be appropriate for secondary osteonecrosis. Patients in whom nonsurgical measures are unsuccessful may be treated with joint-preserving procedures. Joint arthroplasty is required for persons with subchondral bone collapse.

Diagnosis

Clinical Assessment

Diagnosis is based on clinical suspicion and radiographic confirmation. A thorough patient history should identify associated risk factors. The disease is more frequent in men, and the patients with secondary osteonecrosis are often aged more than 45 years and have one or more associated risk factors. Bilateral and multiple joint involvements are seen in more than 90 percent of cases.[2] Pain is the dominant symptom and is usually severe and localized. It is noticed predominantly on active movements and weight-bearing causing significant functional impairment. Physical examination shows tenderness over the involved area with moderate synovial effusion with restricted movements in terminal stages. Several other diseases and conditions may present in a similar manner, such as meniscal or ligamentous injury. Osteonecrosis tends to progress to more advanced disease that requires surgical intervention, hence early diagnosis is important.

Radiographic Assessment

Standard radiography, bone scan and MRI are recommended to evaluate the patient with suspected secondary osteonecrosis (Figs 20.1A and B). AP and lateral radiographs can be used to diagnose advanced disease in persons with signs of impending subchondral fracture or collapse (Figs 20.2 and 20.3). Radiography is an inexpensive modality for staging and monitoring disease progression. Lesions can be detected earliest on MRI because of the ability to assess marrow viability and lesion distribution and to evaluate meniscal and chondral pathology (Fig. 20.4). Many diseases demonstrate bone marrow edema on MRI. This nonspecific finding is associated with ischemia (osteonecrosis, bone marrow edema syndrome, transient osteoporosis, osteochondritis dissecans), mechanical etiologies (bone

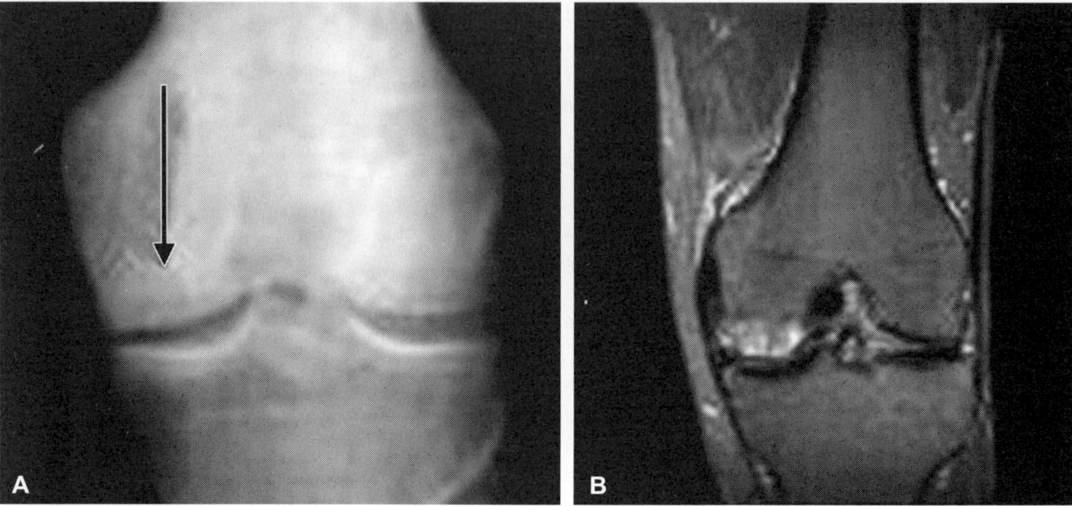

Figs 20.1A and B (A) Plain X-ray showing early radiological signs of osteonecrosis; (B) MRI of the same patient showing charactertic signs of osteonecrosis

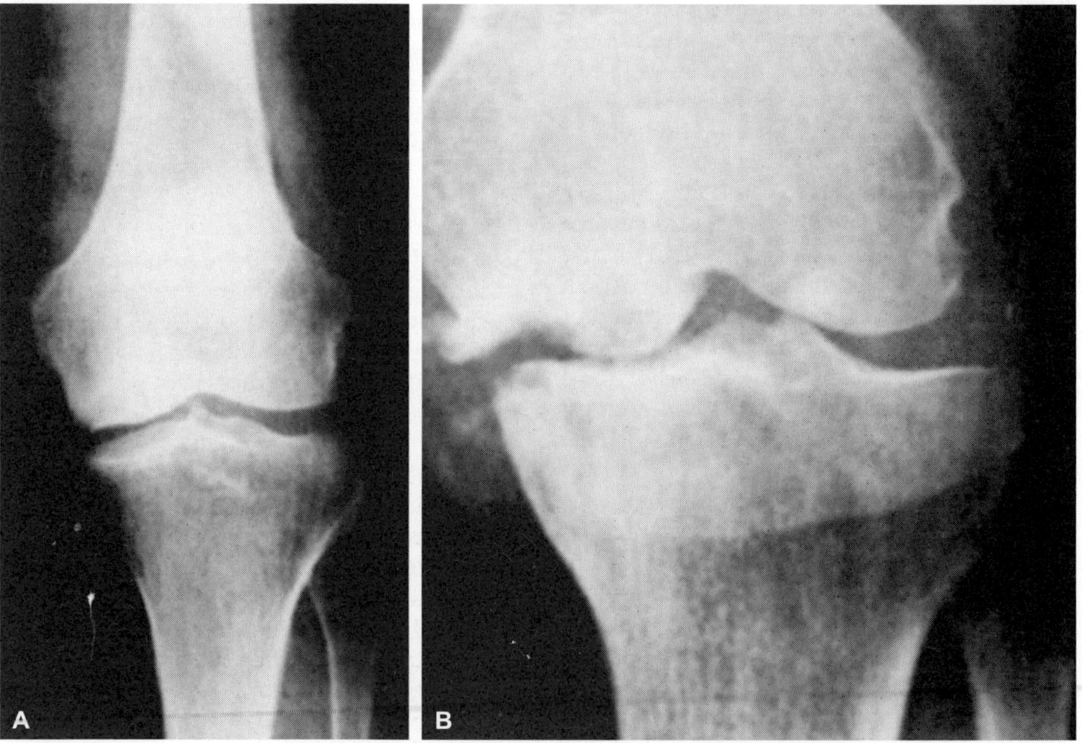

Figs 20.2A and B A woman aged 65 whose disease came on spontaneously and became severe. (A) Radiograph at one year after the beginning of symptoms; (B) Radiograph at two years. There is severe bone collapse, erosion and secondary osteoarthritis

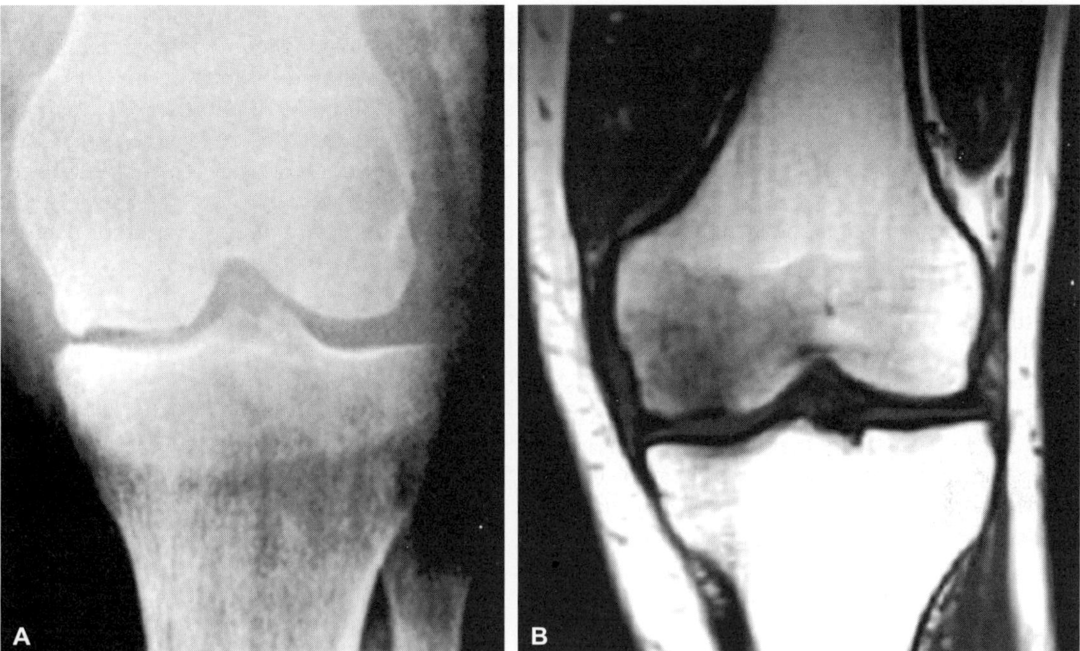

Figs 20.3A and B (A) Standing roentgenogram of the left knee in an sixty three-year-old man who complained of sudden onset of pain, showing flattening of medial femoral condyle; (B) MRI—The medial femoral condyle shows an irregular defect in the articular surface

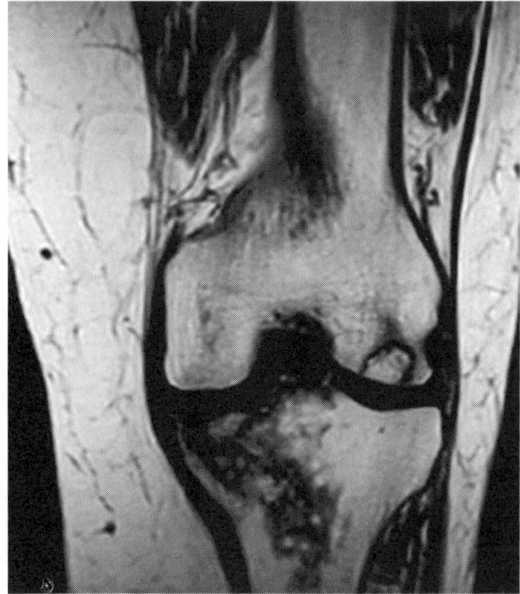

Fig. 20.4 MRI (T1) demonstrating characteristic findings of secondary osteonecrosis, such as multiple hypointense serpentine lesions surrounded by a well-demarcated hyperintense border

bruise, microfracture), and reactive processes (osteoarthritis, postoperative bone marrow edema). MRI findings can be nonspecific; thus, disease-specific findings such as serpentine lesions with a well-demarcated border are necessary to confirm the diagnosis of osteonecrosis.

Patients with secondary osteonecrosis should be screened clinically for other joint involvement. The most frequently affected sites are the hip, shoulder, and contralateral knee. MRI of any other symptomatic joint may be appropriate as the initial screening in patients with secondary osteonecrosis. Evaluation of both hips may be appropriate regardless of the symptoms. Osteonecrosis associated with sickle cell disease progresses to symptomatic disease at a mean follow-up of 14 years (range, 10 to 20 years). This finding reinforces the importance of close patient monitoring, hence regular screening of the knees and hips has been recommended. Some authors prefer bone scintigraphy to detect early knee osteonecrosis. However, Mont et al[5] reported that bone scans identified disease in only 37 of 58 patients (64%), whereas MRI detected all histopathologically confirmed lesions.

Ahuja and Bullogh[6] compared the clinical and pathological features of osteonecrosis of the knee. The pathological findings in the 12 knees with idiopathic osteonecrosis in their series constitute a sequence of changes that ultimately give rise to marked deformities of the joint. These changes consist of fracture of the necrotic bone, fragmentation and collapse of the articular cartilage, breakdown of necrotic segment, fibrillation of the articular cartilage, and subchondral osteosclerosis. A secondary osteoarthrosis was the final result. These changes resemble those seen in so-called idiopathic avascular necrosis of the femoral head.

Several systems are used to stage knee osteonecrosis radiographically. Most were reported in studies that assessed spontaneous osteonecrosis of the knee; however, they can be used to assess secondary and postarthroscopic

osteonecrosis, as well. In all three of the four-stage systems, stage III is characterized by a crescent sign, representing collapsed subchondral bone.[2,7,8] Patients with stage III disease are unlikely to experience regression, and surgical intervention is typically required. Larger lesion size is predictive of disease progression. None of the four methods used to assess lesion size has been validated.

Ficat Staging

Ficat staging of knee osteonecrosis, demonstrating the progression from precollapse lesions to late-stage disease and cortical bone collapse (Figs 20.5A to D).[9-11]

- Stage I, no radiographic evidence of knee osteonecrosis. The femoral condyles appear normal, with no sclerosis and maintained curvature. Symptoms are more intense in the early stage and may continue for six to eight weeks and then may subside. A positive bone scan is necessary to confirm the diagnosis. Treatment at this stage is nonsurgical. The focus is on pain relief and protected weight-bearing.
- Stage II, signs of mottled sclerosis are evident, but the normal curvature of the bone remains intact. It may take several months for the disease to progress to stage II. An MRI or bone scan can be used to diagnose the disease.
- Stage III, the presence of a crescent sign is indicative of subchondral fracture, which defines this stage. By the time the disease reaches stage III (three to six months after onset), it is clearly visible on X-rays and no other diagnostic tests are needed. The articular cartilage covering the bone begins to loosen as the bone itself begins to die. Surgical treatments may be considered at this point.
- Stage IV, collapse of the subchondral bone. At this point, the bone begins to collapse. The articular cartilage is destroyed, the joint space narrows, and bone spurs may form. Severe osteoarthritis results and joint replacement surgery may be necessary.

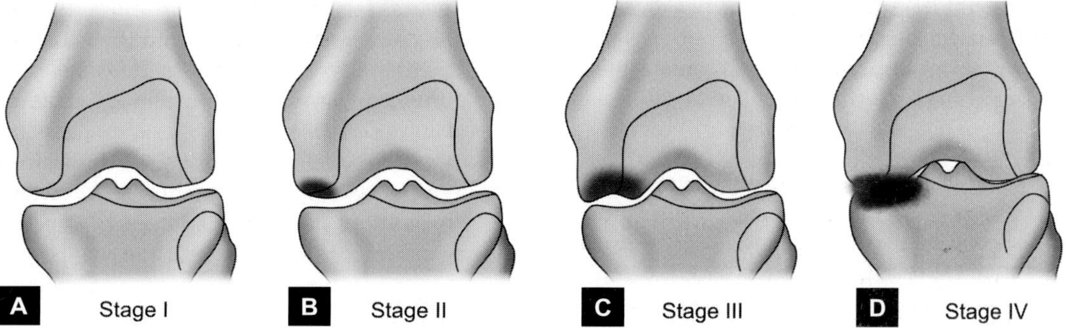

Figs 20.5A to D Ficat staging of knee osteonecrosis, demonstrating the progression from precollapse lesions to late-stage disease and cortical bone collapse. (A) Stage I, no radiographic evidence of knee osteonecrosis. The femoral condyles appear normal, with no sclerosis and maintained curvature; (B) Stage II, signs of mottled sclerosis are evident, but the normal curvature of the bone remains intact; (C) Stage III, the presence of a crescent sign is indicative of subchondral fracture,which defines this stage; (D) Stage IV, collapse of the subchondral bone

Secondary Osteonecrosis: Etiology

The etiology of this lesion remains unknown. Because of the pathological similarity between osteonecrosis of the hip[12-14] and of the knee, two main theories exist, "vascular" and "traumatic". The "vascular" theory implies more than a direct occlusion[15-18] of a small artery, which would seem difficult because of the anastomotic tree in the condyles—it is an alteration in microcirculation with increased bone marrow pressure and decreased flow.[19-22] This mechanism has been studied particularly after cortisone treatment, and probably implies an increased size of the marrow fat cells, and an altered lipid metabolism.

Prognosis

In the natural history and prognosis, two factors seem to be of prime importance: the area of the lesion and the ratio of the size of lesion to that of the condyle. Staging was less important in our study than in a recent paper.[23]

Management

Many treatment algorithms have been proposed for knee osteonecrosis. However, they are primarily supported by limited retrospective reviews with relatively few patients. Prospective randomized studies and multi-center collaboration are needed. Several similar treatment options are available for the management of all three entities with varying degrees of success.[2]

Nonsurgical Treatment

In the early stages of the disease, treatment is not surgical. If the affected area is small, this treatment may be all that is needed. Options include:

- Medications to reduce the pain
- A brace to relieve pressure on the joint surface
- A conditioning program with exercises to strengthen your thigh muscles
- Activity modifications to reduce knee pain.

Surgical Treatment

If more than half of the bone surface is affected, you may need surgical treatment. Several different procedures may be used to treat osteonecrosis of the knee.

Among the surgical options are:

- Arthroscopic cleansing (debridement) of the joint
- Drilling to reduce pressure on the bone surface

- Procedures to shift weight-bearing away from the affected area
- Unicompartmental or total knee replacement.

Surgical

- Surgery of stages I and II—disease is controversial. There have been some studies indicating that drilling of the osteonecrotic area may stimulate revascularization, a new blood supply, to facilitate regeneration of new bone. Cartilage grafting is also considered in stage II disease. Therapeutic benefits of core decompression result in reduction of marrow pressure and increased neovascularization which allows formation of new healthy bone. Recently Marulanda et al.[24] reported the percutaneous approach using a small-diameter drilling technique under fluoroscopic control, and had a success rate of over 90 percent.
- Osteonecrosis is classified stage III—when the joint surface has collapsed and become depressed or flattened. Routine X-rays usually show this collapse and irregularity of the joint surface. The associated damage to the overlying articular cartilage is not visible on routine X-ray but can be seen on MRI scan. Operative treatment such as drilling of the lesion, local bone grafting or placement of a cartilage graft may be considered in younger patients. In older individuals who have progressed to advanced osteoarthritis, joint replacement surgery may eventually be necessary.
- Stage IV disease is when osteonecrosis has progressed to severe damage, osteoarthritis, of the joint. The surface articular cartilage has been destroyed and marked osteoarthritic changes are seen on the X-ray. These patients continue to have symptoms and are treated like typical osteoarthritic patients, which includes symptomatic treatment until such time that knee replacement is necessary.
- The eventual need for surgical intervention in osteonecrosis of the knee is based on several factors, including the area where the osteonecrosis occurs and the extent of the damage to the joint. Small lesions may not go on to extensive collapse and joint damage. Osteonecrosis lesions that are not in the weight-bearing area may cause limited symptoms which resolve when the lesion heals. Patients who develop osteonecrosis in the weight-bearing part of the knee joint with a large area of involvement are more likely to eventually require surgery.
- When conservative measures fail to relieve symptoms, including activity modification, protected weight-bearing using a cane or crutches, the use of braces, and appropriate medications, surgical options are considered.
- For younger patients, typically under the age of 50 and depending on the area and extent of involvement, various surgical procedures may be indicated. Among these are arthroscopic removal of damaged cartilage and/or drilling (to reduce pressure in the bone and re-establish blood supply), and realignment procedures and osteotomies to shift load-bearing away from the damaged surface of the knee. There are also surgical procedures to replace or help regenerate involved bone and cartilage. For the older age population, full or partial knee replacement is the usual surgical treatment.
- Treatment options depend on the extent and location of the osteonecrotic area, patient age, and level of activity. It is important to consult an orthopedic surgeon who is experienced in treating this condition, including all of the surgical options that may result in the best possible outcome.

Nonsurgical

Secondary osteonecrosis progresses to advanced stages in approximately 80 percent of patients treated nonsurgically. Thus, nonsurgical management is not recommended. Use of pharmacologic agents (e.g. diphosphonates, anticoagulants) to manage secondary osteonecrosis has been reported for osteonecrosis of the hip. However, no large randomized trial exists for the use of disphosphonates, iloprost and anticoagulants. Iloprost is a prostacyclin analogue, which might be used in osteonecrosis of the knee. This potent vasodilator may be useful in the management of osteonecrosis by increasing blood flow to the affected region.[2]

Joint-preserving Procedures

In early pre-collapse stages of secondary osteonecrosis, joint-preserving surgical procedures such as core decompression, arthroscopy, osteotomy, and bone grafting may be performed in an effort to avoid arthroplasty. Core decompression may be used in patients with osteonecrosis but without subchondral collapse. It has been suggested that the therapeutic benefit of core decompression is the result of reduced marrow pressure and increased neovascularization, which allows formation of healthy bone. The procedure can be performed by percutaneous approach under fluoroscopic guidance on an outpatient basis, and patients are restricted to weight-bearing with crutches or a cane for the first month after surgery. This technique had a success rate of >90 percent (i.e. Knee Society score ≥80 points) at two to four year follow-up. Core decompression is unlikely to benefit the patient with joint collapse.

Bone grafting has been used in persons with early-stage knee osteonecrosis. Autologous and/or fresh-frozen allografts are incorporated to provide structural support to the subchondral bone and articular cartilage. It is preferred to use a combination of cortical and cancellous allograft introduced through a 1×2 cm extra-articular cortical window. Patients begin with protected weight-bearing and are advanced to full weight-bearing after one month. Evidence supporting these joint preserving procedures is limited. No randomized trials are currently available, and the published studies tend to be small with relatively short follow-up. This bone grafting procedure may delay the need for joint arthroplasty in patients without any collapse.[25,26]

Arthroplasty

Even with early treatment many patients progress to advanced stage of osteonecrosis. Total knee joint replacement is recommended for patients with subchondral collapse and patients in whom the joint preserving surgery has failed. It is desirable to avoid the use of osteochondral grafts in patients with secondary osteonecrosis for two reasons. First, there is the possibility of impaired healing potential of the underlying native bone. Second, the lesions usually involve multiple condyles, which are not amenable to single osteochondral graft. It is not recommended to perform unicompartmental knee arthroplasty (UKA) because of the frequent involvement of multiple condyles. In addition, bone involvement tends to be extensive, which could compromise implant stability. Standard TKA surgical approaches and rehabilitation protocols can be used.

In conclusion, we believe that the regime of treatment for osteonecrosis of the knee should be as follows: for the first six months after the onset of symptoms a period of observation and conservative treatment is desirable. Usually any initially severe symptoms gradually decrease and conservative treatment can be prolonged if the lesion is small (less than five square centimeters) and the ratio low (less than 40%). For larger lesions without resolution of symptoms surgical treatment is indicated. Of the various options, one should consider high tibial osteotomy or knee replacement. Selection between the two should be based upon the same criteria as is customary for osteoarthritis: advanced age and an expected low level of activity favor replacement, and in fact most of our cases are now treated by arthroplasty.

▪ SPONTANEOUS OSTEONECROSIS OF THE KNEE

Very little data exist on spontaneous osteonecrosis of the knee (SPONK), but it is considered to be more common than secondary osteonecrosis (Table 20.1). The prevalence of spontaneous osteonecrosis of the knee may be underestimated because many patients who present with end-stage osteoarthritis may have had occult undiagnosed spontaneous osteonecrosis of the knee. One study indicated

Table 20.1 Comparison of clinical presentation and etiology in knee osteonecrosis

Characteristic	Secondary ON	Spontaneous ON of the knee	Postarthroscopic ON
Age	Typically < 45 years	Typically >50 years	Any
Sex	More likely in men than women	Female to male ratio of 3:1	No predilection
Bilaterality	> 80%	< 5%	Never
Other joint involvement	. 90% (hip, shoulder, ankle)	No	No
Associated risk factors	Direct causes: trauma, Caisson's disease, chemotherapy, Gaucher's disease, radiation, Indirect causes: alcohol abuse, coagulation abnormalities (thrombophilia, hypofibrinolysis), corticosteroid use, inflammatory bowel disease, organ transplant, SLE, smoking	Idopathic, chronic mechanical stress, or microtrauma	Menisectomy, cartilage debridement, anterior cruciate ligament reconstruction, laser or radiofrequency assisted surgery
Proposed pathogenic mechanism	Direct cell injury. Restriction or occlusion of blood supply. Increased intraosseous pressure	Weight-bearing articular surface subjected to altered stresses as the result of sunchondral fracture. Vascular compromise to subchondral bone, resulting in osseous ischemia and subsequent edema. Osteoarthritis variant	Abnormal loading leading to chondral injury, inflammation, edema, and intraosseous pressure. Abnormal loading leading to microfracture and abnormal blood circulation. Direct thermal or photoacoustic injury via laser or radiofrequency assisted arthroscopy
Pathologic findings	Necrotic bone	Fibrotic bone, healing fracture, osteopenia, osteoarthritic, necrosis, found only at the distal end of the fractured segment	Fibrotic bone and healing fracture. Necrotic bone after direct thermal or acoustic injury

a 3.4 percent incidence of spontaneous osteonecrosis of the knee in persons aged >50 years who presented with symptoms in the medial meniscus and an incidence ≤9.4 percent in persons aged >65 years.[27] The medial femoral condylar epiphysis is the most frequent site of spontaneous osteonecrosis of the knee. On MRI, spontaneous osteonecrosis of the knee typically appears as a focal, low-signal finding with linear features in the subarticular bone of the epiphysis (Figs 20.6A and B). The medial tibial plateau is affected in approximately 2 percent of cases.[28] Spontaneous osteonecrosis of the knee rarely occurs in the patella or the lateral femoral condyle. Most cases are unilateral. However, a recent case report demonstrated a patient with bicondylar spontaneous osteonecrosis of the knee.

In such instances, an understanding of the underlying risk factors and radiographic findings associated with secondary osteonecrosis is helpful in diagnosis (Tables 20.1 and 20.2).

Pathogenesis, Etiology, and Associated Risk Factors

Recent studies have attempted to investigate the underlying pathogenesis of spontaneous osteonecrosis of the knee. Early theories suggested a vascular origin, with compromised microcirculation to the subchondral bone resulting in edema, increased intraosseous pressure, and, ultimately, ischemia and necrosis. However, recent pathologic studies have not revealed evidence of necrotic bone.

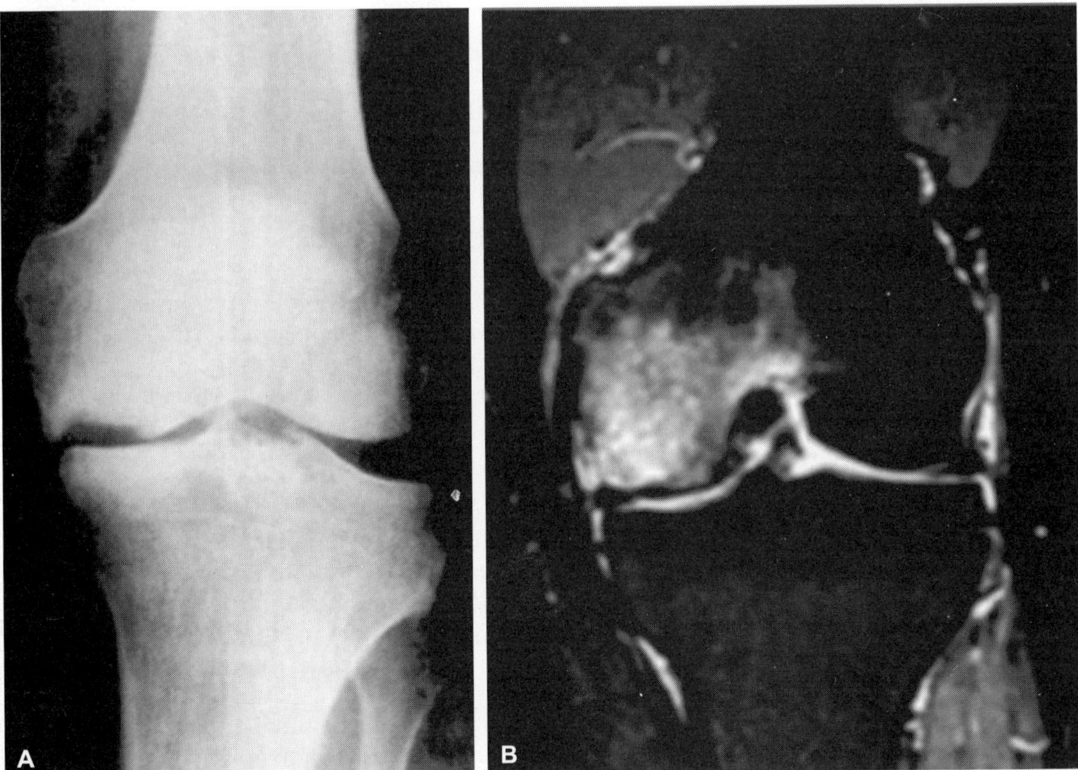

Figs 20.6A and B (A) X-ray in a patient with spontaneous osteonecrosis of the knee demonstrating a lesion; (B) (T2) fat-suppressed magnetic resonance image demonstrating an area of low signal intensity surrounded by high signal intensity caused by edema

Table 20.2 Clinical presentation of SPONK and secondary osteonecrosis

Physical characteristic	SPONK	Secondary osteonecrosis
Age	Typically >55 years	Typically < 55 years
Sex (male-to-female ratio)	1:3	1:3
Associated risk factors	None	Corticosteroids, alcohol, SLE, sickle cell disease, Caisson's disease, Gaucher's disease, fat emboli, thrombus formation
Other joint involvement	Rare	Approximately 75%
Laterality	99% unilateral	Approximately 80% bilateral
Condylar involvement	One (usually medial femoral condyle or either tibial plateau)	Multiple
Location	Epiphyseal to the subchondral surface	Diaphyseal, metaphyseal, epiphyseal
Symptoms	Commonly sudden onset of pain and increased pain with weight-bearing, stair climbing, and at night	Usually long-standing insidious pain; patient may have symptoms and signs of an underlying disorder, such as SLE
Examination	Pain localized to affected area; small synovitis or effusion may occur; ligaments are stable; range of motion may be limited by pain or effusion	Pain is difficult to localize; ligaments are stable; range of motion is grossly intact but may be limited by pain

Radiologic and pathologic evidence suggest that, in some cases, spontaneous osteonecrosis of the knee may be the result of a subchondral insufficiency fracture. As many as 80 percent of patients may present with a meniscal root injury, as well.[29] Some authors have suggested a traumatic origin because spontaneous osteonecrosis is commonly seen in elderly women with osteopenic bone, which is susceptible to microfracture. The authors of one histologic study on whether the disease follows insufficiency fracture reported that many patients had evidence of subchondral fracture, with a reparative reaction consisting of osteoid and immature bone; however, they noted no evidence of necrosis.[30] These findings suggest that "spontaneous osteonecrosis of the knee" is a misnomer and that it is, in fact, a disease that should be defined as an unstable fracture initially, which then becomes true bone death of the displaced fracture fragment in later stages.[32] These findings are supported by Ramnath and Kattapuram,[32] who showed that in 52 subchondral lesions identified as spontaneous osteonecrosis of the knee, patients with a subacute presentation had insufficiency fracture, and patients with chronic disease had osteoarthritis.

Diagnosis

Patients with spontaneous osteonecrosis of the knee typically present with well-defined pain at the medial aspect of the distal femur. This may mimic the pain experienced following tear of the medial meniscus. The pain is often worse at night and on weight-bearing. Women are approximately three times more likely than men to have this pain; most patients present in their late fifties or later.[30]

Recommended imaging modalities are similar to those for secondary osteonecrosis.

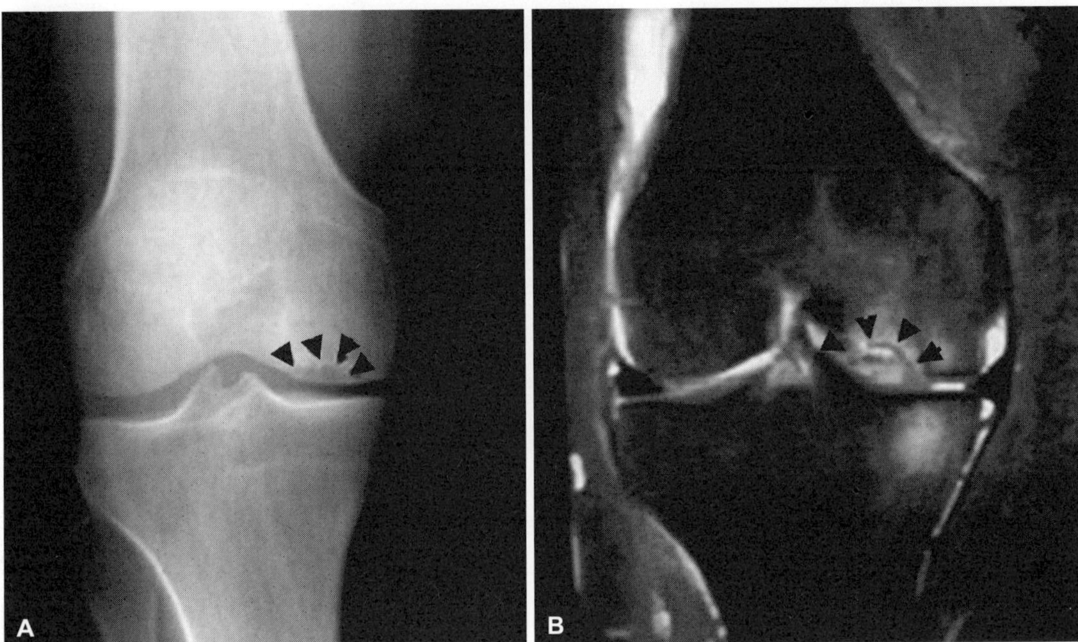

Figs 20.7A and B Plain AP X-ray and MRI (T2-) of the right knee in a patient who developed postarthroscopic osteonecrosis of the medial femoral condyle (arrowheads) following meniscectomy

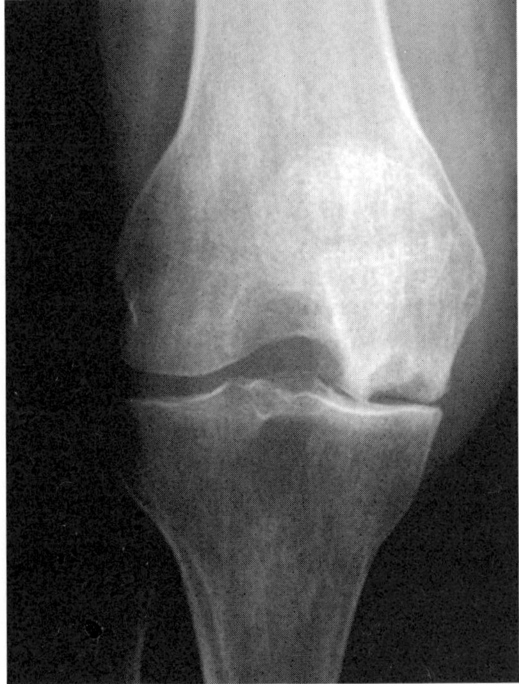

Fig. 20.8 65 years male patient X-ray showing spontaneous osteonecrosis of the medial femoral condyle, which was treated by unicompartment knee replacement

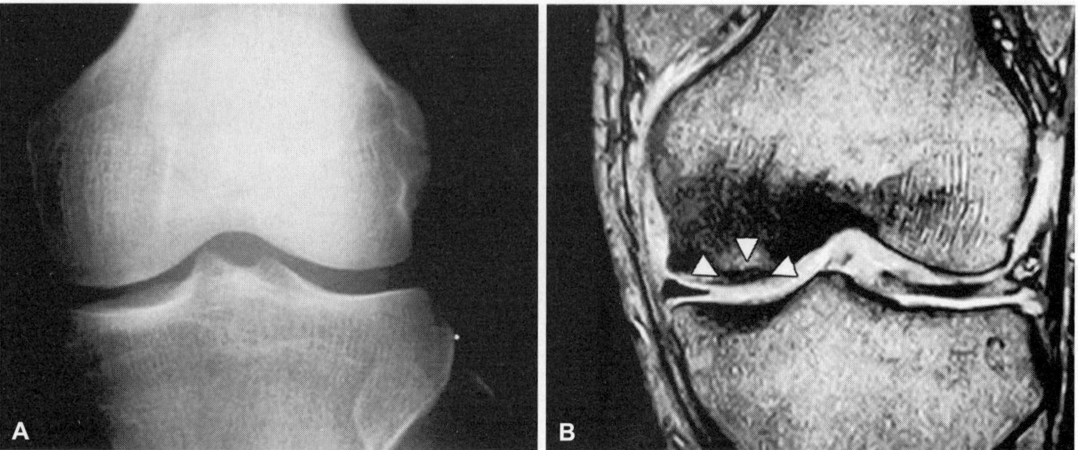

Figs 20.9A and B (A) Plain X-ray of patient showing no radiolucencies, indicating stage-I disease; (B) MR (T2) image showing a low-signal-intensity area in the subchondral portion of the weight-bearing area of the medial femoral condyle, which was surrounded by an oval area of high signal intensity, which was surrounded by a diffuse low-intensity area

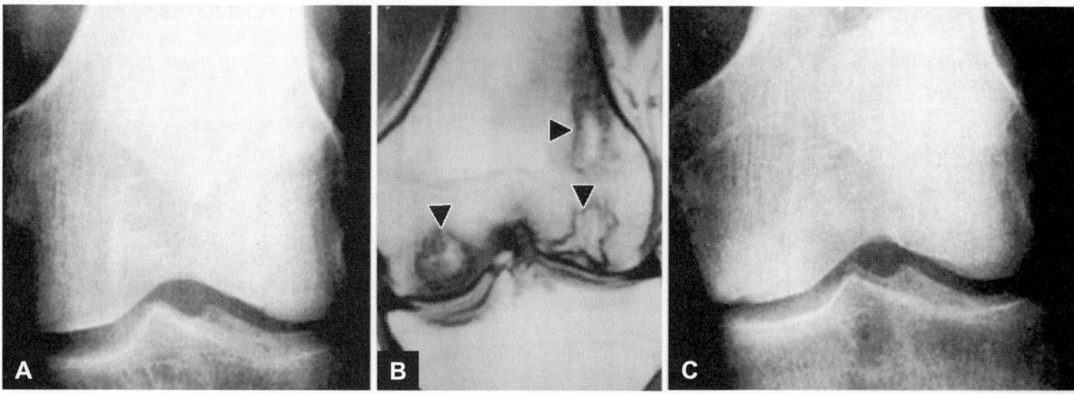

Figs 20.10A to C (A) A sixty-two-year-old woman with pain over the medial femoral condyle. Initial roentgenograms are normal. The patient had a meniscectomy. Pain persisted after the meniscectomy; (B) Same patients scan was markedly positive. The patient had unrecognized osteonecrosis; (C) X-ray six months later shows subchondral collapse and a sclerotic rim, which is the classic early appearance of osteonecrosis of the medial femoral condyle

Table 20.2 lists findings that help distinguish these two entities. Some authors prefer bone scintigraphy for detecting early spontaneous osteonecrosis of the knee. Soucacos et al.[7] noted that bone scans are sensitive in the incipient stage and that MRI may be inconclusive. However, transient bone marrow edema changes cannot be distinguished from osteonecrosis based on bone scans alone. Lecouvet et al.[33] described MRI characteristics that distinguish edema from spontaneous osteonecrosis of the knee. Indications of the latter include the presence of a subchondral area of low signal intensity on T2-weighted magnetic resonance images, a focal epiphyseal contour depression, and

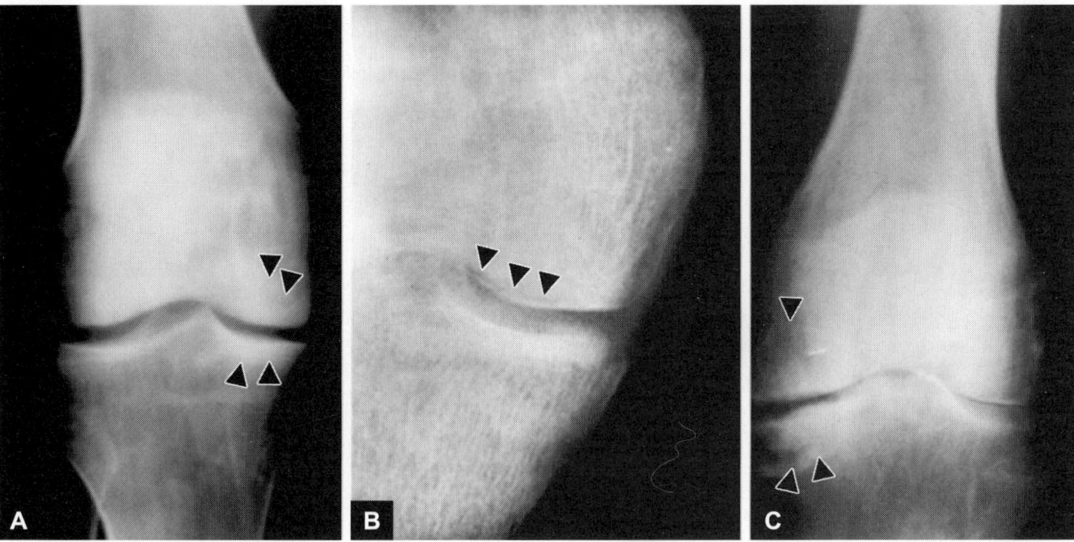

Figs 20.11A to C (A) Plain X-ray showing a stage-II lesion in a thirty-four-year-old woman with systemic lupus erythematosus. Note the sclerotic changes in the distal part of the femur and the proximal part of the tibia (arrowheads); (B) Plain X-ray showing a stage-III lesion in a forty-year-old man with a history of alcohol abuse. The arrowheads denote the area of subchondral collapse; (C) Plain X-ray showing a stage-IV lesion in a twenty-six-year-old man with renal disease. There is joint-space narrowing, and lesions (arrowheads) involving the distal part of the femur and the proximal part of tibia are seen

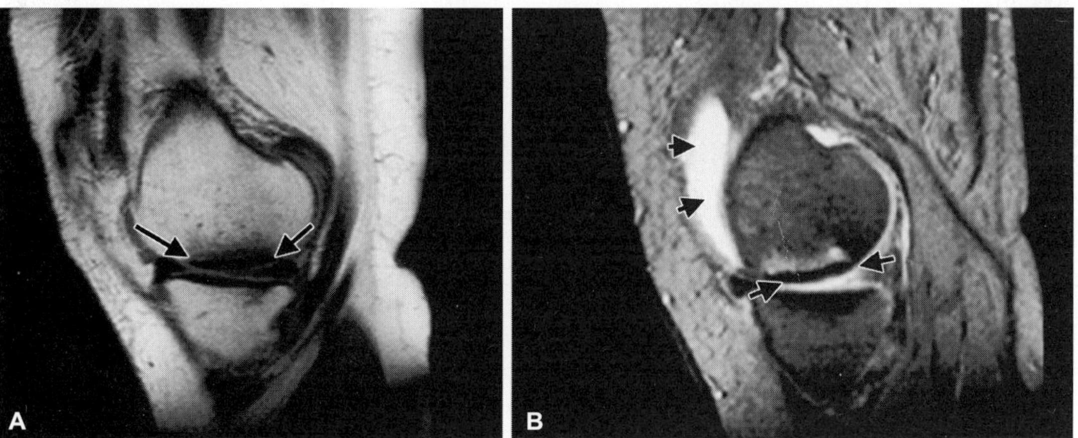

Figs 20.12A and B (A) MRI (T1) scan showing a low-signal subchondral lesion (arrows) of linear morphology. This lesion is associated with ill-defined bone marrow edema; (B) MRI Scan (T2) sequences the subchondral lesion also shows a low signal (arrowheads) and the ill-defined bone marrow edema shows a high signal. Joint effusion (arrows) is also well demonstrated, with a homogeneous high signal

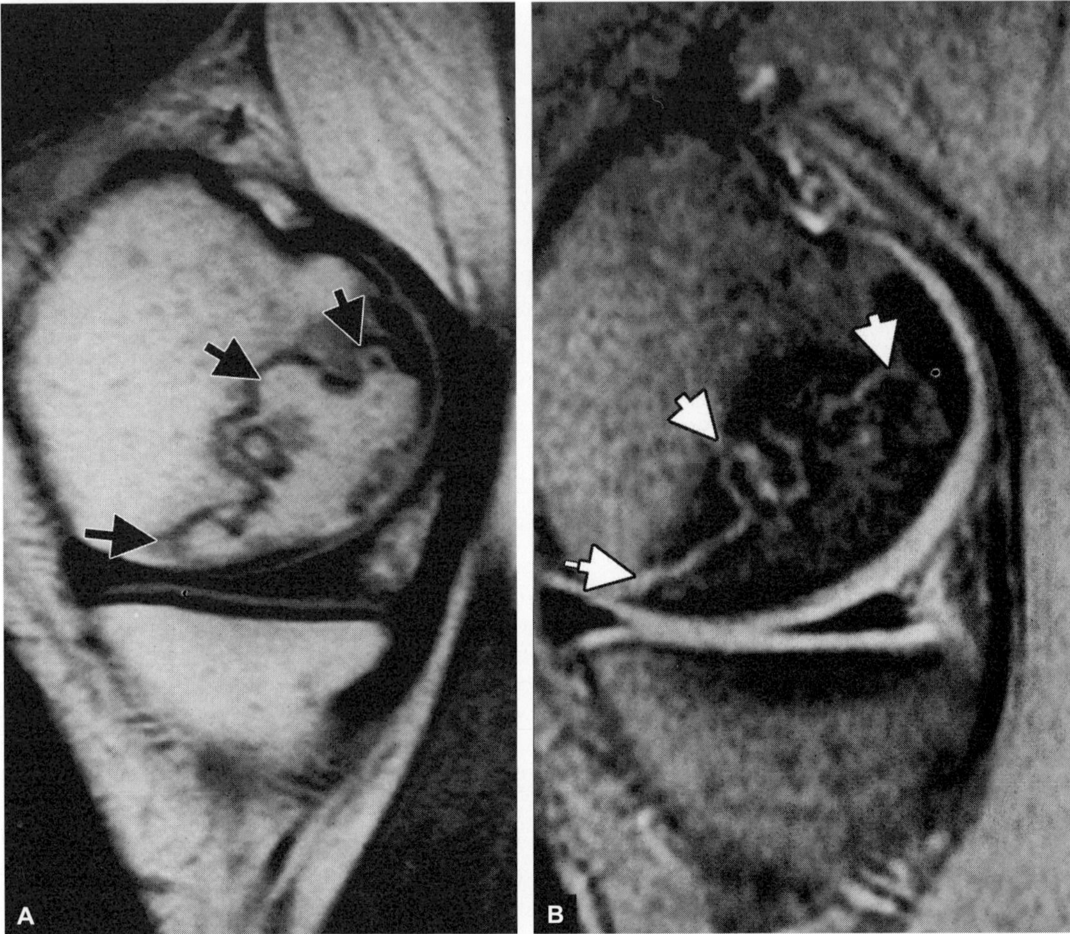

Figs 20.13A and B (A) MRI (T1)-scan demonstrating a large subchondral lesion(arrowheads) isointense with normal fatty marrow and surrounded by a serpiginous low-signal band; (B) MRI (T2) scan sequences this lesion (arrows) is demarcated by a band of high signal intensity inside a hypointense margin—the double halo sign

lines of low signal intensity located deep to the affected condyle.

Differential Diagnosis

Osteonecrosis of the knee is commonly mistaken for osteochondritis dissecans, primary osteoarthritis, meniscal tears, bone bruises, transient osteopenia of the knee, and pes anserinus bursitis. Therefore, it is important to identify osteonecrosis correctly and to differentiate between SPONK and secondary osteonecrosis, by MRI, so as to treat each patient appropriately (Figs 20.11 to 20.13).

Nonsurgical Management

Initial management of pre-collapse spontaneous osteonecrosis of the knee should include protected weight-bearing, analgesics as required, and nonsteroidal anti-inflammatory drugs if tolerated. This approach is believed to reduce stress on the bone, which may halt or reverse disease progression.

Early-stage spontaneous osteonecrosis of the knee responds favorably to nonsurgical management, with resolution of symptoms in ≥89 percent of patients with precollapse disease and no changes on plain radiographs.[34-36] Surgery should be considered for patients who do not improve clinically and/or radiographically (i.e. regression of the lesion size on MRI) by three months following symptom onset.

The favorable natural history of small and midsized lesions associated with spontaneous osteonecrosis of the knee suggests that surgical intervention should be considered only after nonsurgical management fails.

Surgical Management Joint-preserving Procedures

Core decompression may be used in patients who remain symptomatic despite protected weight-bearing; however, outcomes data are limited. Forst et al.[37] reported clinical improvement in 15 of 16 patients with early-stage spontaneous osteonecrosis of the knee, defined as a lack of previous severe knee pain immediately following surgery as well as an improvement in mean Knee Society scores from 74 (SD, 38) points preoperatively to 187 points at the follow-up of 35 months.

Arthroscopy for knee osteonecrosis remains undefined, but it does allow additional assessment of osteonecrosis lesions, and coexisting meniscal tears or chondral lesions can be addressed at the same time. Typically, rehabilitation with protected weight-bearing is recommended for the first month. Miller et al.[38] suggested performing arthroscopic debridement for initial management of spontaneous osteonecrosis of the knee. However, lesion size is ultimately more prognostic. Akgun et al.[39] performed arthroscopic microfracture repair in 26 patients with spontaneous osteonecrosis of the knee who either failed a minimum of four months of protected-weight-bearing or developed mechanical symptoms. Clinical improvement was seen in 96 percent of patients at a mean follow-up of 27 months (range, 12 to 78 months).

Multiple centers have reported on bone grafting for the management of spontaneous osteonecrosis of the knee. Deie et al.[40] treated 12 patients with core decompression and artificial bone graft with an interconnected porous structure. All patients reported a reduction in knee pain and showed no radiographic progression at a mean follow-up of 24.6 months (range, 12 to 42). High tibial osteotomy is rarely used to manage medial femoral condylar lesions and varus knee deformity in persons with spontaneous osteonecrosis of the knee.[23,41] Patients who progress to subchondral collapse may benefit from osteochondral autologous transplantation or mosaicplasty. Localized lesions are filled using autologous osteochondral tissue harvested from uninvolved articular surfaces that undergo less weight-bearing. After four weeks of rehabilitation and protected weight-bearing, patients are allowed to progress to full weight-bearing. Midterm results for repairing defects of the weight-bearing surfaces have been favorable. Duany et al.[42] reported a successful clinical outcome in eight of nine patients who underwent osteochondral autologous transplantation at a mean follow-up of 42 months. These procedures are typically reserved for young patients; however, this technique has been used in patients as old as 76 years. The evidence for the use of joint preserving techniques is limited. Most studies are limited by an uncontrolled retrospective design and a small number of patients. High tibial osteotomy is the only procedure about which results have been reported for ≥30 patients.

Arthroplasty

Unicompartmental knee arthroplasty may be appropriate for some patients with spontaneous osteonecrosis of the knee and end-stage osteoarthritis because the disease typically affects a single condyle (Fig. 20.8). Persons with osteoarthritis in more than one compartment should undergo total knee arthroplasty.

POSTARTHROSCOPIC OSTEONECROSIS

Epidemiology and Anatomic Considerations

Relatively few cases of postarthroscopy osteonecrosis are reported each year, considering the large number of meniscectomy procedures performed. However, one study reported this complication in 2 of 50 patients (4%).[43] Most reported cases of postarthroscopic osteonecrosis occur at the medial femoral condyle. The lateral femoral condyle is the second most frequently affected site. In rare cases, the lateral tibial plateau, medial tibial plateau, or patella is affected.

Pathogenesis, Etiology, and Associated Risk Factors

The etiology of postarthroscopic osteonecrosis likely varies based on whether mechanical surgical instruments or laser probes were used. Most early studies evaluated cases in which disease developed following arthroscopy performed with mechanical surgical instruments only, and it was suggested that occult damage was caused to the cartilage and meniscus.[44] Such damage could lead to altered biomechanics and subsequent bone contact pressure sufficient to cause pathologic fracture of the subchondral bone and synovial fluid leakage. Accumulation of fluid and subchondral edema may be exacerbated by increased absorption of arthroscopy fluids into the pathologic cartilage. Another hypothesis is that "postarthroscopic osteonecrosis" is actually subchondral fracture. MacDessi et al.[45] assessed seven patients (eight knees) with histologic evidence of subchondral fracture characterized by disruption of the trabecular architecture but without osteonecrosis. These findings were similar to the pathology seen in persons with spontaneous osteonecrosis of the knee. Osteonecrosis following radiofrequency or laser-assisted arthroscopic surgery was initially believed to be related to a different pathogenesis. Currently, no consensus exists as to its pathogenesis. Some authors have suggested that thermal energy may directly damage bone tissue or that photoacoustic shock may play a role in osteonecrosis via the formation of a wave generated from expanding gases produced by the rapid vaporization of cellular contents and intracellular water.

Diagnosis

Postarthroscopic osteonecrosis has no age or sex bias, and the lesion is typically localized to the compartment in which the surgery was performed. In one study, patients presented with sudden-onset pain approximately 24 weeks following arthroscopy (range, 4 to 92 weeks). Pain early in the recovery period may be mistaken as normal postoperative healing. MRI as well as AP and lateral radiographs are recommended in patients with suspected postarthroscopic osteonecrosis. The bone marrow edema is located adjacent to the meniscectomized compartment. On T1-weighted magnetic resonance images, these lesions have an appearance similar to that of spontaneous osteonecrosis of the knee, with linear foci of low signal surrounded by diffuse marrow edema in the affected area (Figs 20.7 to 20.10). Patients should have no evidence of bone marrow edema preoperatively.

Management

Protected weight-bearing, analgesics, and nonsteroidal anti-inflammatory drugs may be beneficial. The best outcomes are achieved in patients with small early stage pre-collapse lesions without degenerative articular surface changes. Few reports exist of the use of joint-preserving procedures to manage postarthroscopic osteonecrosis.[46,47] Joint-preserving interventions may be a reasonable approach in persons who have failed nonsurgical treatment. TKA and UKA are recommended for patients with end-stage osteoarthritis. Bonutti et al.[31] performed minimally invasive knee arthroplasty on 19 patients with postarthroscopic osteonecrosis. They reported good to excellent clinical results in 95 percent at a mean follow-up of 62 months (range, 24 to 133 months).

The diagnosis of osteonecrosis about the knee can be difficult, as knee pain is sometimes thought to be referred pain from concurrent hip disease or may be erroneously considered a symptom of an intra-articular disorder such as a meniscal tear. Atraumatic osteonecrosis can also be confused with various other entities, including posttraumatic osteonecrosis, osteochondritis dissecans, and spontaneous osteonecrosis. In post-traumatic osteonecrosis, there is a history of trauma or surgery leading to bone death, usually in an isolated area of the knee. Osteochondritis dissecans is a condition of unknown origin that is usually found in patients younger than twenty-five years of age and is confined to one knee condyle without other joint involvement.[48] It involves a separation of a segment of articular cartilage and subchondral bone from the articular surface of well vascularized bone. Spontaneous osteonecrosis is usually confined to one femoral condyle or one tibial plateau in patients older than the age of 55 years of age, who have no other joint involvement or associated comorbid conditions. It has been described as an entity manifested by a sudden onset of pain of questionable origin. This disease appears similar to an osteonecrotic juxta-articular lesion on radiographic and magnetic resonance imaging, although some authors have questioned whether the disease of osteonecrosis is actually present.[49,50] The prognosis associated with these lesions has been related to their size, with smaller lesions being self-limited and larger lesions leading to joint collapse and the need for total knee arthroplasty.[51-55]

Atraumatic osteonecrosis of the knee has been called secondary, ischemic, idiopathic, or corticosteroid associated necrosis and is usually easily differentiated from the previously described disorders. It is commonly found in patients in their mid-thirties, it involves multiple condyles of the knee, it is usually bilateral, and patients often have osteonecrosis of other large joints. The disease is analogous to the similarly named entity found in the hip with many comorbid conditions. It has been reported in association with systemic lupus erythematosus,[56-60] sickle-cell disease, alcoholism, and use of corticosteroids.[61,62]

Various authors have advocated the use of bone-scanning in the early diagnosis of

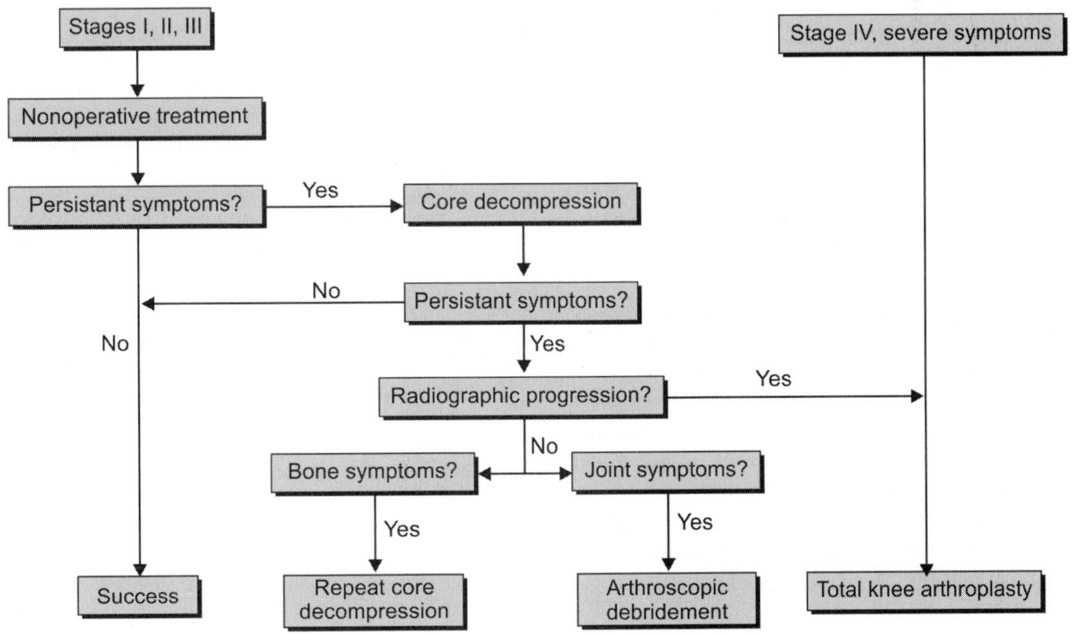

Flow chart 20.1 Treatment algorithm for atraumatic osteonecrosis knee as suggested by M Mont et al 2000[3]

distal femoral osteonecrosis. The advantage of this technique could not be confirmed in the present study, in which only 71 percent of the knees had positive uptake on bone scans, reflecting the lack of sensitivity of this imaging modality with regard to the detection of these lesions. We recommend magnetic resonance imaging as a screening modality.

SUMMARY

In the past several years, three distinct knee osteonecrosis entities have been identified: Secondary osteonecrosis, spontaneous osteonecrosis of the knee, and postarthroscopic osteonecrosis. Although the pathogenesis, associated risk factors, and diagnosis of these entities have been elucidated, none of these conditions is fully understood. MRI is generally accepted as the most sensitive and specific diagnostic tool. Management is based on the stage of disease, as per the protocol suggested by M Mont[3] (Flow chart 20.1). Randomized prospective studies are needed to establish treatment recommendations. Based on recent literature, pre-collapse secondary osteonecrosis should be managed with joint preserving surgical procedures. In contrast, early spontaneous osteonecrosis of the knee and postarthroscopic osteonecrosis should initially be managed nonsurgically. Joint-preserving interventions may be used in patients with recalcitrant disease but without joint collapse. In all three entities, TKA and UKA are the standard management strategies for end-stage disease that has progressed to osteoarthritis.

KEY CONCEPTS IN KNEE OSTEONECROSIS

- Secondary osteonecrosis, spontaneous osteonecrosis of the knee, and post-arthroscopic osteonecrosis are distinct pathologic entities, but they share some similarity in their presentation.
- Secondary osteonecrosis has a multi-factorial etiology and is characterized by loss of bone blood circulation.
- Controversy exists regarding whether spontaneous osteonecrosis of the knee represents insufficiency fracture or is part of the progression of osteoarthritis.
- Postarthroscopic osteonecrosis is associated with subchondral collapse and may be associated with altered knee mechanics.
- MRI is the most sensitive and specific diagnostic tool for all three entities. Disease progression is monitored on standard radiographs.
- Nonsurgical management with analgesics and protected weight-bearing is recommended for early-stage spontaneous of osteonecrosis of the knee and postarthroscopic osteonecrosis, but it may not be appropriate for secondary osteonecrosis.
- Patients in whom nonsurgical measures are unsuccessful may be treated with joint-preserving procedures. Joint arthroplasty is required for persons with subchondral bone collapse.

REFERENCES

1. Ahlback S, Bauer GC, Bohne WH. Spontaneous osteonecrosis of the knee. Arthritis Rheum. 1968;11(6):705-33.
2. Michael A Mont, David R, Marker, Michael G, Zywiel, John A. Carrino: Osteonecrosis of the Knee and Related Conditions. JAAOS. 2011; 19(8):482-94.
3. Michael A Mont, Keith Baumgarten, Aiman Rafai, David Bluemke, Lynne jones, David Hungerford: Atraumatic Osteonecrosis of the Knee. J Bone Joint Surg Am. 2000;82A:1279-90.
4. Uchio Y, Ochi M, Adachi N, Nishikori T, Kawasaki K. Intraosseous hypertension and venous congestion in osteonecrosis of the knee. Clin Orthop. 2001;(384):217-23.
5. Mont MA, Ulrich SD, Seyler TM, et al. Bone scanning of limited value for diagnosis of symptomatic oligofocal and multifocal osteonecrosis. J Rheumatol. 2008;35(8):1629-34.
6. Ahuja SC, Bullogh PG. Osteonecrosis of the knee. A clinico-pathological study in 28 patients. J Bone Joint Surg Am. 1978;6oA:191-7.

7. Soucacos PN, Xenakis TH, Beris AE, Soucacos PK, Georgoulis A. Idiopathic osteonecrosis of the medial femoral condyle: Classification and treatment. Clin Orthop. 1997;(341):82-9.

8. Koshino T. The treatment of spontaneous osteonecrosis of the knee by high tibial osteotomy with and without bone-grafting or drilling of the lesion. J Bone Joint Surg Am. 1982;64(1):47-58.

9. Ficat RP, Arlet J. Necrosis of the femoral head. In: Hungerford DS, (Ed). Ischemia and Necrosis of Bone. Baltimore: Williams and Wilkins; 1980. pp.171-82.

10. Ficat RP. Idiopathic bone necrosis of the femoral head. Early diagnosis and treatment. J Bone Joint Surg Br. 1985;67(1):3-9.

11. Ficat RP. Aseptic necrosis of the femur head. Pathogenesis: the theory of circulation. Acta Orthop Belg. 1981;47(2):198-9.

12. Glimcher MJ, Kenzora JE. The biology of osteonecrosis of the human femoral head and its clinical implications: Part I. Tissue biology. Clin Orthop. 1979;138:284-309.

13. Glimcher MJ, Kenzora JE. The biology of osteonecrosis of the human femoral head and its clinical implications: Part II. The pathological changes in the femoral head as an organ and in the hip joint. Clin Orthop. 1979;139:283-312.

14. Glimcher MJ, Kenzora JE. The biology of osteonecrosis of the human femoral head and its clinical implications: Part III. Discussion of the etiology and genesis of the pathological sequelae; comments on treatment. Clin Orthop. 1979;140:273-312.

15. Jones JP Jr. Concepts of etiology and early pathogenesis of osteonecrosis. In: Schafer M(Ed): Instructional Course Lectures 43. Rosemont, IL, American Academy of Orthopaedic Surgeons; 1994.pp.499-512.

16. Jones JP Jr. Concepts of etiology and early pathogenesis of osteonecrosis. In: Schafer M(Ed): Instructional Course Lectures 43. Rosemont, IL, American Academy of Orthopaedic Surgeons; 1994.pp.499-512.

17. Fisher DE, Bickel WH. Corticosteroid induced avascular necrosis. A clinical study of seventy seven patients. J Bone Joint Surg. 1971;53A: 859-73.

18. Fisher DE, Bickel WH, Holley KE, et al. Corticosteroid induced aseptic necrosis II. Experimental study. Clin Orthop. 1972;84:200-6.

19. Ficat RP. Idiopathic bone necrosis of the femoral head: Early diagnosis and treatment. J Bone Joint Surg. 1985;67B:3-9.

20. Hungerford DS, Jones LC. Diagnosis of osteonecrosis of the femoral head. In: Schoutens A, Arlet J, Gardeniers JWM, et al (Eds): Bone Circulation and Vascularisation in Normal and Pathological Conditions. New York, NY, Plenum Press. 1993.pp.265-75.

21. Wang GJ, Sweet DE, Reger SI, et al. Fat cell changes as a mechanism of avascular necrosis of the femoral head in cortisone treated rabbits. J Bone Joint Surg. 1977;59A:729-35.

22. Solomon L. Drug induced arthropathy and necrosis of femoral head. J Bone Joint Surg Br. 1973;55B:246-61.

23. Koshino T. The treatment of spontaneous osteonecrosis of the knee by high tibial osteotomy with and without bone-grafting or drilling of the lesion. J Bone Joint Surg Am. 1982;64(1):47-58.

24. Marulanda G, Seyler TM, Sheikh NH, Mont MA. Percutaneous drilling for the treatment of secondary osteonecrosis of the knee. J Bone Joint Surg Br. 2006;88(6):740-6.

25. Lee K, Goodman SB. Cell therapy for secondary osteonecrosis of the femoral condyles using the Cellect DBM System: A preliminary report. J Arthroplasty. 2009;24(1):43-8.

26. Rijnen WH, Luttjeboer JS, Schreurs BW, Gardeniers JW. Bone impaction grafting for corticosteroid-associated osteonecrosis of the knee. J Bone Joint Surg Am. 2006;88(suppl 3): 62-8.

27. Pape D, Seil R, Fritsch E, Rupp S, Kohn D. Prevalence of spontaneous osteonecrosis of the medial femoral condyle in elderly patients. Knee Surg Sports Traumatol Arthrosc. 2002;10(4):233-40.

28. Lotke PA, Ecker ML. Osteonecrosis-like syndrome of the medial tibial plateau. Clin Orthop. 1983;(176):148-53.

29. Robertson DD, Armfield DR, Towers JD, Irrgang JJ, Maloney WJ, Harner CD. Meniscal root injury and spontaneous osteonecrosis of the knee: An observation. J Bone Joint Surg Br. 2009;91(2):190-5.

30. Yamamoto T, Bullough PG. Spontaneous osteonecrosis of the knee: The result of subchondral insufficiency fracture. J Bone Joint Surg Am. 2000;82(6):858-66.

31. Bonutti PM, Seyler TM, Delanois RE, McMahon M, McCarthy JC, Mont MA. Osteonecrosis of the knee after laser or radiofrequency-assisted arthroscopy: Treatment with minimally invasive knee arthroplasty. J Bone Joint Surg Am. 2006;88(suppl 3):69-75.

32. Ramnath RR, Kattapuram SV. MR appearance of SONK-like subchondral abnormalities in the adult knee: SONK redefined. Skeletal Radiol. 2004;33(10):575-81.

33. Lecouvet FE, van de Berg BC, Maldague BE, et al. Early irreversible osteonecrosis versus transient lesions of the femoral condyles: Prognostic value of subchondral bone and marrow changes on MR imaging. Am J Roentgenol. 1998;170(1):71-7.

34. Lotke PA, Abend JA, Ecker ML. The treatment of osteonecrosis of the medial femoral condyle. Clin Orthop. 1982;(171):109-16.

35. Yates PJ, Calder JD, Stranks GJ, Conn KS, Peppercorn D, Thomas NP. Early MRI diagnosis and non-surgical management of spontaneous osteonecrosis of the knee. Knee. 2007;14(2): 112-6.

36. Uchio Y, Ochi M, Adachi N, Shu N. Effectiveness of an insole with a lateral wedge for idiopathic osteonecrosis of the knee. J Bone Joint Surg Br. 2000;82(5):724-7.

37. Forst J, Forst R, Heller KD, Adam G. Spontaneous osteonecrosis of the femoral condyle: Causal treatment by early core decompression. Arch Orthop Trauma Surg. 1998;117(1-2):18-22.

38. Miller GK, Maylahn DJ, Drennan DB. The treatment of idiopathic osteonecrosis of the medial femoral condyle with arthroscopic debridement. Arthroscopy. 1986;2(1):21-9.

39. Akgun I, Kesmezacar H, Ogut T, Kebudi A, Kanberoglu K. Arthroscopic microfracture treatment for osteonecrosis of the knee. Arthroscopy. 2005;21(7):834-43.

40. Deie M, Ochi M, Adachi N, Nishimori M, Yokota K. Artificial bone grafting [calcium hydroxyapatite ceramic with an interconnected porous structure (IPCHA)] and core decompression for spontaneous osteonecrosis of the femoral condyle in the knee. Knee Surg Sports Traumatol Arthrosc. 2008;16(8):753-8.

41. Takeuchi R, Aratake M, Bito H, et al. Clinical results and radiographical evaluation of opening wedge high tibial osteotomy for spontaneous osteonecrosis of the knee. Knee Surg Sports Traumatol Arthrosc. 2009; 17(4):361-8.

42. Duany NG, Zywiel MG, McGrath MS, et al. Joint-preserving surgical treatment of spontaneous osteonecrosis of the knee. Arch Orthop Trauma Surg. 2010;130(1):11-6.

43. Cetik O, Cift H, Comert B, Cirpar M. Risk of osteonecrosis of the femoral condyle after arthroscopic chondroplasty using radiofrequency: A prospective clinical series. Knee Surg Sports Traumatol Arthrosc, 2009.

44. Pruès-Latour V, Bonvin JC, Fritschy D. Nine cases of osteonecrosis in elderly patients following arthroscopic meniscectomy. Knee Surg Sports Traumatol Arthrosc. 1998;6(3):142-14717(1):24-9.

45. MacDessi SJ, Brophy RH, Bullough PG, Windsor RE, Sculco TP. Subchondral fracture following arthroscopic knee surgery: A series of eight cases. J Bone Joint Surg Am. 2008;90(5):1007-12.

46. Garino JP, Lotke PA, Sapega AA, Reilly PJ, Esterhai JL Jr. Osteonecrosis of the knee following laser-assisted arthroscopic surgery: A report of six cases. Arthroscopy. 1995;11(4):467-74.

47. Johnson TC, Evans JA, Gilley JA, DeLee JC. Osteonecrosis of the knee after arthroscopic surgery for meniscal tears and chondral lesions. Arthroscopy. 2000;16(3):254-61.

48. Williams JS, Jr, Bush-Joseph CA, Bach BR Jr. Osteochondritis dissecans of the knee. Am J Knee Surg. 1998;11:221-32.

49. Lotke PA, Ecker ML. Osteonecrosis-like syndrome of the medial tibial plateau. Clin Orthop. 1983;176:148-53.

50. Lotke PA, Ecker ML. Current concepts review. Osteonecrosis of the knee. J. Bone and Joint Surg. 1988;70A:470-3.

51. Aglietti P, Insall JN, Buzzi R, Deschamps G. Idiopathic osteonecrosis of the knee. Aetiology, prognosis and treatment. J Bone and Joint Surg. 1983;65B(5):588-97.

52. Ahlbäck S, Bauer GC, Bohne WH. Spontaneous osteonecrosis of the knee. Arthrit and Rheumat. 1968;11:705-33.

53. Al-Rowaih A, Björkengren A, Egund N, Lindstrand A, Wingstrand H, Thorngren KG. Size of osteonecrosis of the knee. Clin Orthop. 1993;287:68-75.

54. Björkengren AG, AlRowaih A, Lindstrand A, Wingstrand H, Thorngren KG, Pettersson H. Spontaneous osteonecrosis of the knee: value of MR imaging in determining prognosis. Am J Roentgenol. 1990;154:331-6.

55. Ecker ML, Lotke PA. Spontaneous osteonecrosis of the knee. J Am Acad Orthop Surgeons. 1994; 2:173-8.

56. Abeles M, Urman JD, Rothfield NF. Aseptic necrosis of bone in systemic lupus erythematosus. Relationship to corticosteroid-therapy. Arch Intern Med. 1978;138:750-4.

57. Hungerford DS, Zizic TM II. The treatment of ischemic necrosis of bone in systemic lupus erythematosus. Medicine. 1980;59:143-8.

58. Jacobs MA, Loeb P, Hungerford DS. Core decompression of the distal femur in the treatment for avascular necrosis of the knee. J Bone and Joint Surg. 1989;71B(4):583-7.

59. Kelman GJ, Williams GW, Colwell CW Jr, Walker RH. Steroid-related osteonecrosis of the knee. Two case reports and a literature review. Clin Orthop. 1990;257:171-6.

60. Mahood J, Bogoch E, Urowitz M, Hastings D, Gladman D. Osteonecrosis of the knee in systemic lupus erythematosus. In: Proceedings of the Canadian Orthopaedic Association. J Bone and Joint Surg. 1990;72B(4):541.

61. Zizic TM, Marcoux C, Hungerford DS, Dansereau JU, Stevens MB. Corticosteroid therapy associated with ischemic necrosis of bone in systemic lupus erythematosus. Am J Med. 1985;79:596-604.

62. Ochi M, Kimori K, Sumen Y, Ikuta Y. A case of steroid-induced osteonecrosis of femoral condyle treated surgically. Clin Orthop. 1995; 312:226-31.

21 SICKLE CELL DISEASE AND OSTEONECROSIS OF THE FEMORAL HEAD

Sickle cell hemoglobinopathy is a genetically transmitted multisystem disease which includes a group of disorders that differ in severity of signs and symptoms. The disease is not uniformly seen everywhere but it has some topographical distribution and is commonly seen in specific communities of scheduled caste and scheduled tribes. In India, it is frequently seen in Central India, in and around the vicinity of Nagpur.[1] The prevalence of osteonecrosis in this population varies from 4 to 20 percent. Despite the fact that sickle cell hemoglobinopathy is infrequently observed, it has great pathological significance considering the high morbidity and mortality resulting from the disease process. The exact etiopathology at both the molecular and genetic level has been extensively studied and deciphered thoroughly, yet there is no cure or established treatment regimen that will arrest the disease. Different modalities of treatment including bone marrow transplant are still in experimental stages and as of today we do not have any satisfactory modality available that will be effective in the treatment of this genetic disorder and its complications.

Hence, early diagnosis and efficient medical supervision for recognition of complications remain the gold standard in management of this inherited disorder.[2,3] The risk of death from complications of sickle cell disease is highest in children under the age of five years and it is suggested that with early detection and appropriate management the mortality in this age group can be reduced to less than five percent. Osteonecrosis of the femoral head is commonly seen in young adults of sickle cell hemoglobinopathy, which is frequently bilateral and in a high percentage of patients, it results in severely disabling, painful, stiff hip (Figs 21.1 to 21.4). The study carried out at our center had the follow-up of osteonecrosis of 352 femoral heads in 224 patients in a duration of 25 years (128 patients had bilateral affection) (Figs 21.5 and 21.6) diagnosed amongst 7380 patients of sickle cell hemoglobinopathy.

Early diagnosis is the key to the success of head-preserving operations, but once there is collapse of head with involvement of more than 60 percent of the weight-bearing surface, and especially when associated with arthritic changes it is necessary to perform total hip replacement of hip joint so as to rehabilitate these disabled patients and provide good quality of life to these sicklers.[1,3]

Lately, it has been observed that the incidence of osteonecrosis of femoral head is steadily increasing amongst the patients of sickle cell hemoglobinopathies. The clinical entity is more important since commonly it is seen in young adults between the ages of 20 to 40 years in the region of Nagpur—Central India and is frequently bilateral. Most of the time the disease results in severely disabling painful stiff hip in the most crucial time of life when an individual's career is supposed to be at the peak. The syndrome of osteonecrosis of the femoral head seen in sickle cell patients initially causes minimal pain and discomfort, and is not noticed in many cases until deformity of the head has already occurred (Figs 21.2 to 21.4).

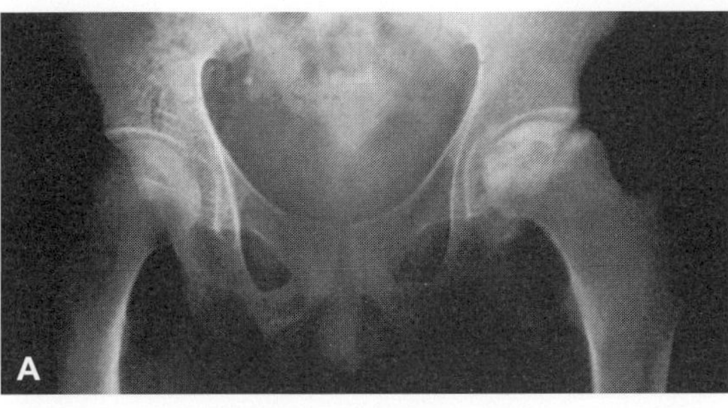
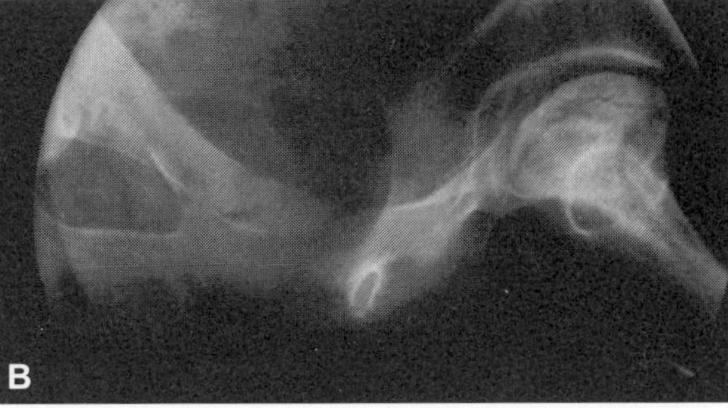

Figs 21.1A and B X-ray pelvis anteroposterior (AP) of a young female patient of 21.5 years old showing osteonecrosis of femoral head with fragmentation and collapse on left side. Lateral view showing classical crescent sign

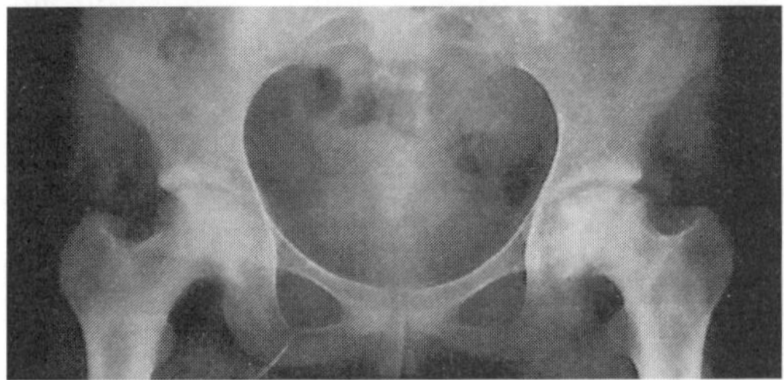

Fig. 21.2 X-ray pelvis AP of a 22-year-old female showing advanced osteonecrosis, with fragmentation and affection of articular surface

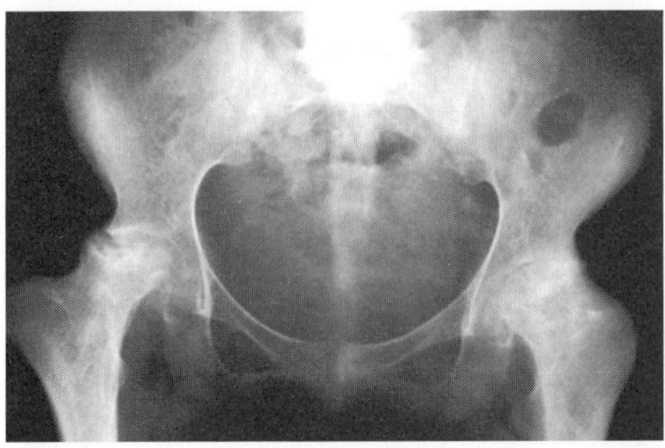

Fig. 21.3 X-ray pelvis AP showing advanced changes of osteonecrosis, both hips with early osteoarthritic changes

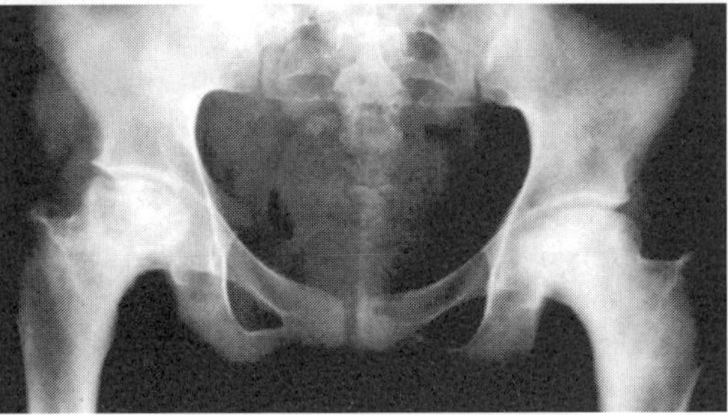

Fig. 21.4 X-ray pelvis of a young 18-year-old boy showing advanced osteonecrosis with secondary osteo-arthritis in right hip and osteonecrosis and deformation of left femoral head

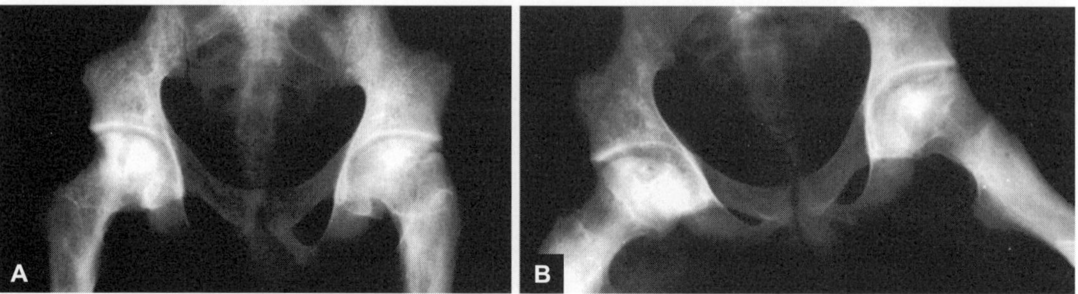

Figs 21.5A and B X-ray pelvis AP and Dunn's view of a young patient 22-year-old patient showing osteonecrosis of both heads with fairly advanced changes of arthritis

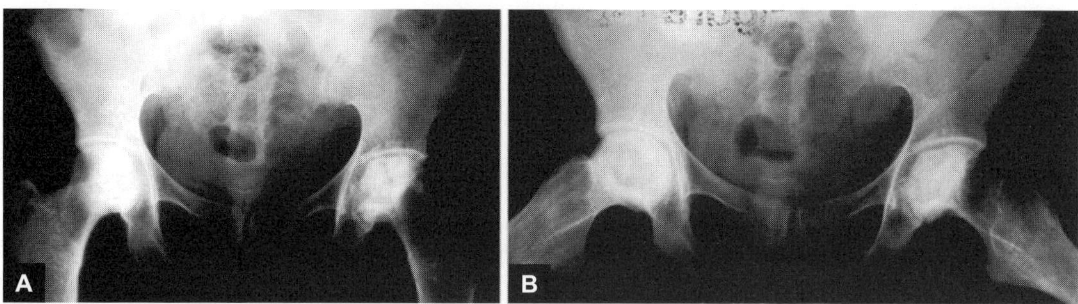

Figs 21.6A and B X-ray pelvis of young patient 28-year-old patient showing osteonecrosis of the left femoral head with fragmentation without any collapse and early changes of osteonecrosis on right side

Osteonecrosis is essentially a vascular disease. The ischemia is either due to occlusion of arteries or obstruction to venous drainage. Interruption of arterial supply or occlusion of venous drainage results in stasis and oxygen starvation. This results in bone cell death, which occurs because of disparity between the oxygen need of the bone cell and the inability of local circulation to meet the need and demand.

CLINICAL MATERIAL AND METHOD

In the duration of 25 years (from 1970 to 1996) 224 patients of osteonecrosis in sickle cell disease affecting 352 femoral heads were studied and followed. Out of this 55 patients were treated conservatively and 169 patients were operated requiring 252 surgeries. There were 136 males and 88 female patients in the age group of 10 to 40 years with about 45 percent patients in the young age group of 20 to 30 years (Table 21.1). In 94 patients 164 head-preserving surgeries were performed. In 60 patients 68 total hip replacements were done and in 15 patients 20 hips were operated for other procedures (Tables 21.2 to 21.5).

Most of the patients of osteonecrosis in sickle cell disease presented with complaints of deep throbbing pain in groin and hip, initially intermittently, later more severe. Subsequently, these patients had complaints of painful limited movements of the hip. A few patients had radiating pain from the groin to the thigh and knee, radiating along with the medial aspect. In some patients the only complaint was discomfort and limp during weight-bearing. In later stages almost all patients had painful stiff hips with grossly restricted movements restricting squatting and sitting cross-legged (Figs 21.1 to 21.7).

Table 21.1 Age and sex incidence in osteonecrosis

Age group	Total number of patients	Sex ratio		Unilateral	Bilateral	Total number of femoral heads
		Males	Females			
10–20	51	38	13			
21–30	99	54	45	96	128	352
31–40	74	44	30			
Total	224	136	88			

Table 21.2 Type and number of surgeries in osteonecrosis

Types of operation	Number of patients	Number of surgeries
1. Head preserving operations	94	164
2. Total hip replacements	60	68
3. Other operations (Bipolar, AMP, Girdlestone, Arthrodesis)	15	20
Total	169	252

Table 21.3 Head preserving surgeries in osteonecrosis in sickle cell disease

Name of operations		Total procedures
I. Core decompression with bone grafting		88
	a. Vascular pedicle iliac graft	18
	b. Phemister (fibular) graft	26
	c. Cancellous iliac graft	14
	d. Meyer's muscle pedicle graft	18
	e. Sartorius muscle pedicle graft	12
II. Osteotomy		76
	a. Ventral rotation osteotomy	42
	b. Flexion osteotomy	16
	c. Valgus/Varus osteotomy	13
	d. McMurray's osteotomy	5
Total head preserving operations		164

Table 21.4 Total hip replacements in sickle cell disease

Name of procedure	Total number of patients	Total hip surgeries
1. Charnley's total hip	36	42
2. Isoelastic hips	24	26
Total	60	68

Table 21.5 Other surgeries—head sacrificing

Name of surgery	Number of patients	Total number of procedures
1. Bipolar hip replacement	6	9
2. Hemiarthroplasty AMP	3	3
3. Girdlestone excision arthroplasty	3	5
4. Arthrodesis	3	3
Total head-sacrificing surgeries	15	20

The activity of patients of sickle cell disease may be impaired by factors other than the hip, therefore other joints that are affected by the disease and other systemic associated conditions must be looked into for final treatment, assessment and evaluation (Fig. 21.7). There is usually association of biliary duct disease, pulmonary insufficiency, osteomyelitis, cardiac abnormalities and so on. The evaluation of hip was done by clinical and radiological assessment. Assessment was done by asking detailed history of symptoms, and level of activity. The clinical examination included function of hips and final outcome which included range of motion of hip, Trendelenburg test and measurement of limb length discrepancy (Table 21.6).

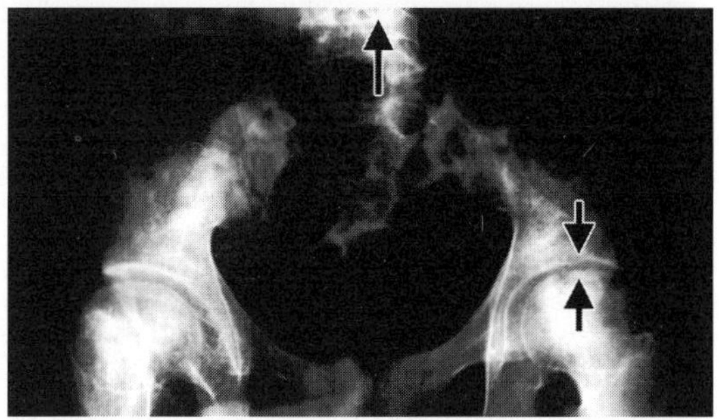

Fig. 21.7 X-ray pelvis AP showing increased density at the periphery in the superolateral segment, but the contour of the femoral head is well preserved on left side with classical radiological changes of hemoglobinopathy in the pelvis and spine

ETIOPATHOLOGY

It has been observed that anterolateral segments of the femoral head superiorly undergo necrosis first and quickly. This is obviously because of occlusion of posterolateral retinacular vessels or by emboli from various sources finding their way through the microcirculation into the subchondral zone of the femoral head. There are various theories for causation of thromboembolic phenomenon resulting in osteonecrosis. However, etiology in sickle cell disease is proved beyond doubt.

Bony changes in sickle cell diseases occur mainly because of hyperplasia of the bone marrow and because of vascular insufficiency resulting in thrombosis and infarction.[1] Because of hyperplasia the multiple erythrocytes cause increase in blood viscosity, stasis, capillary thrombosis and finally infarction of bone. The initial infarcts occur in the most distal portion of the bone, i.e. femoral head, in the subchondral area, where there is maximum sickling and where the circulation through collaterals is very poor and limited. These circulatory changes result in high intraosseous pressure and the femoral head functions as a closed compartment and the eventual infarction of weight-bearing bone is the end stage of progressive compartment syndrome. The blood supply to the cartilage is poor, it is impaired and there is death of bone cells. Continuation of weight-bearing on this femoral head leads to the flattening and irregularities in the contour of the femoral head. Such changes results into weakening of the trabecular structure leading to multiple microfractures and finally collapse in the weight-bearing portion of the femoral head.

Table 21.6 Analysis of results by Merle d'Aubigné and Postel[18] modified by Charnley's system

Operative procedures	Number of patients	Score points		Results	
		Excellent 11–12	Good 9–10	Fair 8	Poor 7 or <
Core decompression and bone frafting	88				
Vascular pedicle graft	18	12	3	2	1
Phamister fibular graft	26	12	5	5	4
Cancellous Iliac graft	14	4	3	4	3
Mayer's muscle pedicle graft	30	15	4	7	4
Total		43	15	18	12
Osteotomy	76				
Ventral rotation osteotomy	42	18	10	8	6
Flexion osteotomy	16	6	4	4	2
Valgus/Varun osteotomy	13	5	3	3	2
McMurray's osteotomy	5	00	1	1	3
Total		29	18	16	13
Total hip replacements	68	58	6	2	2

In later stages proliferative arthritic changes appear in the hip joints. It is said that ischemia provokes bone marrow edema and fibrosis elevating bone marrow pressure, which further decreases the bone blood flow. This cycle of ischemia, edema and increased pressure culminates in bone cell death. The mechanical failure and continued weight-bearing results eventually in collapse of the femoral head and osteoarthritic changes.

Osteonecrosis occurs with greatest frequency in classic homozygous sickle cell anemia in the SS and S-Thal disorders, as well as in heterozygous sickle cell hemoglobinopathy–sickle cell trait (SA). Alterations in the amino acids of hemoglobin S results in confirmational changes in the hemoglobin molecule in the deoxygenated state. Molecular stacking occurs, and hollow, rigid rods or "tactoids" are formed due to regular aggregation of the molecules in the individual cells. Initially these events are reversible when the blood is re-oxygenated. However, the red cells eventually become damaged from repeated sickling and unsickling, and the sickling becomes irreversible. Cells, which are sickled, have difficulty in traversing the small capillaries and it increases the blood viscosity. If a sufficient number of sickled cells come together, they block blood vessels. This sets up a vicious cycle by increasing local hypoxia and promoting further sickling. Eventually, these sickle cells interfere with the blood supply to a small or large area of an organ or tissue, including bone. Such events result in the most common feature of the sickling disorder, the painful vaso-occlusive episode. If these conditions persist, they can lead to infarction and necrosis. The lesions resulting from osteonecrosis are usually accompanied by pain and may cause permanent destruction of articular cartilage, resulting in disability.

EARLY DIAGNOSIS

Since 1983 at our center functional bone investigations were being routinely done but from the year 1993 MRI and CT replaced this invasive procedure. Early diagnosis is important prior to the appearance of radiological changes. Any patient of sickle cell disorder if complains of pain in the hip, is thoroughly investigated by sickling and solubility test and subsequently by hemoglobin electrophoresis.[4] Similarly in patients of osteonecrosis of the femoral head the opposite hip is regarded as "high risk" patient and a close watch is kept on such a patient for at least one year.

Clinical suspicion and bone scanning are of great value if the X-rays are negative in patients of high index of suspicion for osteonecrosis of the femoral head. Limitation of internal rotation and presence of axis deviation test (denoting sectoral involvement) is highly suggestive of osteonecrosis of the femoral head. All the investigations are unnecessary if the X-rays are positive. Although X-ray examination is of limited value in making early diagnosis, it has considerable value in staging.[5-7] If suspicion is very high even with negative bone scan, core decompression and biopsy used to be the routine procedure but with the availability of MRI, these patients are closely observed and one should avoid invasive procedure. There was plenty of opportunities to study asymptomatic, radiologically negative contralateral hip in patients presenting with unilateral osteonecrosis of the femoral head. Presently the philosophy is changed and these patients of sickle cell hemoglobinopathy, who are in extremely high-risk category are closely monitored by isotope bone scanning and sequential MRI studies. Commonly, the patients present after radiographic changes are seen and at times with advanced osteoarthritic changes. If the deformity occurs because of involvement of the subchondral bone or even early collapse of supportive cancellous bone, which is evident radiologically, the prognosis is very poor.

There is no separate classification or staging system for osteonecrosis of the femoral head in sickle cell disease patients and the same classification is used for assessing the condition and for prognostic purposes. Commonly ARCO's classification (1991, 1993)[8] is used which has combinations of:

- Combination of Ficat and Arlet
- Quantification of Steinberg
- Location as per Japanese Investigation Committee.

The success of treatment in osteonecrosis is related to the stage at which disorder it is initiated. Description and knowledge of the various methods used to make an accurate diagnosis early in the disease process (diagnostic modalities currently available) are necessary. After confirmation of sickle cell disease by hematology and finding the amount of fetal hemoglobin percentage the patient is subjected to further radiological investigations.

RADIOGRAPHY

- Scintigraphy
- MRI
- CT
- Plain X-ray pelvis AP and Dunn's view.
  Histopathology confirmation if surgery is decided.

HISTORY AND CLINICAL EXAMINATION

- Pain
- Painful range of movements, especially on forced internal rotation
- Positive axis deviation test
- History of associated risk factor
- High index of suspicion.

The contralateral hip in a patient of unilateral osteonecrosis must be carefully evaluated since the bilateral prevalence is reported to be 50 to 80 percent.

RADIOLOGY

Osteonecrosis of the femoral head generally affects the anterolateral segment, which is placed superiorly in the femoral head. Cancellous bone placed posteriorly is also projected in this area in AP view. It is, therefore, difficult to diagnose osteonecrosis of the femoral head on AP view, when changes are minimal. Routinely Dunn's view in addition to AP and lateral views are taken whenever osteonecrosis of the femoral head is suspected. However, tangential radiographs would delineate the entire femoral head nicely for more accurate assessment of the size of the necrotic segment. Initial X-rays made earlier and latest X-rays during the follow-up periods were used for the assessment of deformity of the hip, abnormalities of the growth of the proximal part of the femur and osteoarthritis. Both Ficat and Arlet classification and ARCO's classification for osteonecrosis of the femoral head were used for clinical assessment and planning the treatment.

In early stages (preradiological) X-ray will not reveal any findings and diagnosis can only be done by isotope bone scanning and MRI, if one suspects osteonecrosis of the femoral head especially in high-risk patients.[9,10] The earliest changes on X-ray are diffuse or spotty osteonecrosis, sclerosis or mixed picture. At times a mixture of osteoporosis, sclerosis and cystic changes are seen. Subsequently small infarct occurs as a rim of increased density at the periphery while the contour is still maintained. This band of increased density results from the repair process. Then the femoral head appears subtly flattened and at this stage crescent sign appears which is caused by fractures through the dead subchondral bone. The fracture is caused by weakening of bone in this region when the rate of bone resorption exceeds the rate of repair. Subsequently, there is fissuring and collapse of the necrotic segment, changing the contour of the the femoral head with a definite step at the margins of the infarcted zones (Fig. 21.8). Finally osteoarthritic changes are seen, initially in the femoral head and subsequently even in acetabular side (Figs 21.9 and 21.10). Kerboul et al.[11] (1974) attempted to evaluate the extent of necrosis by measuring the arc of involvement on AP and lateral radiograph. The extent was considered large when the sum of the area was 200° or small when 160° or less. He reported that when the combined angle is more than 200° the clinical outcome is poorer than when the combined angle is smaller.

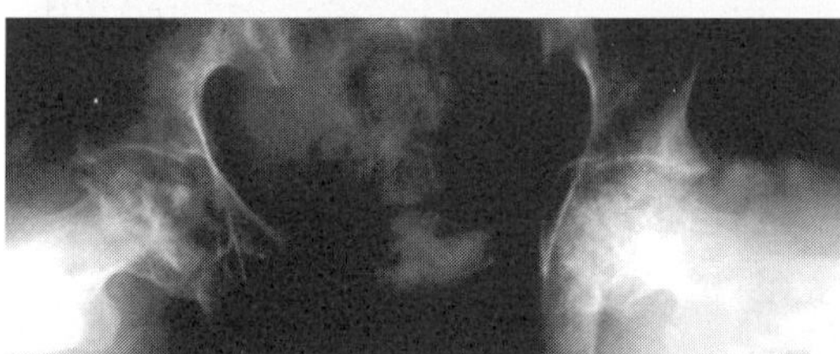

Fig. 21.8 X-ray Dunn's view of pelvis showing fissuring and collapse in a necrotic femoral head of both hips with classical changes of osteonecrosis in a young 24-year-old patient

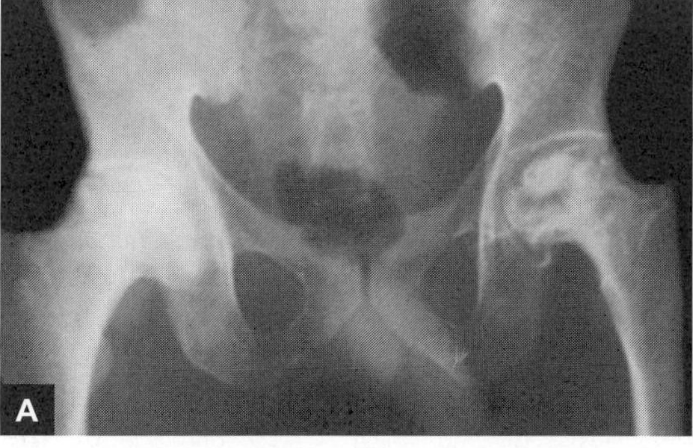
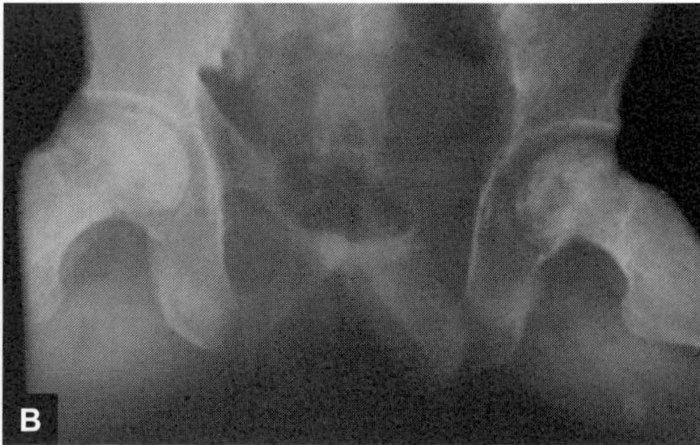

Figs 21.9A and B X-ray pelvis AP and Dunn's view showing bilateral avascular necrosis of the femoral head in a young 25-year-old sickler. The contour of the femoral head is well-maintained on right side but lot of fragmentation, collapse of the femoral head on the left side with arthritic changes

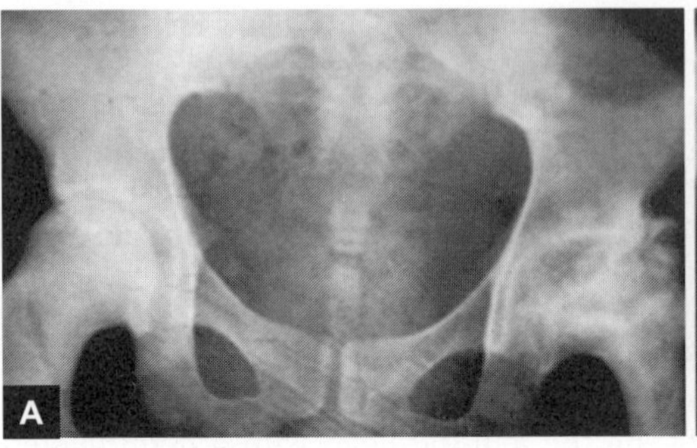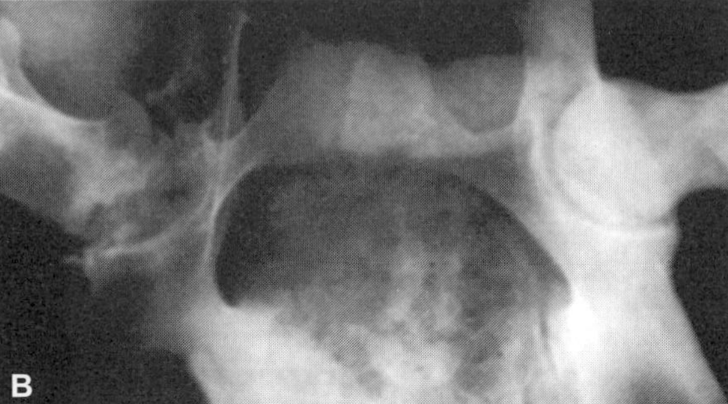

Figs 21.10A and B X-ray pelvis AP and Dunn's view in a 28-year-old sickler with advanced changes of osteonecrosis and osteoarthritis

Osteonecrotic changes are most frequent and severe in the weight-bearing portion, especially in the femoral head. These changes in sickle cell hemoglobinopathy can be subdivided into three groups on the basis of their roentgenographic appearance.

Group I (Legg-Calve-Perthes Type)

Lesions are found in children 8-year-old or less and are similar to those found in Legg-Calve-Perthes disease (Figs 21.11 and 21.12). They usually regenerate without producing significant disability. In teenagers 13 to 18 years old, X-rays may show necrosis involving the entire epiphysis or only a sharply defined, segmental area in the anterosuperior epiphysis. No matter whether the epiphysis is completely or partially involved, the metaphysis is usually spared. The prognosis is not good in older adolescents with extensive epiphyseal involvement, but in younger adolescents spontaneous healing may occur if the epiphysis is only partially involved.

Group II (Osteochondritis Dissecans Type)

Lesions resemble those in osteochondritis dissecans. This type of lesion is rare and was observed in only one teenager and one adult, is restricted to a smaller area of the superior femoral head and, unlike Group I changes in adolescents, does not extend as far as the

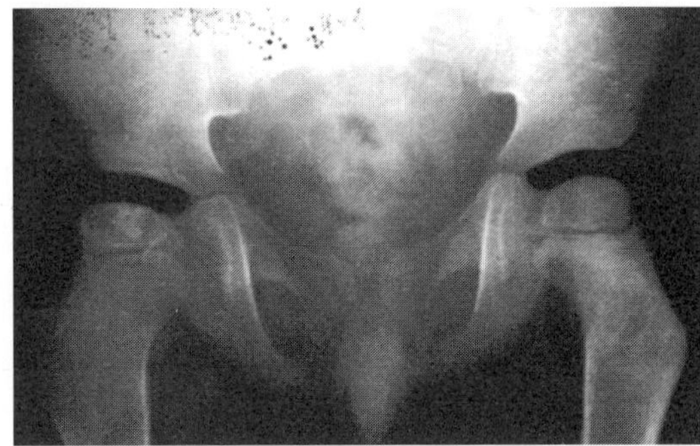

Fig. 21.11 X-ray pelvis of a young 8-year-old boy showing sclerosis and cavitation in the epiphyseal nucleus without any collapse

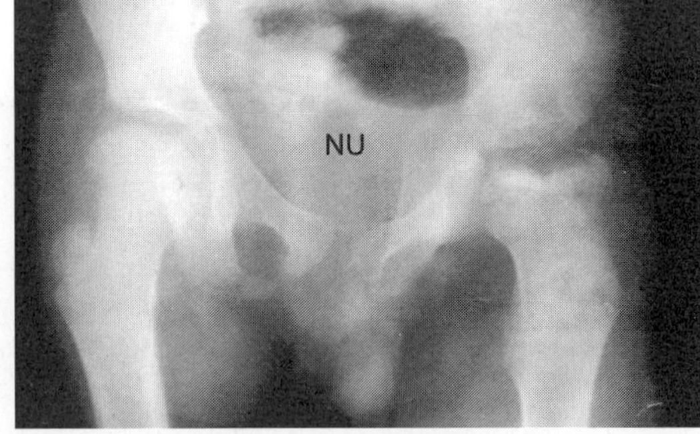

Fig. 21.12 X-ray pelvis showing osteonecrosis. Femoral head on the left side is flattened. The center of the femoral nucleus is affected which is cystic and sclerotic. The patient also had osteomyelitis of same sided femur with growth disturbance

epiphyseal plate. This type of lesion did not heal spontaneously in either case.

Group III (Degenerative Type)

Lesions are characterized by massive necrosis and are restricted to adult patients. X-rays show severe distortion and flattening of the femoral head. The femoral head collapses and, as in younger patients, distortion occurs in the area above the site of the fused growth plate. This suggests persistence of the separation between vascular territories supplying the epiphysis and metaphysis.

Quantifying the extent of osteonecrosis of the femoral head can be a major predictor of future collapse which can be clinically useful in the management of early-stage osteonecrosis of the femoral head (KH Koo and R Kim 1995).[12]

The midcoronal (A) and midsagittal (B) sections which showed the largest diameter of the femoral head were used for the measurement.

$(A/180) \times (B/180)$ = Index of necrotic segment

A = Small necrosis < 33

B = Medium necrosis 34 to 66

C = Large necrosis 67 to 100

The shape of the femoral head and its flattening was evaluated by means of a template with concentric circles. To be classified as spherical (normal) the surface of femoral head on AP and lateral X-rays must follow the circle on the template with variation less than 2 mm. When the variation was more than 2 mm, the head was considered nonspherical but as having coxa plana. Coxa plana was divided into three categories—round, flat and irregular depending upon the shape and regularity of the surface. The changes were labeled as coxa magna when the femoral head was bigger in size by at least 5 mm.

NONINVASIVE TECHNIQUE

Noninvasive techniques like bone scans, CT scan and MRI are useful mainly for screening high-risk patients. However, these investigations offer a unique opportunity (before radiological changes are evident) to diagnose osteonecrosis of the femoral head in its early form.

Bone Scanning

Technetium 99 methylene-di-phosphate (Tc 99m) bone scanning is a useful technique. In general, the reactivity of bone around the infarcted segment shows increased uptake of isotopes on the delayed image. This represents an accumulation of the radionuclide in the area of increased bone turnover at the junction of dead and reactive bone. Scintigraphy with Tc 99m diphosphonate has proven very effective for early detection of osteonecrosis when the routine roentgenograms appeared within normal limits. By obtaining the bone and bone marrow scan in the first several days after the onset of symptoms, it is possible to suspect and diagnose osteonecrosis. The combinations of the large defect on the bone marrow scan and the smaller negative effect on the bone scan appears to be a typical finding in patients with osteonecrosis. Although increased uptake alone can be seen in reflex sympathetic dystrophy, transient osteoporosis, infarction, tumors, etc. a photopenic area surrounded by an area of the increased activity is most consistent with a diagnosis of osteonecrosis.

Since bone scan is a low-cost investigation, its use is recommended in patients who have a negative radiograph for osteonecrosis, no risk factors and unilateral symptoms. If the bone scan is negative, the patient should be observed and followed.

Magnetic Resonance Imaging

Magnetic resonance imaging (MRI) is the most accurate imaging modality for the diagnosis of osteonecrosis. The earliest finding of osteonecrosis is a single density line (a low-intensity signal) on T1-generated image that presumably represents the separation of normal and ischemic bone. Double line on T2-generated image, a signal including line represents hypervascular granulation tissue. Magnetic resonance imaging is used to outline the area of involvement. It can show the revascularization front and can provide objective evidence of changes in the tissues in response to treatment. It also allows sequential evaluation of asymptomatic lesions, which are not seen on plain radiograph. Magnetic resonance imaging is more sensitive and accurate than plain radiography. The extent as measured on an AP radiograph is not the same as in a midcoronal MRI and that in lateral radiograph does not correspond to a mid-sagittal MRI. The extent of necrotic portion at the initial MRI scan predicts the risk of collapse of the femoral head.

Magnetic resonance imaging has replaced all the investigations for early diagnosis of osteonecrosis of the femoral head. Magnetic resonance imaging has been successful in detecting early osteonecrosis of the femoral head in a number of conditions.[13-15] Osteonecrosis in sickle cell disease usually begins in adolescence and in adult life and as such is rare before the age of six to seven years. Eventually the entire femoral head collapses and it may subluxate, the joint space narrows, the head flattens, and the neck becomes wide. Cysts may form in the acetabulum or the femoral head.

Rarely histopathological examination reveals changes of osteonecrosis in patients who had negative MRI.

Computed Tomography

It is expensive and exposes the patient to a considerable amount of radiation and it is usually unnecessary for establishing the diagnosis of osteonecrosis.

Osteonecrosis of the femoral head in sickle cell disease can also be divided in two categories, depending upon the age and presence of femoral capital epiphysis:

A. ***Affection of immature femoral head:***
   - Flattening (widened flattened epiphysis)
   - Epiphyseometaphyseal overlap
   - Metaphyseal lucency with sclerotic border
   - Wide femoral neck

   - Mushroom deformity of femoral head with intact cortex
   - Joint space and articular surface well preserved
   - No disability.

B. ***Affection of mature femoral head:***
   - Segmental involvement, commonly anterosuperior
   - Collapse of femoral head
   - Collapse and disruption of articular surface
   - Sequestration
   - Short cortical discontinuity
   - Upward projection of lateral part of the femoral head
   - Lateral subluxation
   - Lucent subcortical line
   - Lytic defect
   - Osteophytosis and secondary osteo-arthritic changes.

Immature femoral head changes are similar to those seen in Perthes disease. Patchy sclerosis in addition to dense solid shadows, dense layers and rings with lucent centers and osteoporosis were observed in the medulla. Radiologically these two lesions are so similar that differentiation is based on other criteria such as younger age of onset in Perthes, negative sickling test and absence of abnormal hemoglobins.

Osteonecrosis of mature femoral head is typically segmental and frequently affects the AP part of the femoral head. An early radiological sign of this lesion may be lucent subcortical line described by Norman[16] and Bullough[17] in 1963 in Dysbaric Osteonecrosis (crescent sign). This is thought to result from subarticular trabecular fracture and resorption preceding collapse of the articular surface.

After collapse there is subluxation of femoral head and medial part may result in projection lying lateral to acetabular roof and limiting abduction. It is this anterolateral-subluxating portion, which may bring the patient to surgical attention. Early involvement of the femoral head is not painful but once the medial portion begins to collapse the lower extremity is pushed in adduction and a limp due to apparent shortening develops rapidly. Following disruption of the articular surface, clinical outcome depends on the site and degree of destruction of the femoral head and on the development of secondary osteoarthritis.

Treatment

The patient with proven osteonecrosis of the femoral head should be observed closely since 50 to 80 percent of the patients develop bilateral affection.[10,18-20] Any symptoms if it develops in the untreated contralateral hip should be taken as high risk and suspicious of osteonecrosis of the femoral head, especially when seen in sickle cell disease and disorders, which are known to cause osteonecrosis.

The rationale for the treatment of osteonecrosis of the femoral head requires a lot of consideration. Prime importance in this is the age of patients, whether both hips are affected, etiopathology and type of the associated sickle cell disease (the amount of fetal hemoglobin), demands and requirement of the patients and the stage of the disease when the patient presents for the treatment is equally important. (The treatment was planned according to ARCO's classification) (Table 21.7).

Nonweight-bearing conservative management of ischemic necrosis has not been proved to be beneficial and hence various operative procedures are done depending upon the stage of necrosis of the femoral head. Though maximum efforts were taken in performing head-preserving surgeries, on many occasions, young sicklers required total hip replacement. It is believed that once crescent sign appears and there is a collapse of necrotic bone segment, even if it is minimal on X-ray, further collapse is inevitable and hip joints is likely to degenerate.[21] Any procedures like core decompression and bone grafting which are likely to revascularize the dead segment are not going to be useful once the collapse of segment occurs. Hence, in this stage IV the attempts to change the weight-bearing portions by different osteotomies are performed,[22,23] though in some percentage of patients it may fail.

Chung, Alavi and Russel[24,25] 1978 reported the evidence to suggest that osteonecrosis in sickle cell disease in early stages. The changes in early stages are reversible and they reported several patients of osteonecrosis of the femoral head treated by strict nonweightbearing gained both symptomatic and radiographic impairment.

Table 21.7 Details of number of surgical procedures according to the Association research circulation osseous (ARCO's) classification

Type of procedure	Total number of procedures	0 and I	II	III	IV
Core decompression and bone grafting	88				
Vascular pedicle graft	18	04	11	03	Nil
Phemister fibular graft	26	06	12	08	Nil
Cancellous iliac graft	14	Nil	08	06	Nil
Muscle pedicle graft	30	Nil	08	18	04
Intertrochanteric osteotomy	76				
Ventral rotation osteotomy	42	--	08	34	Nil
Flexion osteotomy	16	--	03	13	--
Valgus/Varus osteotomy	13	--	01	12	--
Mcmurray's osteotomy	05	--	--	04	01

Once the changes have advanced to Stage III or further, there is little chance of improvement and surgery is the only option. Amongst the surgery for osteonecrosis of femoral head the patients were graded at the time of presentation, according to stages and divided in two groups:

1. Those requiring head preserving surgery (Early stage).
2. Those requiring head sacrificing surgery (Advanced stage).

Those Requiring Head Preserving Surgeries—Early Stage

Head preserving surgeries were done in Stages I, II, III and rarely in stage IV which included core decompression and bone grafting and various osteotomies (Table 21.7). The aim of the treatment at this stage is to reduce the ischemia, intraosseous tension and perform the procedure, which will cause early revascularization of ischemic head. Only core decompression which was done earlier was always coupled with bone grafting as an additional procedure even in all those cases who had asymptomatic contralateral hip in a known patient of osteonecrosis of femoral head without any radiological changes where the diagnosis was established by MRI and scan. An additional TFL muscle pedicle graft or fibular graft was inserted to protect the core tract similar to the patients, where the changes were evident radiologically before the collapse.

A. ***Prophylactic treatment (stages 0 and I):*** Whenever possible one must prevent the disease from occurring altogether. This can be very well achieved partially in the cases of osteonecrosis of the femoral head following alcohol abuse, dysbarism and by avoiding the use of corticosteroids in conditions, i.e. renal transplantations, skin manifestations, ulcerative colitis and so on. Whereas the situation is different in sickle cell disorder. Sickle cell patients are monitored closely and at the earliest suspicion of a crisis they are hydrated and oxygenated properly and acidosis is corrected. The patient with proven unilateral osteonecrosis of the femoral head should be observed closely since 50 to 80 percent of the patients develop bilateral affection.[10,18-20] Any symptoms if it develops in the untreated hip should be taken as high risk suspicious of osteonecrosis of the femoral head. Wherever, there are no radiographic changes, bone scanning should be done. If the bone scan is negative, patient should be closely observed and followed. May be sequential MRI has a place in this group of patients for early diagnosis.

B. ***Treatment in early stages (before collapse, stages II and III):*** The aim of the treatment at this stage is to reduce the intraosseous tension and perform the procedure which will cause early revascularization of ischemic head. In all these patients the changes were evident radiologically before the collapse (stages II and III). Core decompression and Phemister bone grafting by using long cortical graft from fibula was done on 26 occasions[26] (in six cases on both sides) (Figs 21.13 to 21.18) in 20 patients. Core decompression and bone grafting using cancellous bone graft from iliac crest of the same side was done on 14 occasions where as vascular pedicle grafting from ilium was done on 18 occasions. It is said that cortical graft adds both to the biomechanical and biological advantages during the process of revascularization. Whenever, the crescent sign had appeared without any collapse, it

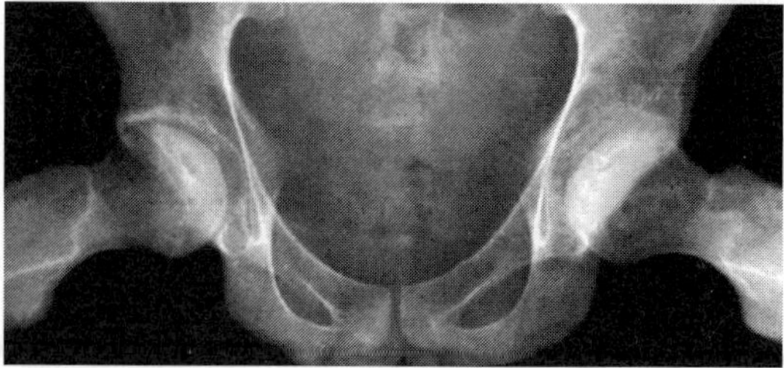

Fig. 21.13 X-ray pelvis Dunn's view showing bilateral osteonecrosis without any collapse but with subtle flattening of right femoral head in a young 20-year-old male with sickle cell trait

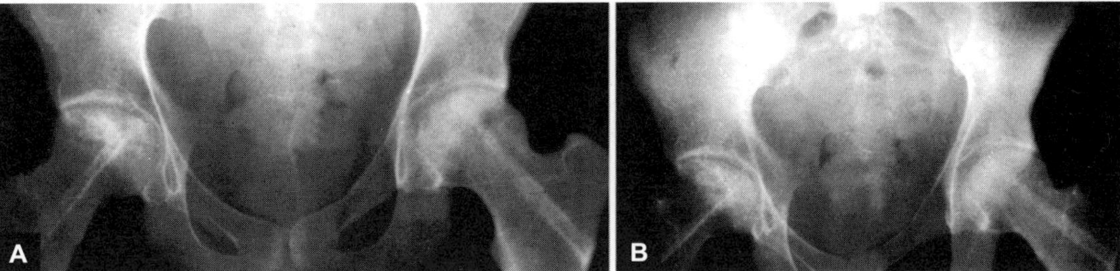

Figs 21.14A and B Postoperative X-ray pelvis 2.5 years of the same patient (Fig. 21.13) after core decompression and Phemister bone grafting using both long fibular graft. Contour of the femoral head is well-maintained even after 2.5 years

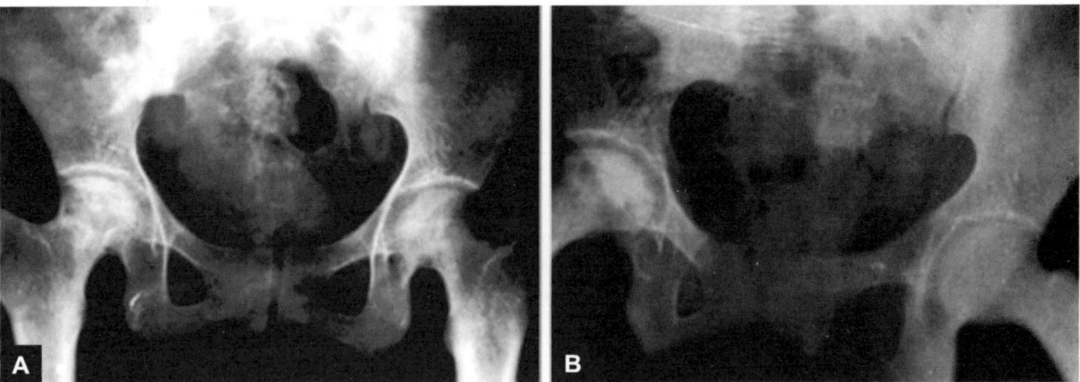

Figs 21.15A and B X-ray pelvis AP and Dunn's view in a young sickle cell disease patient showing osteonecrosis of the right femoral head

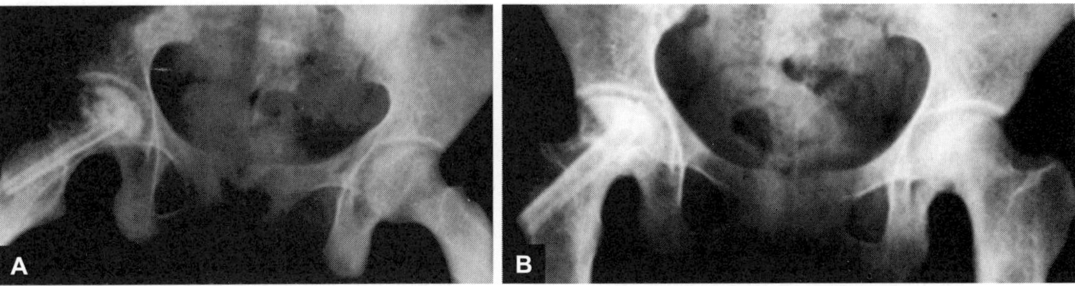

Figs 21.16A and B Postoperative X-ray four months after core decompression and Phemister type free fibular grafting—AP and Dunn's view same patient (Figs 21.15A and B)

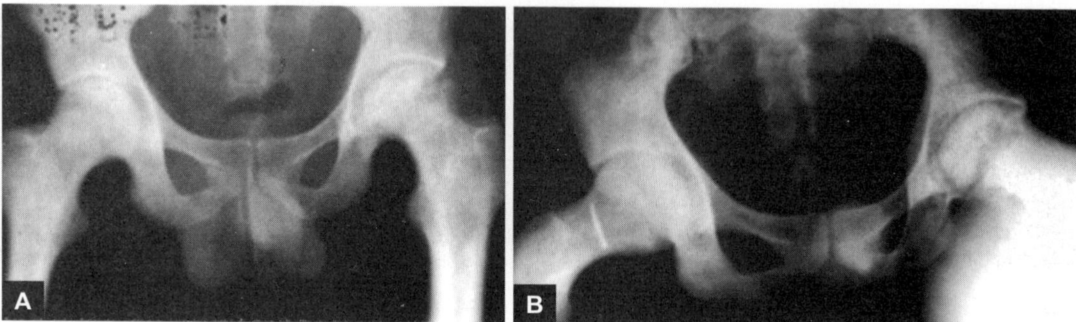

Figs 21.17A and B X-ray pelvis AP and Dunn's view of young sickle cell patient with bilateral osteonecrosis with advanced changes on left side

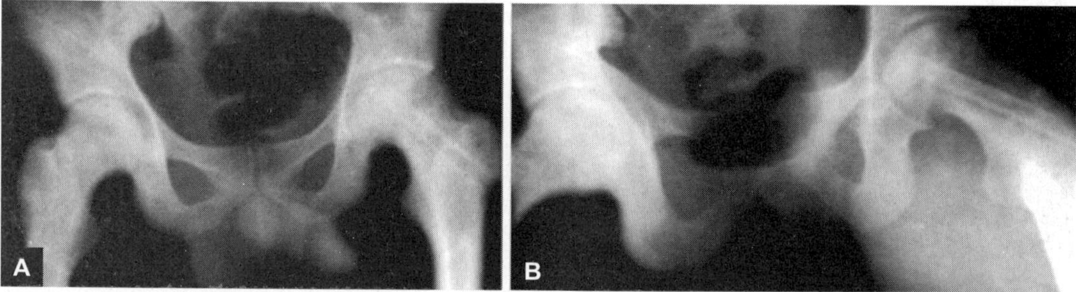

Figs 21.18A and B Postoperative X-ray AP and Dunn's view after core decompression and fibular cortical graft

was taken as the indication of vascular or muscle pedicle grafting in addition to core decompression. On 18 occasions Meyer's (Quadratus femoris muscle pedicle graft)[27] procedure by posterolateral approach was done (Figs 21.19 to 21.22) primarily and on twelve occasions—Sartorius muscle pedicle grafting by anterolateral approach in addition to forage was done (Figs 21.23 and 21.24). Use of vascularized pedicle graft is more advantageous since a high percentage of marrow and osteogenic cells survive within a living graft which helps for early vascularization.[28] This was done by anterior approach on 18 occasions using part of the iliac crest with the deep circumflex iliac vessels. Vascular pedicle is raised from the iliac crest with deep circumflex iliac vessels, which lie above the inguinal ligament opposite the inferior epigastric artery, a branch from the external iliac artery. After achieving the desired length and width of free vascular graft from the iliac crest, the bone graft is swung to the hip region and the graft is tunnelled through the intermuscular plane between the Rectus femoris and Pectineus. Subsequently, a window is made in the neck at the intertrochanteric line and thorough curettage of the necrosed femoral head is done and the graft is trapped and made stable without kinking of vessels (Figs 21.25 to 21.27).

C. ***Treatment following collapse (stage IV):*** It is believed that once crescent sign appears and there is a collapse of necrotic bone segment, even if it is minimal on X-rays, further collapse is inevitable and hip joint is likely to degenerate.[21] Any procedure like core decompression

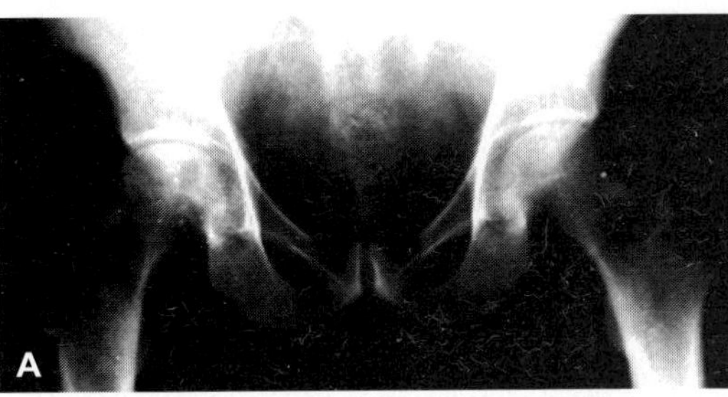 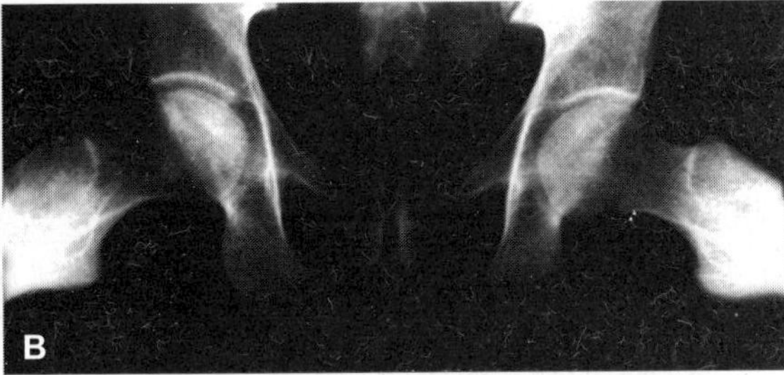

Figs 21.19A and B X-ray pelvis AP and Dunn's view of young lady of 30 years with SS pattern with osteonecrosis of right femoral head without any collapse

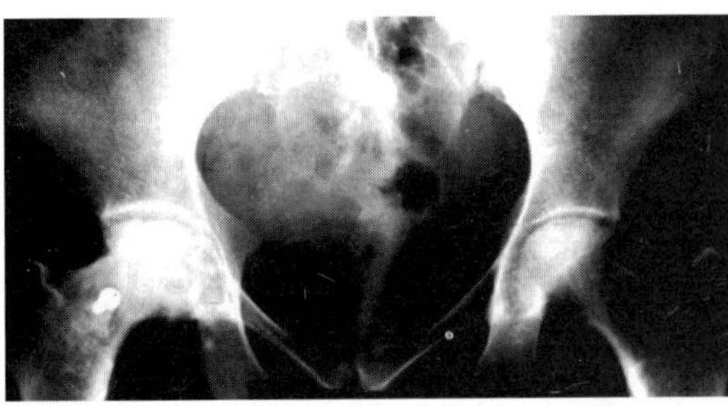

Fig. 21.20 Postoperative X-ray pelvis AP of same patient (Figs 21.22A and B) two years after Meyer's procedure of quadratus femoris muscle grafting showing minimal improvement. But there is no deterioration and no collapse. Contour of femoral head is well-maintained with good hip joint space

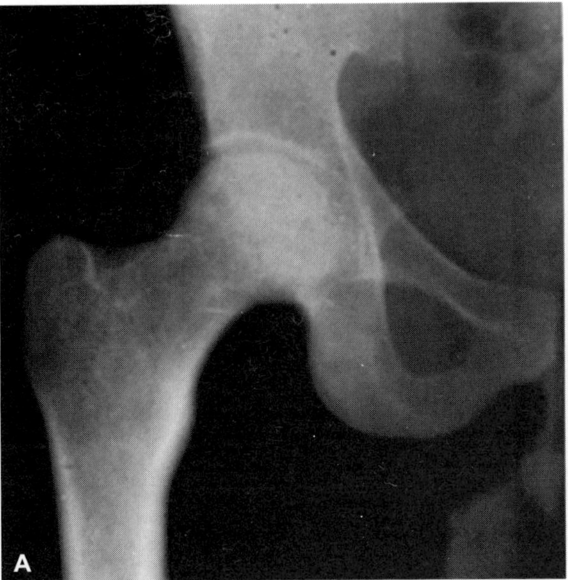 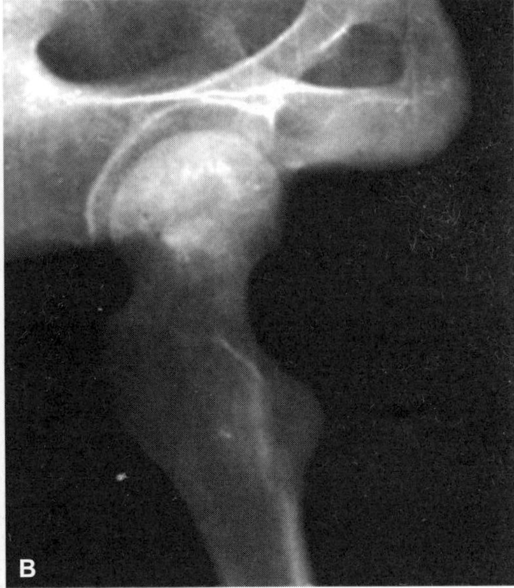

Figs 21.21A and B X-ray right hip AP and lateral view showing osteonecrosis of femoral head in young 36-year-old sickler but without any collapse of necrotic segment

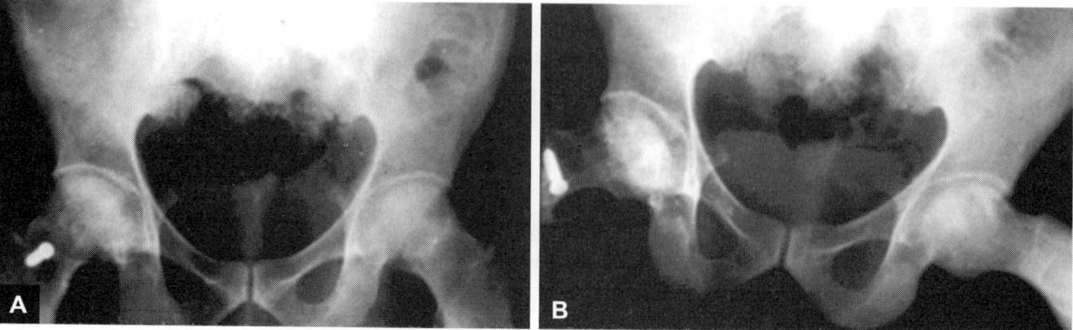

Figs 21.22A and B Postoperative X-ray pelvis AP and Dunn's view of same patient (Figs 21.24A and B) two years after Meyer's operation showing good vascularization of right femoral head without any collapse. Good radiological improvement but early changes of osteonecrosis are seen in contralateral femoral head

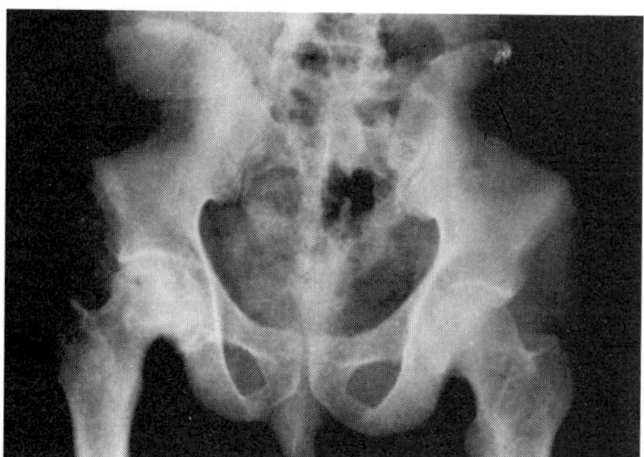

Fig. 21.23 X-ray pelvis AP showing advanced changes of osteonecrosis in right hip with fissuring and minimal collapse in a young 28-year-old with sickle cell trait

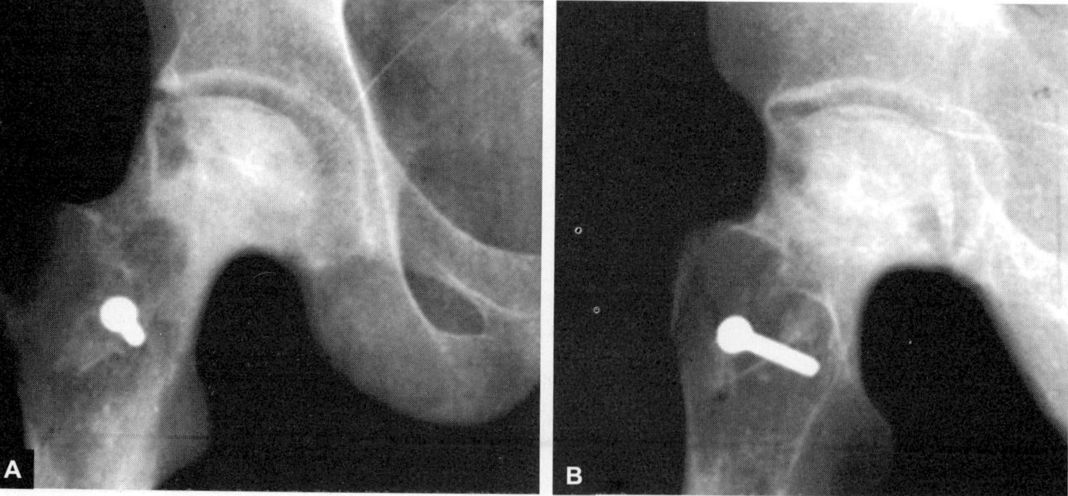

Figs 21.24A and B Postoperative X-ray of same hip (Fig. 21.26) AP and lateral view 1.5 years after core decompression and sartorius muscle pedicle grafting operation, showing revascularization. No progression of osteonecrosis. Hip joint space is well-maintained

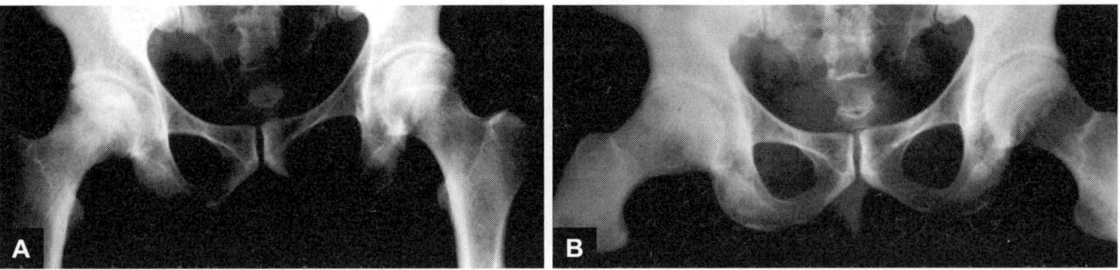

Figs 21.25A and B X-ray pelvis AP and Dunn's view of a young sickler in whom osteonecrosis was suspected but plain X-rays did not reveal any changes

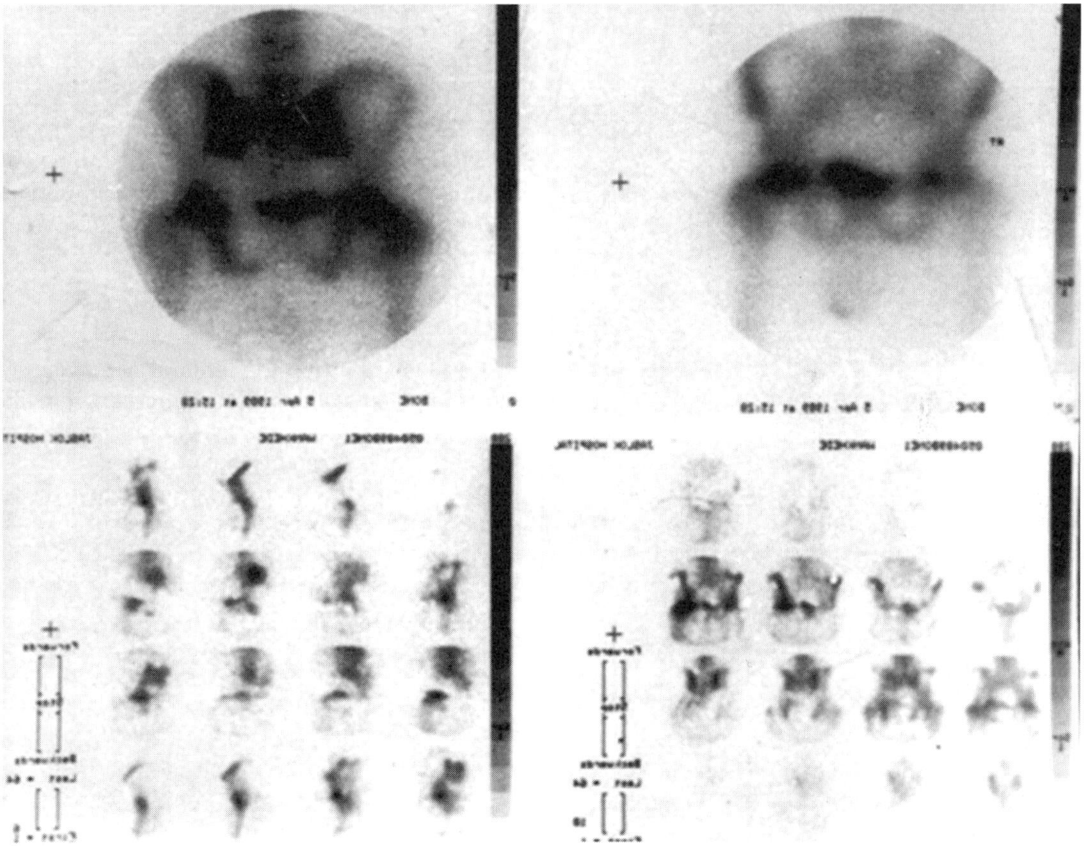

Fig. 21.26 Bone scan of young patient showing increased uptake in right femoral head suggestive of osteonecrosis of femoral in whom the plain X-rays were normal (same patient Figs 21.19A and B)

and bone grafting, which is likely to revascularize the dead segment is not going to be useful once the collapse of segment occurs. Hence, at this stage IV the procedure to change the weightbearing necrotic segment to nonweightbearing portion by different osteotomies, is performed.[22,23]

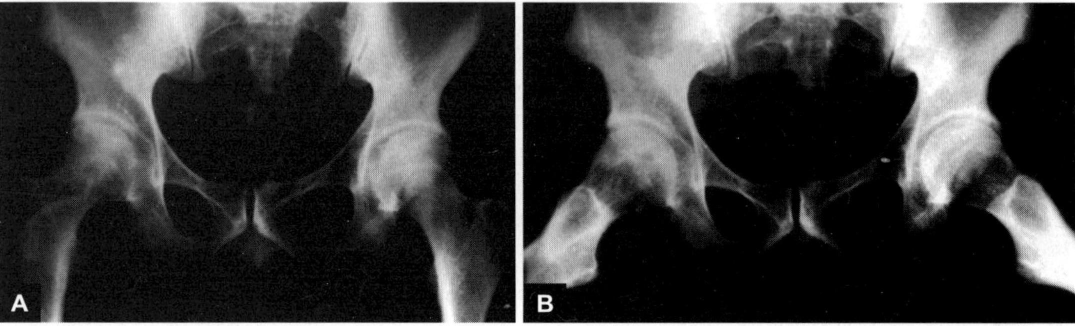

Figs 21.27A and B Postoperative X-ray pelvis AP and Dunn's view, 6 months after core decompression and vascular pedicle grafting from iliac crest showing early revascularization without any collapse or change in the contour of articular surface of femoral head

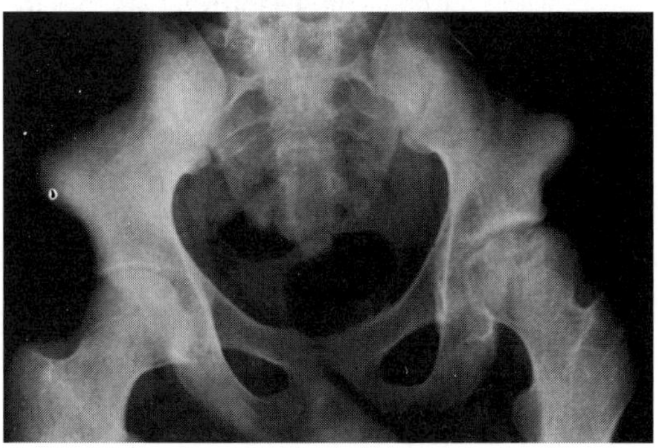

Fig. 21.28 X-ray pelvis AP showing osteonecrosis with collapse of small fragment in the center of left femoral head in young 23-year-old sicker with SS pattern

At our center 37 transtrochanteric ventral rotational osteotomies[22,29] were done primarily in cases with collapse of the femoral head without any degenerative changes (Figs 21.28 to 21.31) and on five occasions secondarily (total 42 operations). On 16 occasions flexion osteotomies were done (Figs 21.32 and 21.33). Basically in both these osteotomies the weight-bearing superolateral necrotic segment is rotated anteromedially in the nonweight-bearing region. Valgus osteotomy was done on five occasions and varus osteotomy was done on eight (Figs 21.34 to 21.36). McMurray's osteotomy frequently done in earlier days was presently not considered as a suitable operation for osteonecrosis of the femoral head though it was done in five cases in very early days. In all these operated patients early mobilization was done but nonweight-bearing was maintained for three to four months.

Those Requiring Head Sacrificing Surgeries—Advanced Stage

In this second group the femoral head was so badly affected, collapsed and fragmented with secondary arthritic changes, that achieving painless, mobile, stable hip was not possible (Figs 21.37 to 21.39). In this group again there were options for three types of surgeries:
1. Girdlestone
2. Arthrodesis
3. Replacement surgery.

Though in earlier days we had performed and promoted many patients for Girdlestone arthroplasty or arthrodesis, presently we encourage the patients more for replacement arthroplasty. Total hip replacement in these patients of sickle cell hemoglobinopathy offers excellent quality of life, since their life expectancy has improved because of better therapy and newer medical care. The patients of sickle cell trait live an almost normal life span as compared to other average patients of sickle cell disease.

In this series following surgeries were performed—68 hip replacement surgeries,

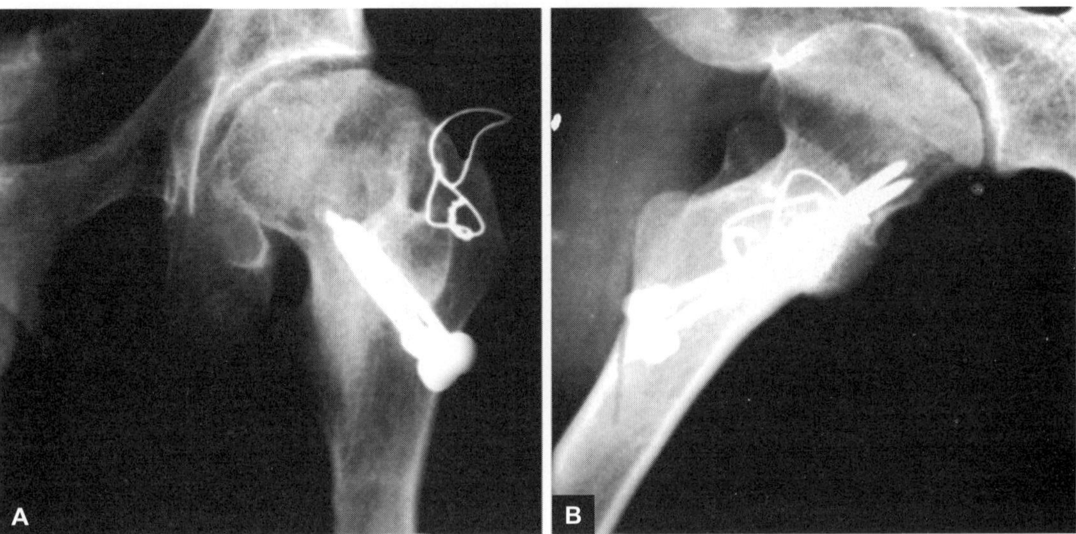

Figs 21.29A and B Postoperative X-ray left hip AP and lateral view two years after ventral rotational osteotomy, showing good revascularization on necrotic segment and smooth articular surface of weightbearing portion of the femoral head

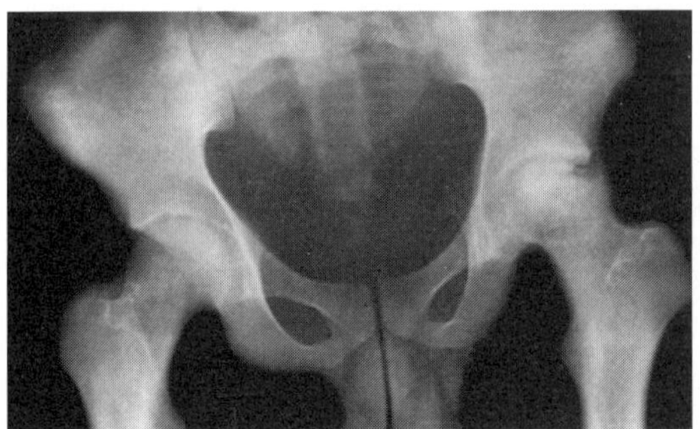

Fig. 21.30 X-ray pelvis AP showing osteonecrosis of left femoral head with collapse of necrotic segment in young 30-year-old sickler

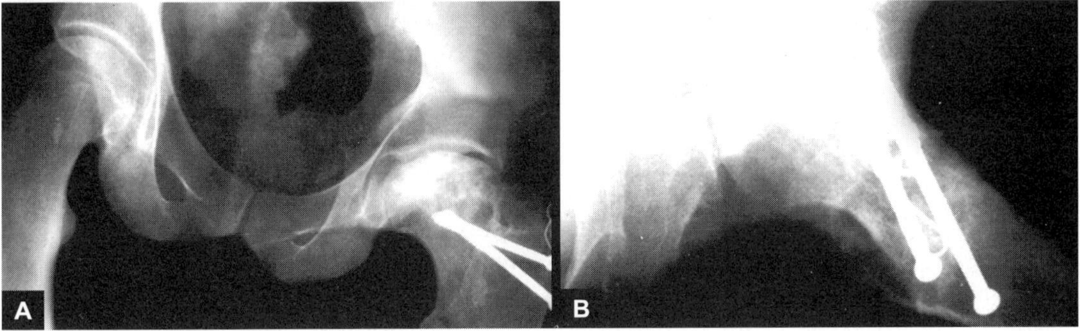

Figs 21.31A and B Postoperative X-ray pelvis (Fig. 21.30) AP and left hip lateral: 14 months after ventral rotational osteotomy showing good revascularization and smooth contour of articular surface

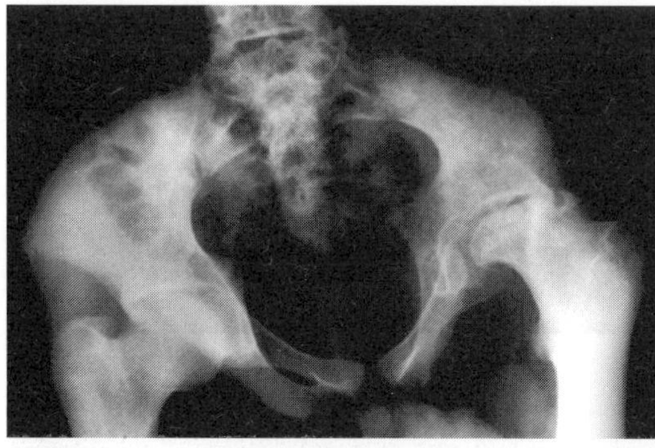

Fig. 21.32 X-ray pelvis AP showing advanced osteonecrosis in a young 19-year-old patient of sickle cell hemoglobinopathy with severe collapse of the femoral head

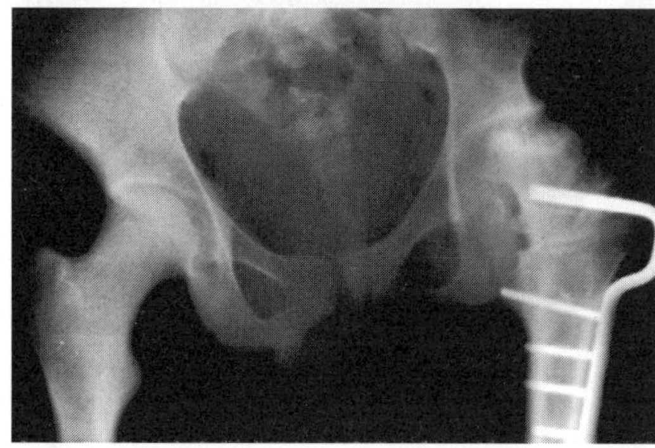

Fig. 21.33 Postoperative X-ray pelvis of the same patient (Fig. 21.32) one year after flexion rotational osteotomy showing improvement, though minimal

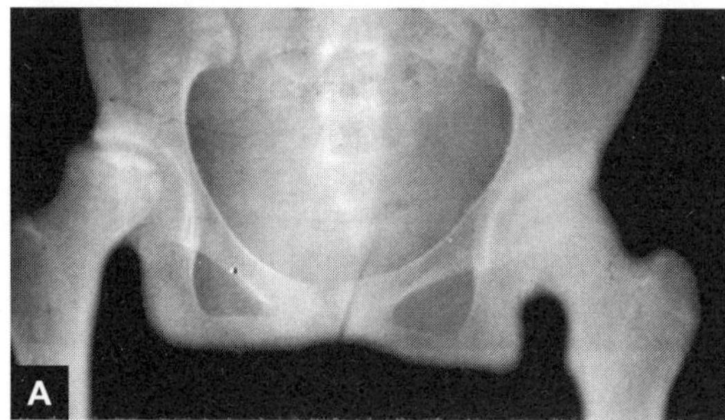

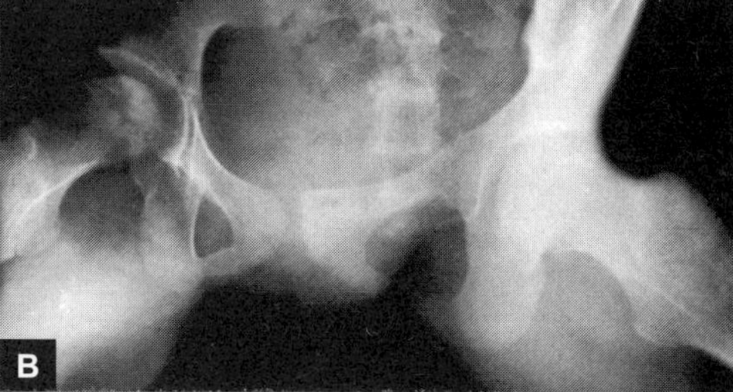

Figs 21.34A and B X-ray pelvis AP and Dunn's view showing osteonecrosis of right femoral head with collapse and lateral subluxation of femoral head in young 20-year-old girl having SS pattern

only five Girdlestone arthroplasty and three arthrodesis (Tables 21.4 and 21.5). Sixty-eight total hip replacements were done in 60 patients who were suitable for surgery. These 60 patients form the part of this study: 34 hips were classified as Charnley Functional Class A (unilateral disease) 9 as Class B (bilateral disease) and 17 as Class C (systemic disease affecting the ability to walk). Amongst these patients the younger 20 patients had isoelastic hip replacement (noncemented femoral and acetabular components) and the physiologically older 38 patients had Charnley's type of hip replacement (cemented femoral and acetabular components). Amongst other replacement we did bipolar prosthesis on nine occasions, hemiarthroplasty on three occasions. We had no experience of

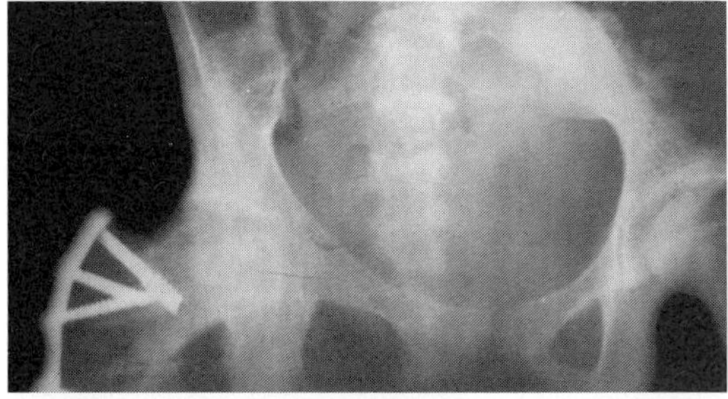

Fig. 21.35 Postoperative X-ray pelvis of the same patient of (Figs 21.34A and B) two months after varus osteotomy showing good containment and attempt towards revascularization

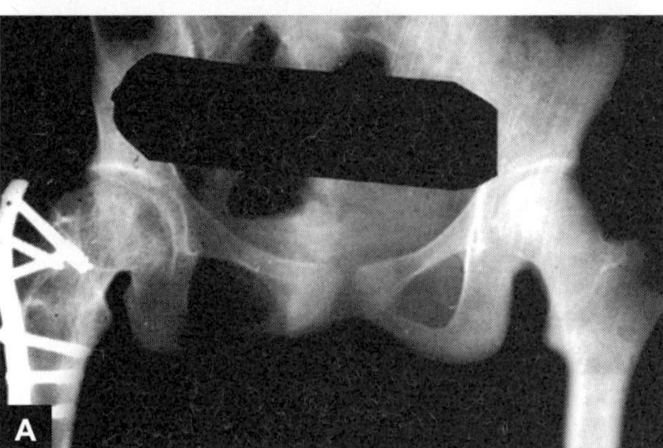

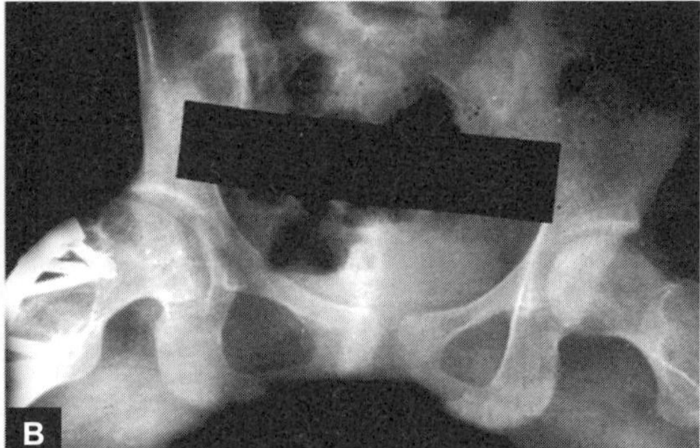

Figs 21.36A and B Postoperative X-ray pelvis AP and Dunn's view of same patient (Figs 21.34A and B) eight months after surgery showing good containment, revascularization and smooth articular surface of the right femoral head

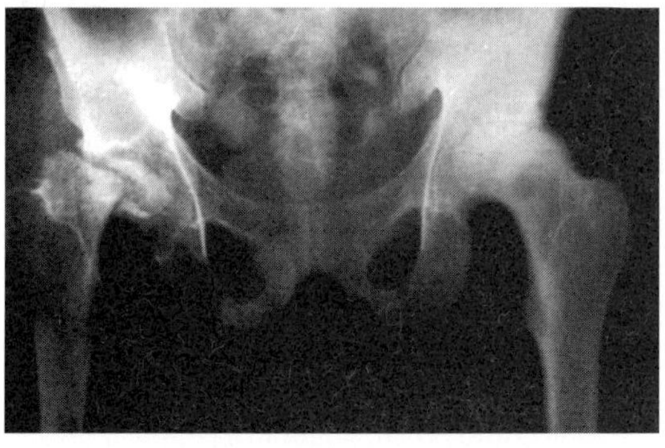

Fig. 21.37 X-ray pelvis showing gross collapse of the femoral head on the right side with fairly advanced changes on the left side

osteochondral allograft[27] or spongioplasty or vascular bundle transplantation (Hori) or electrical stimulation (Steinberg et al. 1984, 1985). The patients were evaluated pre-operatively and postoperatively with the use of the system of Merle d'Aubigne and Postel[18] as modified by Charnley for the assessment of pain and walking ability. Although, the scores for pain and walking were prospectively evaluated for each patient each year, only the results of the most recent postoperative assessment were analyzed for this study (Table 21.6). The scoring system awards 6 points each for pain and walking, with the maximum score being 12 points. A combined score of 11 or 12 points was considered to indicate an excellent

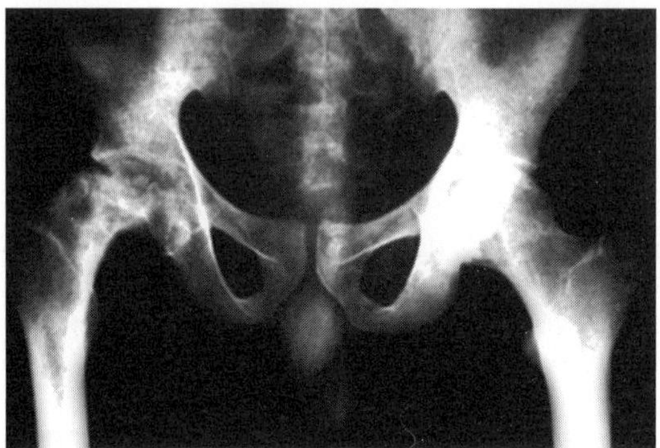

Fig. 21.38 X-ray showing collapse of femoral head, with subluxation and arthritic changes

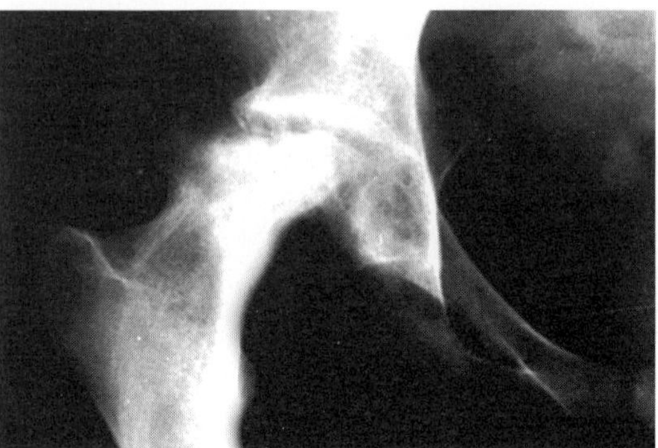

Fig. 21.39 X-ray of the hip showing advanced necrosis with subluxation and arthritic changes

result: 9 or 10 points, a good result: 8 points, fair and 7 points or less a clinical failure. Any pain score of 3 points or less at the time of the most recent evaluation was also considered to represent a failure. This clinical scoring system was used at yearly intervals for the first five years post-operatively and then at two year intervals.

PERIOPERATIVE MANAGEMENT

The management of a patient of sickle cell disease, who has to undergo surgery demands a planned control of various factors, which can precipitate sickling or aggravate the already existing anemic state. The management aims at maintenance of a steady state of hemo-globin and avoidance of factors that are known to precipitate sickling like hypoxia, acidosis, hypotension, peripheral circulatory stasis, hypothermia, dehydration, respiratory depression.

Blood Transfusion

Preoperatively or during surgery, transfusion with packed red cells is sometimes necessary but is not without risk. The rationale for preoperative transfusion is to achieve reduction in the level of HbS by diluting with HbA blood. By their presence normal red cells limit the maximum increase in viscosity resulting from the condition of lower pH and decreased oxygen tension. This raises the Hb level to normal, and thereby live sickle cells to be removed from the circulation. Such a procedure simultaneously dilutes the sickle cells with normal cells and increases the blood volume and thus without producing circulatory overload.

Anesthesia

Wherever possible, general anesthesia should be avoided and spinal anesthesia or epidural block should be used.

Hypoxia

Hypoxia can be prevented by taking the following precautions during surgery and postoperatively:

- Before inducing a patient 100 percent oxygenation for 3 to 5 minutes
- Intubation should be smooth without any episode of breath holding or laryngeal spasm
- Maintenance with gas (N_2O) or Halothane should be combined with proper oxygen concentration (30–50%) in the inspired air
- Extubation should be preceded by 100 percent oxygenation
- Postoperatively oxygen supplementation under supervision should be continued till full recovery of the patients from anesthesia.

Acidosis

This can be prevented by preoperative oral soda bicarb 0.5 to 1 g/kg/day. Intraoperatively administration of intravenous soda bicarb 3.3 mEq/kg/h over a period of 90 minutes is recommended. It should be continued after surgery for 24 to 48 hours.

Hypotension, Peripheral Stasis and Dehydration

This can be avoided by encouraging oral intake preoperatively and proper intravenous fluid infusions intraoperatively. Tourniquets should be avoided as far as possible. Their use should be kept limited to only those situations where their omission will jeopardize the surgical safety or success. Low molecular weight dextran to prevent hypotension is given intraoperatively.

Hypothermia

Hypothermia has a two-fold effect:
1. Vasoconstriction leading to peripheral stasis and thus precipitating sickling.
2. Shivering leading to increased oxygen demand.

Measures to prevent hypothermia include:
- Prevention of excessive cooling of the theater.
- Judicious use of halothane intraoperatively because halothane is known to cause post-operative shivering.
- Infusing intravenous (IV) fluids of optimum temperature.

Drugs

1. Zinc orally preoperatively and post-operatively.
2. Folic acid orally.
3. Low molecular weight dextran intra-operatively to replace the fluid loss is recommended.
4. Sodium bicarbonate orally and IV preoperatively, during surgery and postoperatively.
5. Hydroxyurea 500 mgm daily.

Complications

Postoperative hematoma was commonly observed and was seen in 21 patients. Nine patients had deep-seated infection. In two patients the femoral head had to be excised, out of which total hip replacement was done in one patient after a year. Mechanical loosening was noticed in the acetabular component in one patient of total hip replacement (THR), which required revision. Bacteremia with generalized spread of infection occurred in these patients of sickle cell disease. No other complications were noticed. Though sickle cell crises was precipitated on 11 occasions, total complications were observed in 36 patients in this study of 169 patients treated surgically (Table 21.8).

Follow-up and Results

One hundred and sixty-nine patients were followed who required surgery on 252 hips. Amongst 164 head-preserving surgeries on 88 occasions core decompression and various types of bone grafting were done. And on 76 occasions different types of intertrochanteric osteotomies were done to change the site of the necrotic segment into nonweight-bearing portion. Whereas in 75 patients surgery to preserve the integrity of the femoral head was not possible and were subjected to head-sacrificing surgery. The patients were routinely followed every month and the results were analyzed by Merle d' Aubigné and Postel[18] modified by Charnley's system at the end of 12 months (Table 21.6).

In 60 patients 68 THR's were done, where as in 15 patients 20 surgeries of Girdlestone, hemiarthroplasty, bipolar and arthrodesis were done.

DISCUSSION

The need to treat ischemia of the femoral head is becoming more common since many cases are

Table 21.8 Postoperative complications

Name of complication	Number of patients	
	A Head preserving group	B Head sacrificing group
1. Hematoma	19	2
2. Infection	8	1
3. Mechanical loosening	--	2
4. Septic loosening	--	1
5. Bacteremia	3	--
Total	30	6
6. Precipitation of hematological crisis	8	3
7. Post-traumatic fracture of the tip of stem	--	--

detected in early stages in young patients. One must consider the possibility; of osteonecrosis if individual who has history of sickle cell disease, has pain in the vicinity of the hip. Osteonecrosis of the the femoral head is a common skeletal manifestation and complication observed in sickle cell disease. Osteonecrosis affecting the femoral head might be the first presentation of the sickle cell disease. The symptomatology varies depending upon whether it is a trait or disease and the stage of the osteonecrosis. Once there is a collapse of the articular surface by and large patients are likely to require replacement arthroplasty. Obviously if segmental collapse is minimal one could consider head-preserving surgery, whereas if collapse of the articular surface is more and if more than 60 percent of the weight-bearing surface is involved replacement arthroplasty is the surgery of choice. Hypoxia, hypotension, circulating stasis, hypothermia, hypovolumia, respiratory depression, acidosis are all possible causes of sickle cell crisis which can cause and lead to complications of anesthesia and surgery which can predispose and precipitate sickling. Unless these patients are given plenty of parenteral fluids, (they cannot tolerate preoperative oral fluid) restoration due to renal concentrating defects is difficult and they become dehydrated leading to a vaso-occlusive crisis.

Nonweight-bearing conservative management of ischemic necrosis has not been proved to be beneficial and hence various operative procedures are done depending upon the stage of necrosis of the femoral head. Core decompression offers the opportunity to study histological changes of early bone ischemia. It also achieves reduction in the symptoms of the precollapse stage of ischemic necrosis. With this study it is emphatically agreed that core decompression is the effective treatment in preradiological and precollapse stage of osteonecrosis of femoral head[9,10,30] but it is necessary to add cortical graft at the tract of the core to avoid iatrogenic fracture. Certainly early diagnosis is the key to the success of head preserving operations. Once the crescent sign appears it is desirable to couple the bone grafting procedure in addition to the core decompression preferably vascular pedicle grafting. In patients with ischemic necrotic segment without crescent sign, Phemister[26] bone grafting is superior since it provides biomechanical and biological graft, where as once crescent sign appears without any collapse vascular or muscle pedicle graft is a good procedure. Once the collapse of ischemic segment occurs all the procedures of core decompression and bone grafting are not expected to do any more good, and at this stage various osteotomies amongst head preserving operative groups are indicated.[22,23,31] In such situations one must analyze the possible future development in osteonecrosis, so that failed osteotomy does not affect or worsen the situation for performing total hip replacement. However, this does not reduce the importance of the effectiveness of osteotomies, since at this stage, this is the only group of operations in which relatively young patients do not undergo joint replacement and a benefit of 10 to 15 years can be easily drawn from osteotomy. Various intertrochanteric osteotomies are performed to preserve the joint as an important and efficient method to treat the cases of ischemic necrosis of femoral head, which usually threatens the younger patients with its rampant destruction of joint, which may result in severe disability. Basically, in osteonecrosis of the femoral head, which is common in the young age group, a conservative approach is chosen (Kerboul et al. 1974)[11] rather than a radical approach of reconstructive surgery. Essentially the results depend on the preoperative condition of the joint and the site of necrotic focus. If the ischemic necrosis of the femoral head is diagnosed early in stages 0 and I, core decompression by and large gives very good results. Head-preserving operations certainly gives satisfactory results in stages II, III and few selected cases of stage IV. The prognosis of stages II and III is fairly good where as in stage IV it is satisfactory, since about one third of this group are likely to progress further and may require joint surface or total hip joint replacement or resurfacing operations[32] (Dutton RO and Amstutz HC et al. 1982). If there is a collapse of the articular surface, head preserving operation may be considered but with >60% articular surface involvement and degenerative changes total hip replacement is the treatment of choice. Replacement of the femoral head with a metal prosthesis may restore function and aid in rehabilitation of bed-ridden patients. This procedure has not been tried on a sufficient number of patients to appraise its work and its risk. The relatively short life of patients with sickle cell anemia and the inability of these patients to be gainfully employed should be taken into consideration in planning major elective operative procedures.

Joint replacement is being done in an increasing number of patients with the advent of general medical care of these sickler patients and advances in anesthetic agents and techniques. The relatively short life span of these patients should be taken into consideration before planning such a major surgical procedure. Haddad[33] presented several cases and recommended hemi-arthroplasty, and not arthrodesis, Girdlestone or total joint replacement. The clinical outcome of total joint replacement performed within the last 20 years has been excellent. The result has been disappointing in younger patients combined with the traditional older technique of cementing which has resulted into poorer results thus bringing noncemented joint replacement into vogue. The theoretical advantage is biological ingrowth of bone thus leading to less likelihood of mechanical failure at implant bone interface. However, two potential problems challenge this theory, i.e. stress shielding of the proximal femur and osteolysis due to particulate debris.

Dorr et al.[34] reviewed the results of 108 hip arthroplasties performed with cement in 81 patients who had been less than 45 years old. After four and a half years follow-up, they found a 19 percent of revision, a 29 percent of impending failure in hips that were not revised, and radiolucent lines at the bone-cement interface in 95 percent cases. In a more recent review of the same patients after nine years of follow-up, the rate of revision had almost tripled to 33 percent of hips, the rate of impending failure had risen to 56 percent in the hips that had not been revised and radiolucent lines were present in all but one hip. Chandler et al.[35] reviewed results of 33 total hip arthroplasties performed with cement in 29 patients who were 30 years old or less. After an average follow-up of 67 months, 21 percent of patients had a revision, 33 percent an impending failure, and 97 percent radiolucency at the bone-cement interface.

In the present study of 68 hips in which cemented and noncemented both varieties were used with satisfying results in either group, but it seems better to use noncemented in the physiologically younger patients and to use cemented in physiologically older patients based on a better survivorship. The overall rate of revision compares quite favorably with the earlier reported series. With the modern cementation techniques the earlier known complications of cementation can be avoided in the long-term.

Gunderson reported results after joint replacement and enumerated the complications like hematological crisis, infected hematoma, bacteremia, and post-traumatic fracture of the tip of the stem. Epps and Castro,[36] 1978; Sebes and Kraus,[37] 1993 reported the results of arthroplasty in sickle cell disease. Sickle cell disease patients are at considerable risk of postoperative morbidity including infection, early mechanical and septic loosening. In this study the patients complicated with deep infections belonged to Charnley Class C. High rate of failure of joint replacement combined with high incidence of complications in patients of sickle cell disease suggested that the risk to benefit ratio of this procedure should be assessed carefully for each patient.

Hanker (1988), suggested perioperative care of patients of sickle cell disease and these recommendations should be followed to minimize postoperative complications. These patients must have adequate hydration and oxygenation to avoid acidosis, hypoxia and vascular stasis. They may require preoperative transfusion to raise the hematocrits to more than 30 percent and to lower the level of hemoglobin S.

To improve the quality of life, to achieve painless mobile hip it is necessary to perform total hip replacement, even if the rate of complications is very high in these young patients of sickle cell hemoglobinopathies once the collapse of the femoral head has occurred.

◼ CONCLUSION

After the study, observation and follow-up of these patients of osteonecrosis of the femoral head the surgical treatment was streamlined. The stage wise treatment options for these patients of osteonecrosis has been suggested (Table 21.9). However, early diagnosis is the key to the success of head preserving operations in these sickler patients. Presently we advocate the following surgical procedures according to the stage of involvement in these patients of sickle cell hemoglobinopathy.

Table 21.9 Stagewise treatment option

Stage 0 and I	II/III	III/IV	IV and V

Core decompression and bone grafting
• Phemister fibular graft
• Vascular Pedicle graft.
	Core decompression and bone grafting
	• Phemister fibular graft
	• Vascular pedicle graft
	• Muscle pedicle grafting
	  – Quadratus femoris
	  – Sartorius
	  – TFL
		• Intertrochanteric osteotomy (Various types)
		• Vascular pedicle graft.
		• Muscle pedicle graft
			• THR
			• Hemiarthroplasty
			  – AMP
			  – Bipolar
			• Girdlestone arthroplasty of arthrodesis

◼ REFERENCES

1. Babhulkar Sudhir. Orthopaedic manifestations and bone changes in sickle cell haemoglobinopathy. Monogram by CBS Publishers;1997.pp.78-93.

2. Babhulkar SS. Osteonecrosis of the femoral head (in young individuals). Indian Journal of Orthopaedics. 2003;37(2):77-86.

3. Babhulkar SS. Osteonecrosis of the femoral head: treatment by core decompression and vascular pedicle grafting. Indian Journal of Orthopaedics. 2009;43(1):27-35.

4. Daland GA, Castle WB. A simple and rapid method of demonstrating sickling of red blood cells, the use of reducing agents. J Lab Clin. Med. 1948;33:1082.

5. Marcus ND, Enneking WF, Massam RA. The silent hip in idiopathic aseptic necrosis: treatment by bone grafting. J Bone Joint Surg Am. 1973;55A:1351-66.

6. Steinberg ME, Hayken GD, Steinberg DR. A new method for evaluation and staging of avascular necrosis of the femoral head. In: Arlet J, Ficat RP, Hungerford DS (Eds). Bone Circulation. Baltimore, MD, Williams and Wilkins; 1984. pp.398-403

7. Ficat RP. Idiopathic bone necrosis of the femoral head: Early diagnosis and treatment. J Bone Joint Surg Br.1985;67B:3-9.

8. Gardeniers JWM. ARCO international classification of osteonecrosis. ARCO News 1993;5:79-82.

9. Hungerford DS. Bone marrow pressure, venography and core decompression in ischaemic necrosis of femoral head. Hip Society Meeting, proceedings.1979;pp.218-37.

10. Ficat RP. Treatment of avascular necrosis of femoral head "The Hip". The Hip Society 1983. pp.279-95.

11. Kerboul M, Thomine J, et al. The conservative surgical treatment of idiopathic aseptic necrosis of femoral head. J Bone and Joint Surgery Br 1974;56B:291-6.

12. Koo KH, Kim R. Quantifying the extent of osteonecrosis of the femoral head: A new method using MRI. J Bone and Joint Surgery Br. 1995;77B:875-80.

13. Totty WG, Murphy WA, Ganz WI, et al. Magnetic resonance imaging of the normal and ischaemic femoral head. AJR. 1984;143:1273-80.

14. Mitchell DG, Kressel HY, Arger PH, et al. Avascular necrosis of the femoral head: morphologic assessment by MR imaging, with CT correlation. Radiology. 1986;161:739-42.

15. Mitchell DG, Rao VM, Dalinka MK, et al. Femoral head avascular necrosis: correlation of MR imaging, radiographic staging, radionuclide imaging, and clinical finding. Radiology. 1987; 162:709-15.

16. Norman A, Bullough P. The radiolucent crescent line: An early diagnostic sign of avascular necrosis of the femoral head. Bull Hosp Joint Dis. 1963;24:99-104.

17. Bullough PG. The morbid anatomy of subchondral osteonecrosis. In: Urbaniak JR, Jones JP (Eds). Osteonecrosis: Etiology, diagnosis, and treatment. Rosemont, IL: American Academy of Orthopaedic Surgeons: 1997. pp.69-72 (Monogram by AAOS 1997).

18. Marle D'Aubigne R, Postel M, Mazabraud A, et al. Idiopathic necrosis of femoral head in adults. J Bone and Joint Surgery Br. 1965; 47B: 612-33.

19. Boettcher WG, Bonfiglio M, Smith K. Nontraumatic necrosis of the femoral head. Part I. Relation of altered haemostasis to etiology. J. Bone Joint Surgery Am. 1970.pp.312-9.

20. Boettcher WG, Bonfiglio M, Smith K. Nontraumatic necrosis of the femoral head. Part II experiences in treatment. J Bone and Joint Surgery Am. 1970;52A:322-9.

21. Kenzora JE, Glimcher MJ. Accumulative Cell Stress: The multifacatorial etiology of idiopathic osteonecrosis. Orthopaedic Clinics of North America. 1985;16(4) 669-79.

22. Sugioka Y. Transtrochanteric anterior rotational osteotomy of the femoral head in treatment of osteonecrosis affecting the hip. Clin Orthop. 1978;130:191-201.

23. Kempt I, Karger C. Post rotational osteotomy of femoral head in avascular necrosis. Rev Chir Ortho. 1984;70:271-82.

24. Chung, Ralston. Necrosis of femoral head in Sickle cell disease. J Bone and Joint Surgery Am. 1969;51A:33-58.

25. Russel J. An essay on necrosis - "The Classic" Clin Orthop. 1978;130:5-7.

26. Phemister DB. Treatment of necrotic head of femur in adults. J. Bone and Joint Surgery Am. 1949;31A:55-6.

27. Meyer's MH. The treatment of osteonecrosis of hip with fresh osteochondral allografts and with the muscle pedicle graft technique. Clin Orthop. 1978;130:202-9.

28. Babhulkar SS. Osteonecrosis of femoral head: Treatment by core decompression and

vascular pedicle grafting. Indian Journal of Orthopaedics. 2009;43(1):27-35.

29. Sugioka Y. Transtrochanteric rotational osteotomy in treatment of idiopathic femoral head necrosis, Perthes disease, osteoarthritis. Clin Orthop. 1984;184:12-23.

30. Camp JF, Colwell CW. Core decompression of the femoral head for osteonecrosis. J Bone and Joint Surgery Am. 1986;68A:1313-9.

31. Simonnet JH, Aubaniac JM. The results of intertrochanteric flexion osteotomy in idiopathic avascular necrosis of femoral head - 52 cases. Rev Chir Ortho. 1984;70:219-29.

32. Dutton RO, Amstutz HC, Thomas BJ, Hedley AK. Tharies surface replacement for osteonecrosis of femoral head J Bone Joint Surgery Am. 1982; 64:1225-37.

33. Haddad RJ, Jr. Sickle cell disease involvement of the hip and its surgical treatment. Clin Orthop. 967;55:135-149.

34. Dorr LD, Luckett M, Conaty JP. Total hip arthroplasties in patients younger than 45 years: a nine to ten year follow-up study. Clin Orthop. 1990;260:215-9.

35. Chandler HP, Reineck FT, Winson RL, McCarthy JC. Total hip replacement in patients younger than thirty years old: a five-year follow-up study. J Bone Joint Surg Am. 1981;63A:1426-34.

36. Epps CH Jr, Castro Oswaldo. Complications of the total hip replacements in sickle cell disease. Orthop Trans. 1978;2:236-7.

37. Sebes Jeno I, Alfred P Kraus. Avascular necrosis of the hip in the sickle cell hemoglobinopathies. Journal of the Canadian Association of radiologist 1993;34:136.

▣ BIBLIOGRAPHY

1. Acurio MT, Richard J. Friedman. Hip arthroplasty in patient with sickle cell haemoglobinopathy. J Bone and Joint Surgery Br 1992;74B:367-71.

2. Ballas SK, Talacki CA, Rao VN, Steiner RM. The prevalence of avascular necrosis in sickle cell anaemia, Haemoglobin. 1989;13(7-8):649-55.

3. Baumgard SH, Leach RE. Avascular necrosis of the femoral head secondary to sickle cell disease. Case reports of the two Caucasian Sisters. Clin Orthop. 1970;69:207-12.

4. Bishop AR, Roberson JR, Eckman JR, Fleming LL. Total hip arthroplasty in patients who have sickle cell haemoglobinopathy. J Bone and Joint Surgery Am. 1988;70(6):853-5.

5. Blau S, Hamerman D. Aseptic Necrosis of Femoral head in sickle cell anaemia. Arthitis Rheum. 1967;10:397-402.

6. Bomelberg D, Ehringhaus C, Zeigler R, von Lengerke HJ, Timm C. Femur head necrosis in sickle cell anaemia. Monatsschr Kinderheilkd. 1986;134[4]:212-5.

7. Brooks BJ Jr, et al. Erythropoietin therapy for sickle cell anaemia in Jehovah's witnesses (letter); South Med Jr. 1991;84(11):1416-7.

8. Charache, Samuel, Page DL. Infarction of bone marrow in the sickle cell disorders. Ann.Intern. 1967;67:1195-1200.

9. Clarke HJ, Jinnah RH, Brooker AF. Total replacement of hip for avascular necrosis in sickle cell diseas. J Bone and Joint Surgery Br 1989;71[3]:465-70.

10. Clark Gunderson, Robert DD'Ambrosia, Hiromu Shoji. Total hip replacement in patients with sickle cell disease JBJS. 1977;59-A(6):760-2.

11. Diggs LW. Bone and joint lesions in sickle cell disease. Clin Orthop. 1967;52:119.

12. Diggs LW. Sickle Cell Crisis. The American Journal of Clinical Pathology, 1965;44(1):1-19.

13. Donald G Mitchell, Herbert Y, Kressel, Peter H Arger, Murrey Dalinka, Charles E. Spritzer, Marvin E. Steinberg. Avascular necrosis of the femoral head. Radiology. 1986;161(3):739-42.

14. Donald G. Mitchell, Michael Fallon, Herbert Y Kressel, Vijay M Rao, Murray K Dalinka, Charles E. Spritzer, Abbas Alavi, Marvin E. Steinberg; Femoral head avascular necrosis, corelation of MRI, radiographic staging, radionuclide imaging and clinical findings, Radiology. 1987;162(3):709-15.

15. Edward O'Hara. Roentgenographic osseous manifestation of the anemias and the Leukemias, Clin Orthop No. 52, May-June 1967, Pg.63

16. Ebong WW. Avascular necrosis of the femoral head associated with hemoglobinopathy. Tropical and Geographical Medicine. 1977;29:19-23.

17. Ebong WW, Kolawole TM. Aseptic necrosis of the femoral head in sickle disease. Br J Rheumatol. 1986;25(1):34-9.

18. Elke R, Morscher E. Total prosthesis arthroplasty in femoral head necrosis, Orthopade. 1990;19(4):236-41.

19. Emilio S Musso, Sharon N Mitcheel, Marry Schink Ascani, C Andrew Barett. Results of conservative management of osteonecrosis of the femoral head. Clin Orthop. 1986;207:209-5.

20. Ficat RP. Idiopathic bone necrosis of femoral head. Early diagnosis and treatment. J Bone and Joint Surgery [Am.] 1985;67-B:3-9.

21. Genin P, Vouge M, Bloch P. Osteonecrosis of the femoral head caused by sickle cell anaemia in benign epidemiologic and radiological aspect. Bull Asso Pathol Exot. Filiales. 1985;78(2):249-55.

22. Golding JSR. Conditions of the hip associated with hemoglobinopathies. Clinical orthopaedics and related reasearch. 1973;90:22.

23. Golding JSR. Bone changes in sickle cell anaemia. Ann Roy Colle Surg. England 1956;19: 296-314.

24. Golding JSR, MacIver JE, Went LN. The bone changes in sickle cell anemia and it's genetic variant. J Bone and Joint Surgery Br. 1959;41B: 711-8.

25. Gregory J Hanker, van Nuys, Herlan C. Amstutz. Osteonecrosis of the hip in the sickle cell disease. J Bone and Joint Surgery [Am.]. 1988;70A(4):499-506.

26. Hawker H, Neilson H, Hayer RJ, Sergaent GR. Haematological factors associated with avascular necrosis of the femoral head in homozygous sickle cell disease. British J Haematal. 1982;50:29-34.

27. Hanker GJ, Amstutz HC. Osteonecrosis of the hip in the sickle cell diseases. J Bone and Joint Surgery [Am.]. 1988;70(A):499-506.

28. Herold HZ. Avascular necrosis of the femoral head in children under the age of 3; Clin Orthop. 1977;126:193-5.

29. Hernigou P, Galacteros F, Bachir D, Goutallier D. Deformities in the hip in adults who have sickle cell disease and had avascular necrosis in childhood. J Bone and Joint Surgery [Am.]. 1991;73(1):81-92.

30. Hernigou P. Avascular necrosis of the femoral head in sickle cell disease.Treatment of collapse by the injection of acrylic cement. J. Bone and Joint Surgery Br. 1993;75 B(6):875-80.

31. Hernigou P, Bachir D, Galacteros F. Hip dysplasia, a complication of Sickle cell disease; Rev Rhum Ed Fr. 1993;60[7-8]:505-13.

32. Hernigou P, Galacteros F, Bachir D, Goutellier D. Natural history of hip necrosis in sickle cell disease; Rev Chir Orthop 1989;75[8]:542-57.

33. Hungerford DS, Zizic TM. Pathogenesis of ischaemic necrosis of the femoral head. "The Hip": The Hip Society; 1983:pp.249-62.

34. Hungerford DS, Dennis W Lennox. The importance of increased intraosseous pressure in development of avascular necrosis of femoral head; Implication for treatment - Orthopaedic Clinics of North America, 1985;16:4635-68.

35. Iwegbu CW, AF Fleming. Avascular necrosis of the femoral head in sickle cell disease. J Bone and Joint Surgery Br. 1985;67B:29-32.

36. Jones JIP, Sakovich L. Fat embolism of bone. J Bone Joint Surgery Am. 1966;48A:149-63.

37. Jones JIP, Jamenson RM, Engelman EP. Alcoholism, Fat embolism and avascular necrosis of femoral head. J Bone and Joint Surgery, Am. 1968;50A:1065.

38. Jones JP. Fat embolism and osteonecrosis. Orthopaedic Clinics of North America. 1985;16(4):595-633.

39. Kanoley and Ahulum FID, Lancet, 999, 1970.

40. Kauichi R Tanaka, George O Clifford, Arnold R Axerold. Sickle cell anaemia (homozygous S) with aseptic necrosis of femoral head. J Bone and Joint Surgery 1956;11:998-1007.

41. Kenzora JE, Steele RE, Yosipovitch ZH. et al. Experimental osteonecrosis of femoral head in adult rabbits. Clin Orthop. 1978;130:8-46.

42. Kenzora JE, Glimcher MJ. Pathogenesis of idiopathic osteonecrosis. The ubiquitous crescent sign. Orthopaedic Clinics of North America 1985;16(4):681-96.

43. Kenzora JE. Treatment of idiopathic necrosis: Orthopaedic Clinics of North America 1985;16(4):717-25.

44. Koren A. Avascular Necrosis of bones in children with sickle cell anaemia. Pediatr Hematol Oncol. 1993;10(4):385-7.

45. Khermosh O, Weissman SL. Coxa vara, avascular necrosis and osteochondritis dessicans complicating solitary bone cysts of the proximal femur. Clin Orthop. 1977;126:143-46.

46. Lifeso RM. Total Joint replacement in sickle cell disease. Orthop Trans. 1985;9:453.

47. Lee REJ, Golding JSR, Serjeant GR. The radiological features of avascular necrosis of the femoral head in homozygous sickle cell disease. Clinical Radiology. 1981;32:205-14.

48. Mijiyawa M, Pfudie S, Pitche V, N'Dakena K, Amedegnato MD, Doury P. Coxofemoral pathology in rheumatology. Med Trop. 1994;54(1):38-42.

49. Milner PF, Kraus AP, Sebes JI, Sleeper LA, Dukes KA, Emry SH, Bellebue R, Koshy M, Moohr JW, Smith J. Sickle cell disease as a cause of osteonecrosis of femoral head. N. Engl. J. Med. 1991;325(21):1476-81.

50. Moseley JE, Manly JB. Aseptic necrosis of bone in sickle cell disease, Radiology/Roentgenology. 1953;60:656.

51. Moran MC, Huo, Garvin, Pellicci, Salvati; Total hip arthroplasty in Sickle cell haemoglobinopathy. Clin Orthop. 1993;[294]:140-8.

52. Matthew D Mitchell, Harold L Kundel, Marvin E Steinberg, Herbert Y Kressel, Abass Alavi, Leon Axel. Avascular necrosis of the Hip. AJR. 1986;147:67-71.

53. Mitchell DG, Kressel HY, Arger PH, et al. Avascular necrosis of the femoral head: morphologic assesment by MR imaging, with CT correlation. Radiology 1986;161:739-42.

54. Mitchell DG, Rao VM, Dalinka MK, et al. Femoral head avascular necrosis: correlation of MR imaging, radiographic staging, radionuclide imaging, and clinical finding. Radiology. 1987;162:709-15.

55. Musso ES, Mitchell SN, Schink-Ascani M, Basset CAL. Result of conservative management of osteonecrosis of the femoral head: a retrospective review. Clin. Orthop 1986;207:209-15.

56. Ndugwa CM. Aseptic necrosis of the head of femur among sickle anaemia patients in Uganda. East African Medical Jr. 1992;69(10):572-6.

57. Omojala MF, Annobil S, Adzaku F, Addae SK, Mohammad S. Bone changes in sickle cell anaemia; East African Med. Jr. 1993;70(3):184-8.

58. Pierce RO, Jr. Aseptic necrosis of the hip in sickle cell disease. J Nat. Med. Assan, 1979;71:45-8.

59. Rand C, et al. Avascular necrosis of femoral head in sickle cell syndromes: a report of 5 cases. Acta Hematol, 1987;78(2-3):186-92.

60. Rijke AM, Pope TL Jr, Kent TE. Bilateral protrusio acetabuli in sickle cell anaemia. South Med. Jr. 1990;83(3):328-9.

61. Roesingh GE, James J. Early phase of avascular necrosis of femoral head in rabbits. J Bone and Joint Surgery [Br.] 1969;51B:165-76.

62. Rand C, Pearson TC, Heatley FW. Avascular necrosis of femoral head in sickle cell syndrome. Acta Haematol, 1987;78(2-3):186-92.

63. Reich RS, Rosenberg NJ. Aseptic necrosis of bone in caucasians with sickle cell anemia. J. Bone and Joint Surgery [Am.]. 1953;35A(4):894-904.

64. Rutt A, Kusswetter W. Sickle cell anaemia and it's skeletal and joint changes as an orthopaedic problem; Z Orthop. 1986;124(2):140-3.

65. Sadat M. Ali Avascular necrosis of the femoral head in sickle cell disease. An integrated classification. Clin. Orthop. 1993;290:200-5.

66. Sennara H, Gorry F. Orthopaedics aspects of sickle cell anaemia and haemoglobinopathies. Clin Orthop. 1978;130:154-7.

67. Sebes JI, Diagnostic imaging of bone and joint abnormalities associated with sickle cell haemoglobinopathies. AJR Am J Roentgenol. 1989;152(6):1153-9.

68. Smith EW, Conley CL. Clinical features of genetic variants of sickle cell disease. Bull. John hopkins Hosp. 1954;94:289.

69. Sebes Jeno I. Diagnostic imaging of bone in joint abnormalities associated with sickle cell haemoglobinopathies. AJR Am. J Roentgenol. 1989;152(6):1153-9.

70. Sherman Mary. Pathogenesis of disintegration of the hip in sickle cell anaemia. South Med. J. 1959;52:632-7.

71. Sheldon Blau, David Hamerman. Aseptic necrosis of the femoral heads in sickle-A Haemoglobin disease. Arthritis and rheumatism. 1967;10(4): 397-400.

72. Soloman L. Mechanism of idiopathic osteonecrosis; Orthop. Clinic. North Am. 1985;16(4): 655-67.

73. Stanley MK, Chung, Edgar L. Ralston necrosis of the femoral head asociated with Sickle cell anaemia and its genetic variants, J Bone and Joint Surgery Am. 1969;51A(1):33-58.

74. Stanley MK Chung, Abass Alavi, Marie O. Russell management of osteonecrosis in sickle cell anemia and it's genetic variants. Clin. Orthop. 1978;130:158.

75. Steinberg ME, Brighton CI, et al. Treatment of avascular necrosis of the femoral head by combination of bone grafting, decompression and electrical stimulation. Clin Orthop. 1984; 186:137-53.

76. Sugioka Y. Transtrochanteric rotational osteotomy of femoral head - Proceeding of Hip Society;1980.pp.3-23.

77. Taylor PW, Thorpe WP, Trueblood MC. Osteonecrosis in Sickle cell trait. J Rheumatol 1986;13(3):643-6.

78. Tanaka KR, George O, Clifford, Arnold R. Axelrod: Sickle cell anemia (Homozygous S) with aseptic necrosis of Femoral head. Blood 1956;11:998-1008.

79. Theis JC, Owen R. Skeletal complications in Sickle cell disease in the UK. J R Coll Surg Edinb 1988;33:306-10.

80. Totty WG, Murphy WA, Ganz WI, et al. Magnetic resonance imaging of the normal and ischaemic femoral head. AJR 1984;143:1273-80.

81. Wang CJ, Seet DE, Roger SI, Thomson EC. Fat cell changes as a mechanism of avascular necrosis of the femoral head in cortisone treated rabbits. J Bone and Joint Surgery [Am.] 1977;59A:729-35.

82. Wang CJ, Dughman SS, et al. The effect of core decompression of femoral head blood flow in steroid induced avascular necrosis of femoral head. J. Bone and Joint Surg. [Am.] 1985;67A:121-4.

83. Ware HE, Brooks AP, Toye R, Berney SI. Sickle cell disease and silent avascular necrosis of the Hip. J Bone and Joint Surgery Br. 1991;73(6):947-9.

84. Washington ER, Root L. Conservative treatment of sickle cell avascular necrosis of the femoral head. J Paediatr Orthop. 1985;5(2):192-4.

85. Wayne Alen S, Steven B Zelicof, Clement B Saldge, Total hip arthroplasty in Beta Thallassemia. Clin Orthop. 1993;294:149-54.

22

OSTEONECROSIS OF TALUS

Whenever osteonecrosis involves the bones of a joint (e.g. the talus), especially weight-bearing it often leads to destruction of cartilage, resulting in arthritis and pain. In the case of the talus, three joints can be affected; the ankle joint, the talonavicular joint, and the subtalar joint. The ankle joint allows up and down, flexion-extension movement of the foot, while the subtalar and talonavicular joints allow in and out, inversion-eversion movement of the foot. The normal function of the subtalar joint is to allow walking on uneven surfaces, inclined surfaces, ladders, etc. without falling. Osteonecrosis can be caused by two large categories—trauma and nontraumatic. In the case of trauma, a fracture of the bone disrupts the blood supply to the bone leading to osteonecrosis. There are many causes of nontraumatic osteonecrosis. These include idiopathic, steroid-induced, where high dose corticosteroids are given for such diseases as rheumatoid arthritis, lupus, and cancer, excess alcohol consumption, sickle cell anemia, radiation treatments, and chemotherapy. Osteonecrosis of the talus can be quite devastating, and can lead to total loss of the ankle joint with arthritis, deformity and pain (Figs 22.1A and B). The development of traumatic osteonecrosis is determined to a large extent by the type of the talus fracture. In

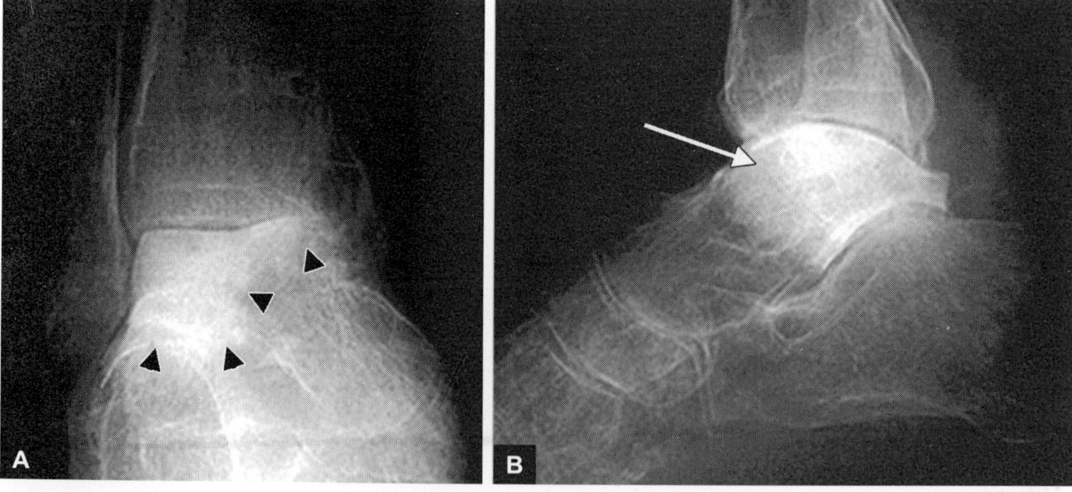

Figs 22.1A and B (A) Osteonecrosis of the talus. AP radiograph shows marked sclerosis of the talar dome and body (arrow heads); (B) X-ray (Lateral view) shows marked sclerosis of the entire talar dome and throughout the lateral talar region

the fractures, which are not very severe (they do not shift or displace much), the incidence of osteonecrosis is lower (Fig. 22.2). However, when the talus dislocates out of the ankle socket, the incidence of vascular necrosis is very high, almost 100 percent.[1]

The development of osteonecrosis is related to the type of the fracture, and not the manner in which it is treated. This is because of the blood supply to the talus, which is damaged with certain fracture types, and not with others, and regardless of how the talus is put back together, the blood supply cannot change. Interestingly however, the presence of osteonecrosis does not change the rate of healing of the fracture. If the fracture does not heal at all, this can result commonly in "non-union", and the fracture healing in a poor position, a "mal-union" is infrequently seen. Even in fractures where osteonecrosis does develop, the fractured bone invariably goes on to union. There seems to be just enough blood supply left coming across the fracture to heal it, but not enough to maintain the blood supply for a totally viable talus (Figs 22.3A to C: showing vascular supply of talus). This point is

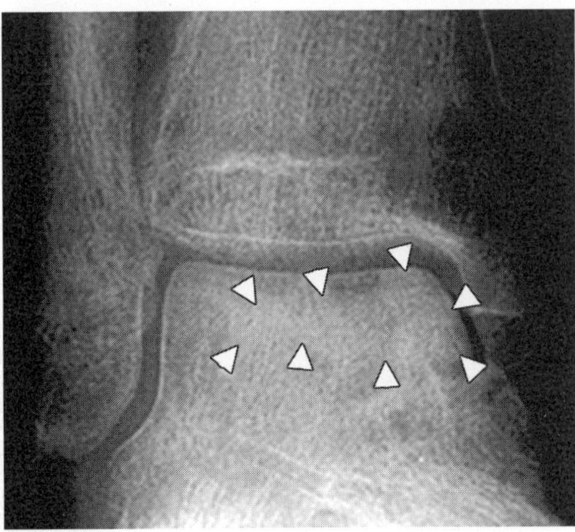

Fig. 22.2 X-ray (mortice view) shows an area of increased opacity in the medial talar dome that extends laterally toward the lateral talar dome (arrowheads), a finding that represents an osteonecrotic segment

important when planning treatment following treatment of the fracture.

The fracture of the talus has a high incidence of osteonecrosis, where one is concerned about the consequences of bone healing if it occurs. In that situation, the talus can break up into small pieces, fragment and collapse. This is not however predictable. The majority of fractures which develop osteonecrosis do not go on to collapse, and the avascular necrosis is limited to small segments of the talus (Fig. 22.2). Once osteonecrosis is suspected, it limits the patient from walking on the leg at all; worrying about the possibility that avascular necrosis would progress and lead to collapse of the bone. In fact, this has never been demonstrated to be necessary, and once the fracture has healed, bearing of weight on the leg is actually permissible. When considering osteonecrosis of the talus, it is convenient to classify the amount of bone that is involved by distinguishing small (osteochondral lesions), partial, and total involvement of the talus (Figs 22.4A and B). The osteochondral lesion of the talus can be considered to be a partial osteonecrosis.

A fracture of the talar neck can heal in the presence of avascular necrosis of the talus. It makes sense to distinguish between early- and late-stage osteonecrosis: - 'late' is more than 9 to 12 months after injury. In the late stages only a few options remain; one is arthrodesis and the other is talectomy. In the early stages it is important to notice whether the osteonecrosis has developed secondary to a fracture. The Hawkins' sign is the most helpful radiographic sign, the MRI also is useful, but may be too sensitive to offer any prognostic value or assist in algorithms that are used for treatment.[2,3] If subchondral atrophy in the talar dome is not present at six weeks or more weeks after fracture (absent Hawkins' sign) and the fracture has healed radiographically, the concern shifts to avoiding late segmental collapse of the talus. Creeping substitution of the talar body can take up to 36 months to complete.

There are few diseases, which causes osteo-necrosis of talus, commonly seen in sickle cell

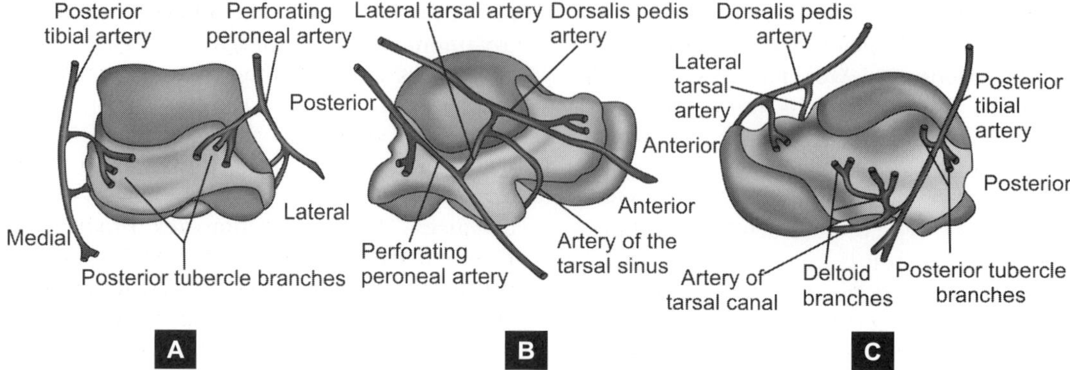

Figs 22.3A to C Drawings illustrate the blood supply of the talus. (A) Medial talar blood supply. The first branches of the posterior tibial artery are the posterior tubercle branches. More distally, the posterior tibial artery gives off the tarsal canal artery with its deltoid branches. This artery courses through the tarsal canal; (B) Lateral talar blood supply. The lateral tarsal artery connects the dorsalis pedis artery to the perforating peroneal artery. It also branches to form the tarsal sinus artery; (C) Inferior talar blood supply. The tarsal sinus artery and the tarsal canal artery form an anastomotic loop within the tarsal canal. Posterior talar blood supply. The posterior tubercle branches of the posterior tibial artery and perforating peroneal artery supply the medial and lateral tubercles

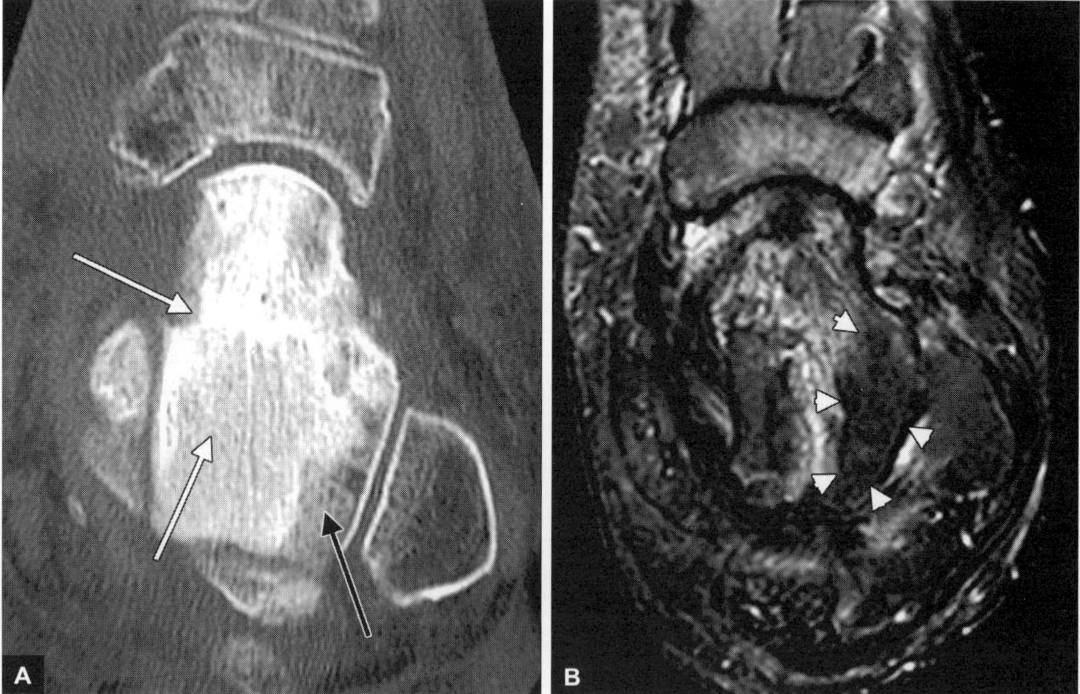

Figs 22.4A and B Osteonecrosis of the talus in a 42-year-old man following fracture talus after accident (A). Axial CT scan through the talus shows diffuse sclerosis involving the majority of the talus (white arrows), with focal sparing of the lateral talar dome (black arrow); (B) Axial fat-saturated T2-weighted MR image shows diffuse high signal intensity in the majority of the talus. The lateral talar dome demonstrates normal bone marrow signal intensity (arrowheads), a finding that corresponds to the normal region seen at CT

disease or after consumption of corticosteroid, etc. Lately it is also observed after organ transplantation. We have seen many patients of osteonecrosis of talus with sickle cell disease, after corticosteroid consumption (Figs 22.5 and 22.6) and few patients after renal transplantation (Figs 22.10 to 22.12), but the large bulk is after injury – Fracture or fracture dislocation of talus (Figs 22.7 to 22.9).

Controversy exists concerning the best way to treat patients who have a healed fracture and an absent Hawkins' sign that indicates osteonecrosis of the talar body. Penny and Davis[4] concluded that weight-bearing on a sclerotic and avascular talus poses no real danger for dome collapse, especially when the subsequent revascularization occurs slowly.

If, however, revascularization occurs rapidly, it will proceed to a profound structural weakness within the trabecular bone and result in gross collapse of the talar dome. There is no way to determine the period and speed with which the talus will revascularize; it has not been proven that non-weight-bearing prevents talar collapse. Therefore, some investigators suggest non-weight-bearing until fracture healing and until revascularization is complete,[5-8] whereas others propose protected weight-bearing in a patellar tendon-bearing (PTB) brace until revascularization has occurred.[9-11] A third group believes that it is impossible to keep the patients non or partially weight-bearing sufficiently; they concentrate instead on treating the sequelae symptomatically.[2,3,11] Poor results with osteonecrosis of the talus could not be correlated with the methods of treatment or time off from weight-bearing.[3] If the fracture is healed and there is no pain, progressive weight-bearing is accepted and is recommended (also for bone remodeling).[12] There is no evidence to suggest that the patient has to remain off the foot using crutches for an indefinite period of time to prevent the talus from collapsing further. The foot may need

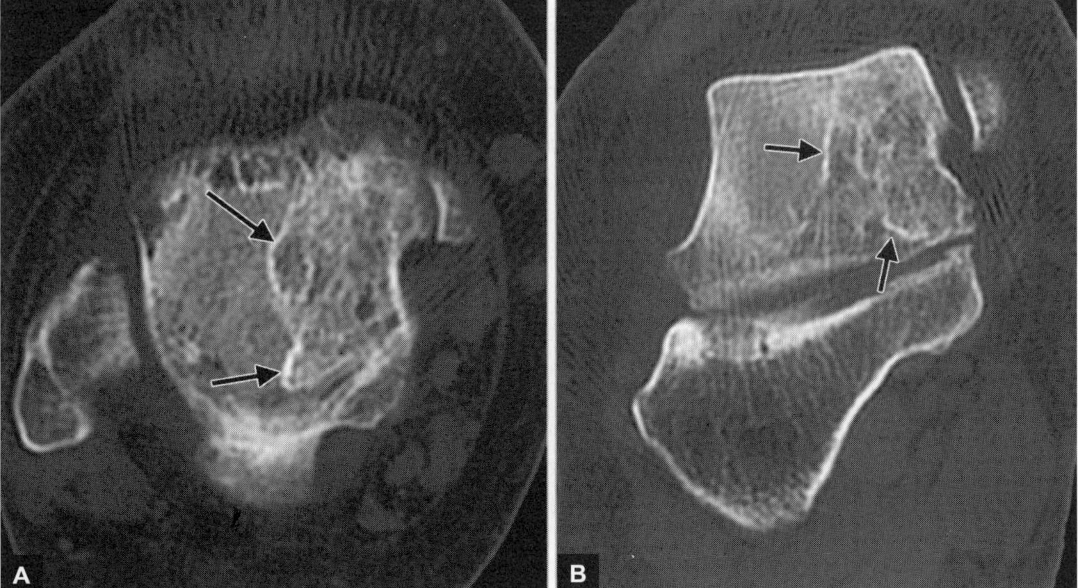

Figs 22.5A and B Osteonecrosis of the talus in a 51-year-old woman who had received steroids. (A and B) CT scans through the right talus show a mixed hypoattenuating-sclerotic pattern along the medial half of the talar dome that is outlined by a serpiginous sclerotic line (arrows). The mixed imaging pattern is consistent with osteonecrosis

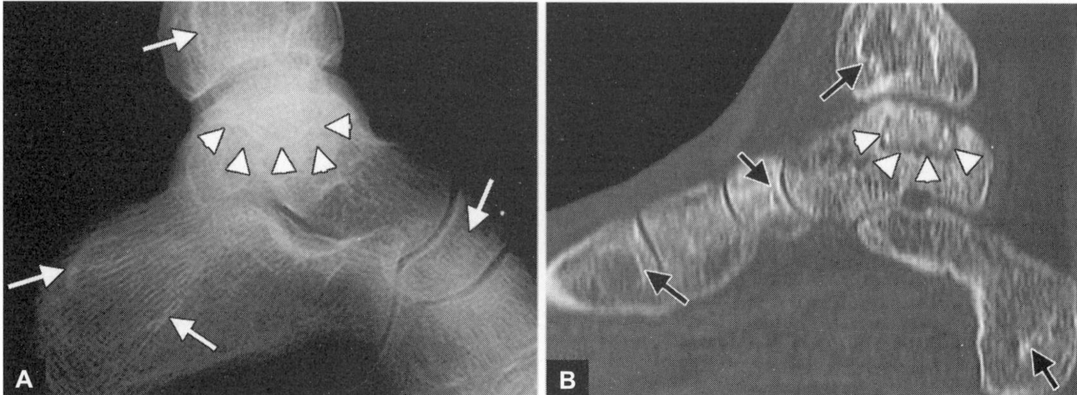

Figs 22.6A and B Osteonecrosis of the talus in a 42-year-old man who was receiving steroids for collagenosis. (A) Lateral X-ray of the ankle shows a large, curvilinear radiolucent cleft extending from the talar dome into the talar body (arrowheads). In addition, there is serpiginous sclerosis within the distal tibia, calcaneus, and navicular bone (arrows); (B) Corresponding CT image of the ankle shows a hypo attenuating area (arrowheads) surrounding a collapsed fragment of the talar dome. Areas of serpiginous sclerosis within the distal tibia, calcaneus, navicular bone, and base of the first metatarsal bone are again evident (arrows), findings that are consistent with medullary infarcts

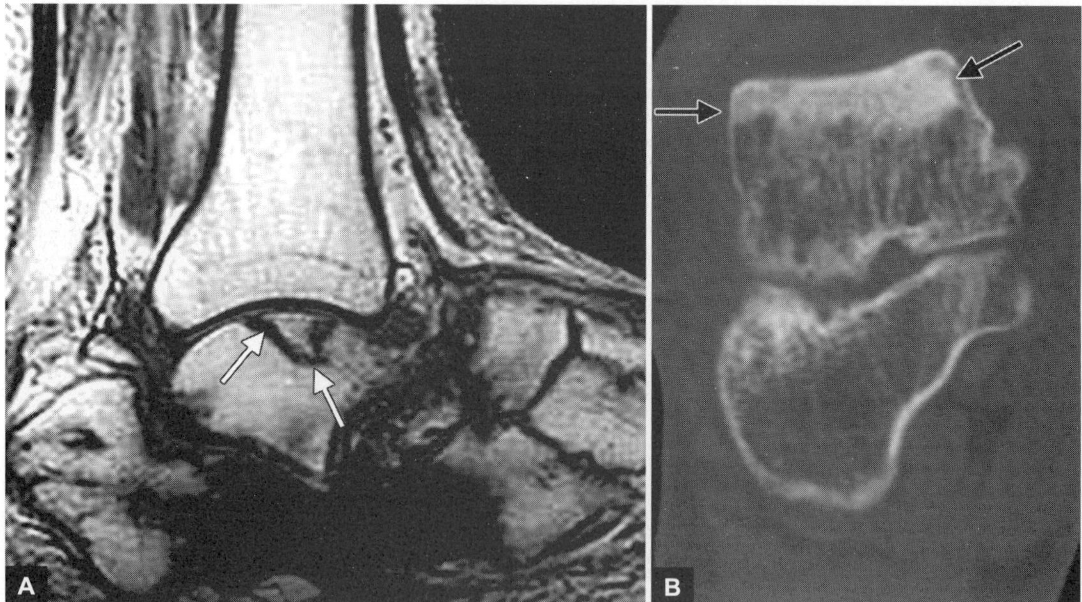

Figs 22.7A and B (A) Post-traumatic osteonecrosis of the talus in a 42-year-old man, MRI (T1) scan through the ankle demonstrates a serpiginous low-signal-intensity line in the talar dome (arrows); (B) Osteonecrosis of the talus in a 33-year-old man with a talar neck fracture: CT scan through the talar dome shows an irregular, approximately 1 cm-thick region of subchondral sclerosis spanning the entire width of the dome (arrows)

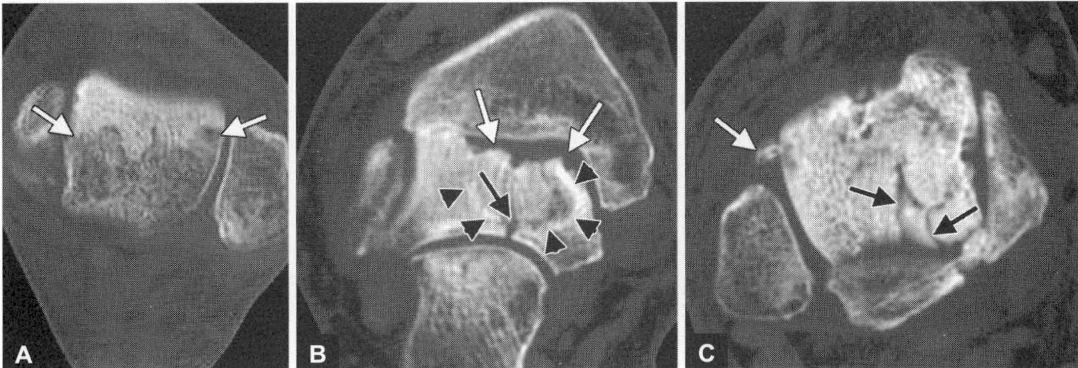

Figs 22.8A to C (A) Showing osteonecrosis of the anterior talus in a 33-year-old male after injury. CT scan through the talar dome reveals focal sclerosis in the anterior part of the dome (arrows), a finding that corresponds to an osteonecrotic segment; (B and C) Collapse and fragmentation of the talus in a 61-year-old man who had sustained minor trauma. (B) Coronal CT scan of the ankle shows collapse of the articular surface of the talar dome (white arrows) and a vertical split fracture extending from the talar dome into the subtalar joint (black arrow). In addition, there is a curvilinear sclerotic line within the talar body (arrowheads) that represents necrotic bone. (C) Corresponding axial CT scan through the talar dome shows linear fractures through the posterior aspect of the dome (black arrows). The bone attenuation of the talar dome looks diffusely increased compared with that of the distal tibia and fibula. In addition, there is a small, ossific hyperattenuating area at the lateral aspect of the talus (white arrow), likely due to prior trauma

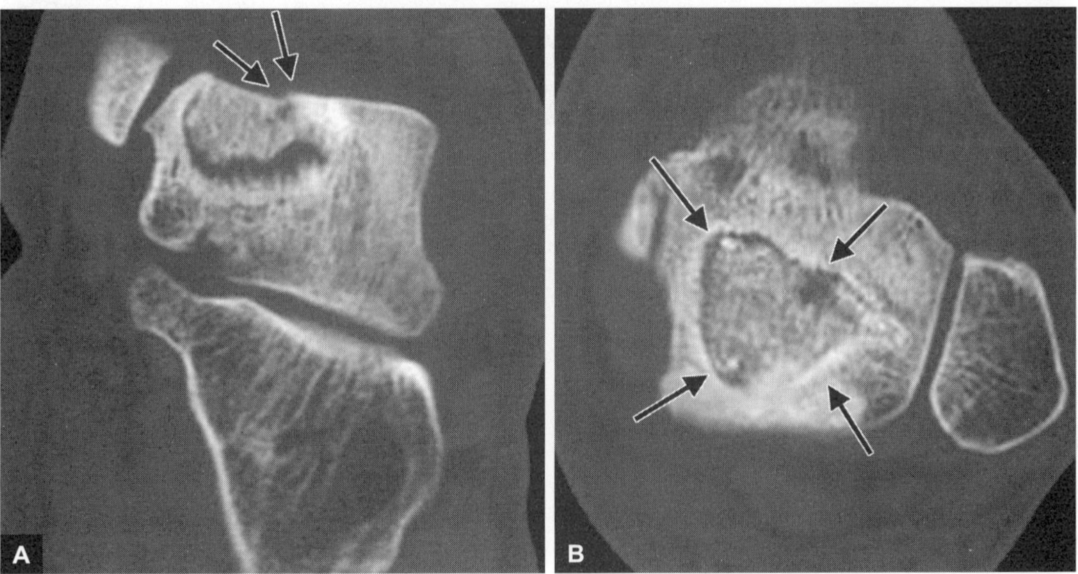

Figs 22.9A and B Severe osteonecrosis of the talus with collapse of the talar dome. (A) Coronal CT scan through the talus shows a large hypoattenuating area surrounding an osteonecrotic segment of the medial talar dome, with a 1 mm articular step-off due to collapse of the medial articular surface (arrows); (B) Axial CT scan through the talar dome clearly depicts the large osteonecrotic segment (arrows), a finding that corresponds to the collapsed fragment seen

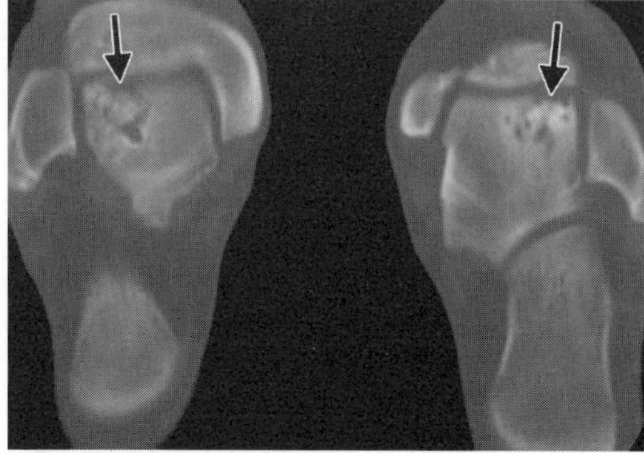

Fig. 22.10 Bilateral osteonecrosis of the talus in an 18-year-old man who had undergone renal transplantation. Coronal CT scan of both ankles shows collapse of the articular surface of the lateral talar domes bilaterally (arrows), with underlying mixed hypoattenuating sclerotic regions of necrotic subchondral bone

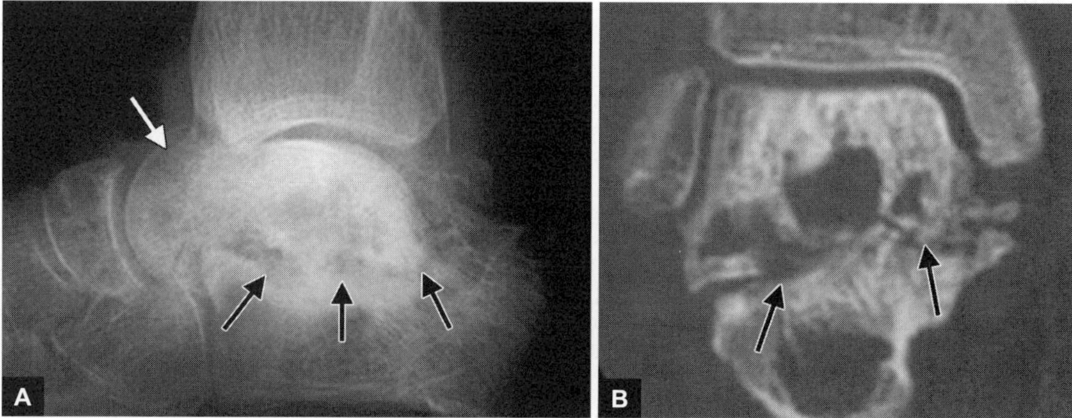

Figs 22.11A and B (A) Osteonecrosis of the talus in a female patient who had undergone renal transplantation. Lateral X-ray of the right ankle shows diffuse sclerosis of the entire talus due to osteonecrosis, with sparing of the superior aspect of the talar head (white arrow). The inferior aspect of the talus shows irregular radiolucency (black arrows), with severe narrowing and anterior subluxation of the subtalar joint; (B) Coronal CT scan through the ankle shows sclerosis of the talar dome due to necrosis, along with multiple cystic hypoattenuating areas and fragmentation of the inferior articular surface of the talus (arrows)

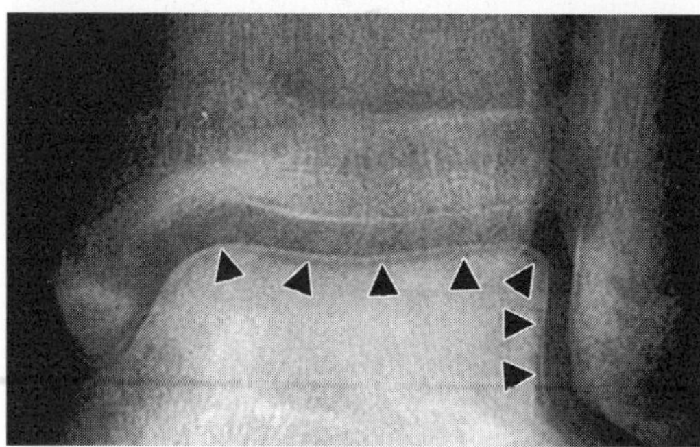

Fig. 22.12 X-ray of the ankle reveal striking subchondral radiolucency (arrowheads), a finding that indicates talar viability, called as Hawkins' sign

to be protected, using a boot or a brace, and certain activities with impact on the leg may need to be restricted, but walking should be acceptable. Once collapse of the talus occurs, then problems begin, including arthritis and deformity. The two best courses of the disease are spontaneous resolution or the wearing of a PTB and continuing to a complete resolution. If that does not occur, the orthopedic surgeon has two options-core decompression and bone grafting. These are very difficult problems to correct surgically, but with the newer methods of reconstructive surgery, results and final outcome have been very successful.

TREATMENT OPTIONS

Core Decompression

One of the surgical options is core decompression. The principal behind this technique is to drill a hole in the talus, which may lead to decompression of the bone and resultant healing of the talus because it increases the blood supply to the talus. This has been successfully used for osteonecrosis of other joints and bones. It can only be used at the early stages of osteonecrosis of talus (Figs 22.13 and 22.14).

The theory behind core decompression-to decrease intraosseous pressure and to enhance revascularization is well known. It is only recommended in Stages I and II of osteonecrosis of the talus. We use either a small, 1.5 to 2 mm drill or a 4.0 mm drill to perforate the area of the necrotic lesion. With the small drill it is preferred to put several holes (8–10), whereas with the 4.0 mm drill only use 2 to 4 holes. It is easy to use the posterolateral approach between the peroneal tendons and the Achilles tendon (Fig. 22.14). Rarely, other approaches are used (e.g. a lateral or medial one, through small incisions with a little dissection). Typically, 70% of patients have reduced pain and increased motion and would be considered to have a good result. Postoperatively, the patients are put in a short leg cast for two weeks and start range of

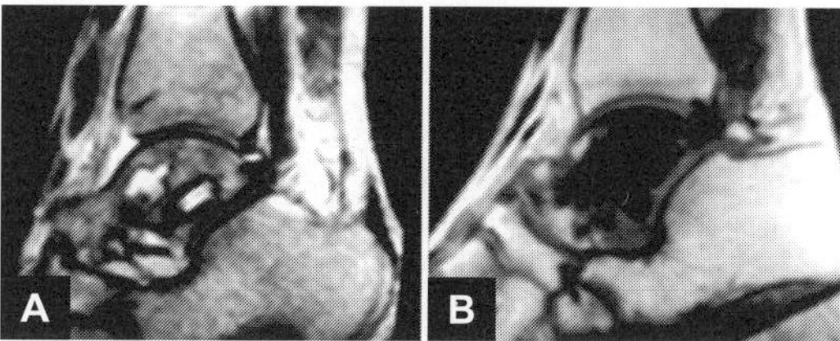

Figs 22.13A and B MRI showing presence of irregular shadows in the middle of talus – suggesting osteonecrosis

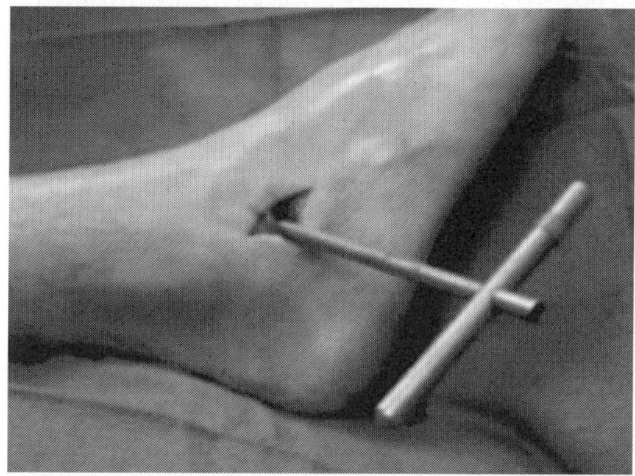

Fig. 22.14 Operating room picture showing a large bore for decompression *(For color version, see Plate 5)*

motion exercises after wound healing. Most patients are treated with a PTB brace. After six weeks, partial weight-bearing is allowed and is increased individually to full weight-bearing.

Mont et al.[13] reviewed 11 patients (17 ankles) who had core decompression for symptomatic osteonecrosis of the talus before collapse. The Mazur grading system was used to assess function preoperatively and at final follow-up; radiographs were graded according to the Ficat and Arlet classification that was modified for the ankle. At a mean follow-up of seven years (range, 2 to 14 years) 14 ankles (82%) had an excellent or good outcome [Mazur scores N 80 points; pain scores N 40 points (range, 41 to 50)]. The other three ankles required tibiotalar fusion at a mean of 13 months (range, 5 to 20) after core decompression. The investigators concluded that core decompression is a viable method for the treatment of symptomatic osteonecrosis of the talus before collapse.

In 1998, Delanois et al.[14] reviewed 37 ankles in 24 patients who were treated at their institution between July 1, 1974, and December 31, 1996 for atraumatic osteonecrosis of the talus. The mean duration of symptoms before the patients were seen was 5.4 months (range, 2 months to 2 years). The mean ankle score at the time of presentation was 34 points (range, 2 to 75 points), according to the system of Mazur et al.[15] A radiographic review revealed-according to the system of Ficat and Arletthat eight ankles had Stage III or IV disease of the talus at presentation. The remaining 29 ankles had Stage II disease.

Thirty-two ankles that remained severely symptomatic were treated with core decompression, which was useful in the treatment of precollapse (Stage II) disease. Twenty-nine of these ankles had a fair to excellent clinical outcome at a mean of 7 years (range, 2 to 15 years) postoperatively; the remaining 3 ankles had an arthrodesis after the core decompression failed. Three ankles were treated initially with an arthrodesis for postcollapse (Stages III or IV) disease. All 6 of the ankles that had an arthrodesis fused at a mean of 7 months (range, 5 to 9 months) postoperatively. When patients who have a history of osteonecrosis of the hip, are seen because of pain in the ankle, the diagnosis of osteonecrosis of the talus should be considered. Early detection may allow the ankle to be treated nonoperatively or with core decompression, and thus, reduce the need for arthrodesis.

If the pain disappears after core decompression, they are allowed full-weight-bearing, and are followed-up for reassessment every 3 months. If there is no segmental collapse and no pain, it is considered favorable and problem appears to be resolved. In cases of increasing pain when weight-bearing is progressed, bone grafting is the next reasonable option. Generally four types of bone graft are available for these cases non-vascularized auto or allograft and vascularized pedicle or free autograft. There are no long-term results with large bone substitutes and has no personal experience.

Muscle Flap

Another option is a vascularized muscular transfer. The principle behind this technique is to swing a muscle to this area which brings a blood supply with it.

Bone Grafting

Nonvascularized Autograft

The non-vascularized autograft from the iliac crest is probably the most widely used bone graft, followed by the allograft (e.g. talus, femoral head). With the increasing symptoms one may decide to treat osteonecrosis surgically. One may use a tricortical iliac crest bone graft as a scaffold and additional cancellous bone graft after excising the necrosis. The approach is a lateral one with a fibular osteotomy. Postoperatively, the rest of the void is filled with cancellous bone graft. Postoperatively, the patient should be nonweight-bearing for six weeks and then started on protected partial weight-bearing in a Controlled Ankle Motion with walker with mobilization exercises.

Vascular Bone Graft

Another option is a vascularized bone transfer. The principle behind this technique is to place a bone with its blood supply to the talus. In 1989, Hussl et al.[16] reported a vascularized bone graft from the iliac crest that was used for revascularization of the talus in post-traumatic osteonecrosis in a 16-year-old patient. The first cuneiform was found to be supplied by the middle pedicle branch of the distal medial tarsal artery. This is a short pedicle that can be used for navicular pseudarthrosis but is too short for the talus. Basically, the same is true for the next pedicle of the transverse branch to the third cuneiform off the distal lateral tarsal artery. The fourth potential vascular pedicle was a transverse segment of the anterior lateral malleolar artery to the lateral malleolus. This pedicle also is approximately 4 cm long but usually is an extremely small vessel.

Shock Wave

Yet another option for talar osteonecrosis is the use of shock wave (extracorporeal shock wave therapy-ESWT). It is a high-intensity acoustic application (also used to break up kidney stones). No surgery is required, but you do have to be put to sleep in the operating room. The application of shock wave therapy in certain musculoskeletal disorders has been around for approximately 15 years, and the success rate in non-union of long bone fracture, calcifying tendonitis of the shoulder, tennis elbow and plantar fasciitis ranged from 65 to 91 percent. The complications are low. Recently, shock wave therapy was extended to treat other conditions including osteonecrosis of the femoral head, patellar tendonitis (jumper's knee), osteochondritis dessicans and non-calcifying tendonitis of the shoulder. Shock wave therapy is a novel therapeutic modality without the need of surgery and it's risks. It is convenient and cost-effective. The exact mechanism of shock wave therapy remains unknown. Shock wave induces blood vessel formation, which can treat the underlying cause of talar osteonecrosis.

▮ SALVAGE PROCEDURES: ARTHRODESIS

What are the options if the aforementioned methods do not work? There are several salvage possibilities (e.g. ankle arthrodesis, subtalar arthrodesis, tibiotalocalcaneal arthrodesis). All of these arthrodeses are disabling to the patient. Although they may revascularize the body of the talus to some extent, the patient is left with a pronounced gait abnormality and the expected future complication of arthritis in the surrounding joints.

Fusion

The classical way to treat talar osteonecrosis is with an ankle fusion. It is recommended to place the ankle in neutral dorsiflexion-plantarflexion, 0 to 5 of hindfoot valgus, and 5 to 10 of external rotation with the talus translated posteriorly.[17-19] If possible, the talus should be positioned exactly under the tibia. The surgeon always should examine the contralateral side for individual modifications in position; generally, the hindfoot is realigned with the leg and the foot is positioned plantigrade. Many techniques can be used that combine a preferred approach with a preferred method of arthrodesis and fixation. Special circumstances, however, might necessitate alteration of a preferred approach or the use of different fixation techniques. In general, there are surgical principles to be followed (e.g. creating broad, congruent cancellous bone surfaces and stabilizing with rigid internal fixation). If there is no or little malalignment of the ankle joint, it is possible to perform an arthroscopic ankle arthrodesis.[20] Using the anterolateral, medial, and posterolateral portals, the surgeon performs an anterior synovectomy and debridement of the ankle with a full radius shaver. Then the articular surfaces are denuded of cartilage with the periosteal elevator followed by a power burr. The medial and lateral gutter are also denuded to expose bleeding subchondral bone, while maintaining the contour of the bony surfaces. Internal or external fixation *in situ* is accomplished by two or three percutaneous, cannulated or non-cannulated cancellous screws that are parallel or converging. The advantages of this method are less blood loss, a shorter time to union, and an increased union rate because of the minimal interruption of the surrounding soft tissue with subsequent better blood supply. Furthermore, there are fewer complications in patients who have compromised healing potential (e.g. vascular disease, diabetes, rheumatoid arthritis, history of corticosteroid use, previous skin or soft tissue flaps). The main disadvantages are that deformities cannot be corrected if they are more than a few degrees and severe bone deficiencies cannot be addressed well.

The mini-open technique is similar to the arthroscopic technique but the portals are extended to an anterolateral and anteromedial 1.5 to 2 cm incision. The advantages and disadvantages correspond with those of the arthroscopic technique. It is important to close the anterior capsule meticulously. With this technique it is possible to perform additional iliac crest grafting. Several investigators have offered modifications of the open technique. Simin et al.[21] described a technique with a distal tibial inlay graft without fixation that may be used as a primary or secondary salvage procedure. Lionberger et al.[22] reported a 28 percent pseudarthrosis rate and fibrous ankylosis secondary to prolonged immobilization. They developed a modified Blair fusion and suggested using a pediatric hip compression screw and a modified Stone staple for fixation. Morris[23] modified Blair's technique by placing a screw in the tibial inlay and using a longitudinal Steinmann pin. Patterson et al.[24] described a technique with an anterior sliding graft to provide fixation and fusion. They used an anterolateral approach and limited the periosteal elevation to the anterior aspect of the tibia in the region of the graft site. The joint is debrided of cartilage and fibrous tissue while maintaining its shape. The anterior tibial graft (1.2 cm wide, 1.5 cm depth, 5 cm long) is cut out with a saw and removed. After positioning the ankle in the desired position, the quadrilateral area in the talar dome is marked through the tibial defect with the talus positioned posterior in the tibia plafond. The bone is removed from the talus in a plantar flexed position. One 6.5 mm screw is inserted from the posterior medial malleolus directed anteriorly and one 6.5 mm screw is inserted from the anterior lateral tibia into the posterior talus. The tibial graft is implanted and fixed with two 4.5 mm screws. The postoperative treatment includes six weeks of nonweight-bearing and six weeks in a short leg cast with weight-bearing as tolerated. There is a moderate risk of an anterior stress fracture of the tibia.

The technique that was proposed by Mann and Rongstad[25] in 1998 includes a transfibular approach with resection of the distal fibula; this allows good joint visualization. They did not propose to maintain joint shape but preferred two matched parallel cuts on the distal tibia and the talar dome. This is especially necessary to correct massive malalignment or angular deformities. Two parallel interfragmentary compression screws are inserted from the sinus tarsi into the tibia with the screw tip engaging the medial tibial cortex. The screw heads are buried in the sinus tarsi. A partial or total resection of the medial malleolus may be necessary. In cases of total resection, an additional screw or another fixation device should be considered. Rarely does the surgeon need to augment with medial staples.

Another described technique is the "*In situ* dowel grafting" method, which consists of using a rotated bone plug in patients who have rheumatoid arthritis or painful, non-deformed ankles. This technique includes using a hollow trocar to create a plug of bone that is approximately 8 mm in diameter and is cut across the ankle parallel to the joint surface. The plug is then rotated 90°.

Besides fixing the arthrodesis site with screws, the surgeon can use different external fixators (e.g. monoplanar, multi-planar) or plate fixation. If using a lateral plate, a large or small fragment T-plate is applied to the lateral side (compression type) or a pediatric 90° osteotomy compression plate can be used. The other possibility is to use a double T-plate fixation, that is stronger than the fibular strut fixation (lateral fibular strut is fixed with two 4.5 mm screws in the tibia)—with the crossed screw fixation (6.5 mm).

Total Ankle Replacement

Traditionally, when arthritis of the ankle joint occurs after osteonecrosis and talus fracture, a fusion of the ankle has been recommended (Fig. 22.15). This fusion is a complicated operation, and the results of the fusion are not always predictable and ankle motion is lost. For this reason, alternative treatments are desirable. In particular, instead of the fusion of both the ankle and the subtalar joint, an ankle joint replacement can be performed (Figs 22.16A to C). This is an exciting alternative, and many workers are gaining more experience with this surgery over time. Now, with newer

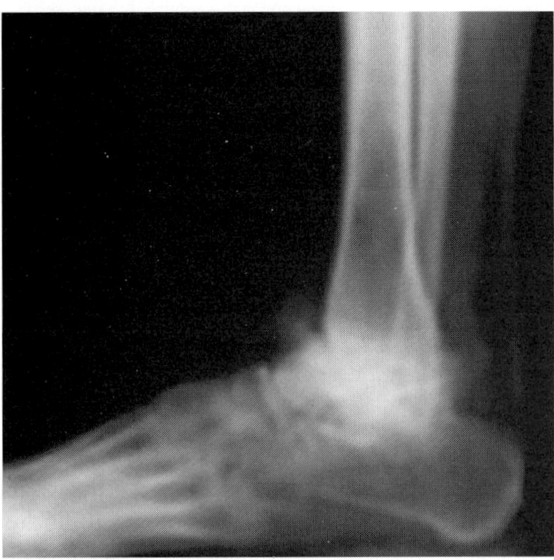

Fig. 22.15 Osteonecrosis of talus showing the collapse of talus with secondary arthritis

total ankle replacement implants, one can make custom implants when necessary.

Total Talus Replacement

Lastly, a complete total talus replacement can be used.

Summary of the Treatment of Osteonecrosis of the Talus

Osteonecrosis of the talus is a challenging disease process with respect to pathophysiology and treatment.

As always in medicine, the treatment needs to be individualized. Arthrodesis always should be the last option and is a challenging procedure.

1. ***Fusion of the ankle:*** This has been a treatment recommended but of course glues together the ankle and limits the flexion and extension range of motion permanently. The fusion is not easy to accomplish, and the success rate of this type of surgery can be unpredictable.

2. ***Total ankle replacement:*** Total ankle replacement is now an accepted treatment for ankle arthritis, but cannot always be performed if osteonecrosis is present. The ankle replacement must have a good bone to sit on, and if the necrotic lesion is extensive, it cannot be performed. However, if a fusion of the subtalar joint is performed first (sometimes using a custom implant), there is often sufficient bone underneath the talus then to support the ankle prosthesis.

3. ***Drilling of the talus (Core decompression):*** There is a lot of evidence that by creating a hole with either a drill or a device that looks like a kitchen tool used to core an apple, one can increase the blood supply to the talus. The drilling creates little holes and channels that allow tiny little blood vessels to grow and improve the blood supply to the talus.

4. ***Muscle flap:*** All muscle has a blood supply to it in order to stay alive. Frank Horst

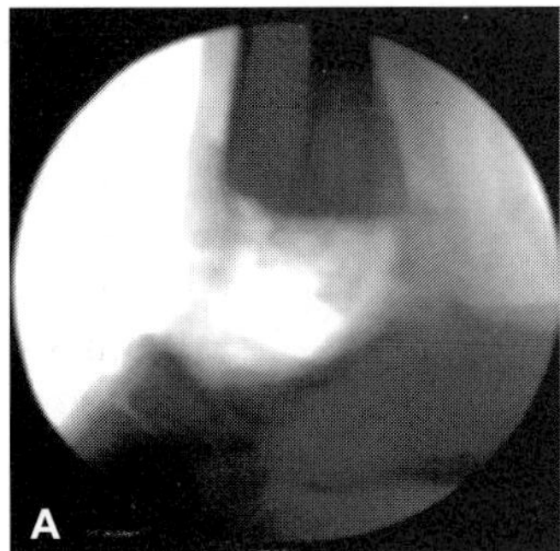
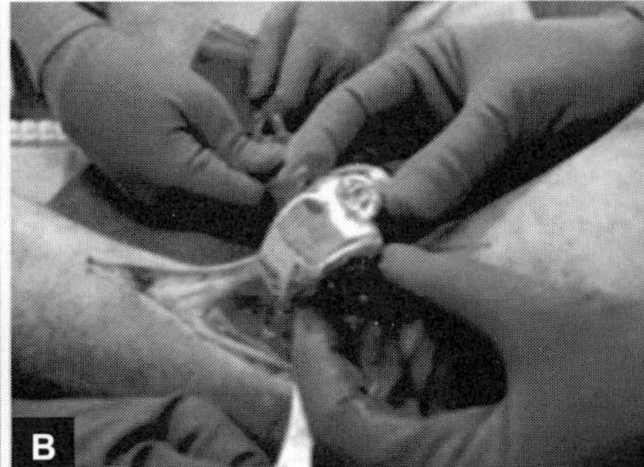
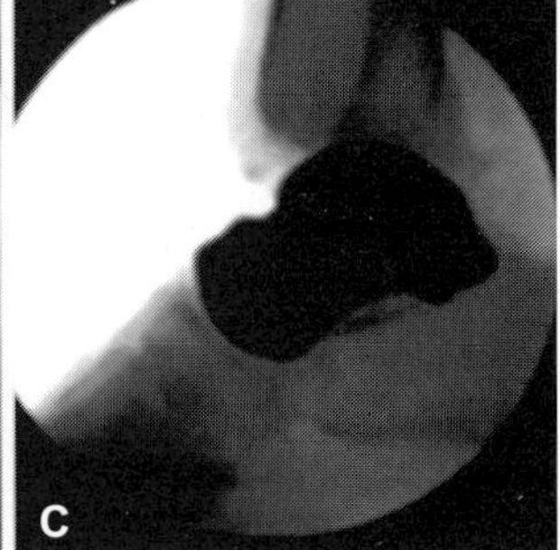

Figs 22.16A to C (A) Operating room X-ray after removal of talus; (B) Clinical picture showing talar prosthesis; (C) X-ray in OT after implantation of talar prosthesis (*For color version of Figure 22.16B, see Plate 5*)

et al.[17] developed an operation which moves a small muscle on the side of the outside of the foot into the talus. This is a new procedure, and with the short-term follow-up of these patients, the results seem to be good.

5. ***Free vascularized bone graft:*** It is possible to take a tiny blood vessel attached to a piece of bone and using the microscope, to transplant this into the talus.

6. ***Shock wave therapy (SWT):*** This is a nonsurgical method that increases the blood supply to the talus.

7. ***Total talus replacement:*** This is a novel technique of replacing the talus with a metal implant.

REFERENCES

1. Canale ST, Kelly Jr FB. Fractures of the neck of the talus. Long-term evaluation of seventy-one cases. J Bone Joint Surg Am. 1978;60:143–56.
2. Hawkins LG. Fractures of the neck of the talus. J Bone Joint Surg Am. 1970;52:991-1002.
3. Henderson RC. Post-traumatic necrosis of the talus: the Hawkins sign versus magnetic resonance imaging. J Orthop Trauma. 1991;5(1): 96–9.
4. Penny JN, Davis LA. Fractures and fracture-dislocations of the neck of the talus. J Trauma. 1980;20:1029–37.
5. Adelaar RS. The treatment of complex fractures of the talus. Orthop Clin North Am. 1989;20: 691–707.
6. Canale ST. Fractures of the neck of the talus. Orthopedics. 1990;10:1105–15.
7. Kenwright J, Taylor RG. Major injuries of the talus. J Bone Joint Surg Br. 1970;52:36–48.
7a. Wright DG, Adelaar RS. Avascular necrosis of the talus. Foot Ankle Int. 1995;16:743–4.
8. Comfort TH, Behrens F, Gaither DW, Denis F, Sigmond M. Long-term results of displaced talar neck fractures. Clin Orthop. 1985;199:81–7.
9. Grob D, Simpson LA, Weber BG, Bray T. Operative treatment of displaced talus fractures. Clin Orthop. 1985;199:88–96.
10. Szyszkowitz R, Reschauer R, Seggl W. Eighty-five talus fractures treated by ORIF with five to eight years of follow-up study of 69 patients. Clin Orthop. 1985;199:97–107.
11. Rammelt S, Zwipp H, Gavlik JM. Avascular necrosis after minimally displaced talus fracture in a child. Foot Ankle Int. 2000;21:1030–6.
12. Trauth J, Blasius K. Talusnekrose und ihre Behandlung. [Talus necrosis and its treatment]. Aktuelle Traumatol. 1988;18:152–6. [in German].
13. Mont MA, Schon LC, Hungerford MW, et al. Avascular necrosis of the talus treated by core decompression. J Bone Joint Surg Br. 1996;78:827–30.
14. Delanois RE, Mont MA, Yoon TR, Mizell M, Hungerford DS. Atraumatic osteonecrosis of the talus. J Bone Joint Surg Am. 1998;80:529–36, Rec #: 140.
15. Mazur JM, Schwartz E, Simon SR. Ankle arthrodesis. Long-term follow-up with gait analysis. J Bone Joint Surg Am. 1979;61(7): 964–75.
16. Hussl H, Sailer R, Daniaux H, Pechlaner S. Revascularization of a partially necrotic talus with a vascularized bone graft from the iliac crest. Arch Orthop Trauma Surg. 1989;108: 27–9.
17. Horst F, Gilbert BJ, and Nunley JA. Avascular necrosis of the talus:current treatment options. Foot Ankle Clin N Am. 2004;9:757-73.
18. P, Morrey BF, Chao EY. The optimum position of arthrodesis of the ankle. A gait study of the knee and ankle. J Bone Joint Surg Am. 1987;69: 1052–62.
19. Horst F, Nunley JA. Ankle arthrodesis. J Surg Orthop Adv. 2004;13(2):81–90.
20. Myerson MS, Quill G. Ankle arthrodesis. A comparison of an arthroscopic and an open method of treatment. Clin Orthop. 1991;268: 84–95.
21. Simin RM, O'Neil Jr CJ, Karlin JM, Silvani SH, Scurran BL. Fractures of the neck of the talus and the Blair fusion: a review of the literature and case report. Clin Pediatr Med Surg. 1988;5: 393–420.
22. Lionberger DR, Bishop JO, Tullos HS. The modified Blair fusion. Foot Ankle. 1982;3:60–2.
23. Morris HD, Hand WL, Dunn AW. The modified Blair fusion for fractures of the talus. J Bone Joint Surg Am. 1971;53(7):1289–97.
24. Patterson BM, Inglis AE, Moeckel BH. Anterior sliding graft for tibiotalar arthrodesis. Foot Ankle Int. 1997;18:330–4.
25. Mann RA, Rongstad KM. Arthrodesis of the ankle: a critical analysis. Foot Ankle Int. 1998; 19:3–9.

23

HAND-FOOT SYNDROME

Sickle cell dactylitis, hand-foot syndrome is a frequently misdiagnosed condition occurring in infants and young children with sickle cell disease and is supposed to be a acute presentation of osteonecrosis of smaller bones of the hand and feet. On many occasions this is the earliest and only clinical manifestation. This syndrome of temporary ischemia is clinically presented as swelling of hand and feet of acute onset. It usually occurs before the age of five years and is commonly seen in infants. The clinical picture of acute swelling of both hands and feet is accompanied by severe anemia, fever and leukocytosis and may be associated with crisis or respiratory infection. Skeletal manifestations of sickle cell hemoglobinopathy were seen in 944 patients, 46 out of which had hand-foot syndrome.[1] All the 46 patients were admitted in the stage of sickle cell crisis. The workup of these patients involved hematological investigations and radiology of the involved part.

OBSERVATIONS

All these children were very sick and most of the time in sickle cell crisis. The radiological picture of this syndrome is quite characteristic and is commonly observed between 7 and 14 days after the onset of symptoms.[1,2] After the onset of swelling of hands and feet (Figs 23.1 and 23.2), the earliest radiological change is appearance of subperiosteal new bone formation in one or multiple metacarpals or phalanges. There is cortical thinning and there are multiple irregular intramedullary deposits,

areas of spotty destruction and periosteal destruction is commonly seen (Figs 23.3 to 23.5). Usually, the symptoms are bilateral and

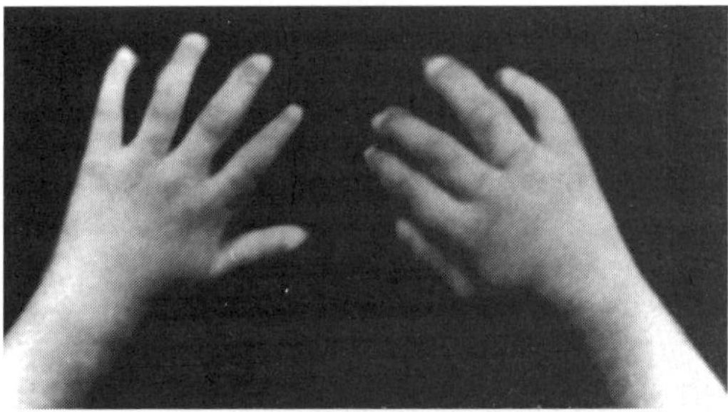

Fig. 23.1 Clinical photograph of a three-year-old child of sickle cell disease with SS pattern showing marked swelling of both the hands with fusiform swelling of fingers. Patient was admitted with acute illness in the stage of sickle cell crisis

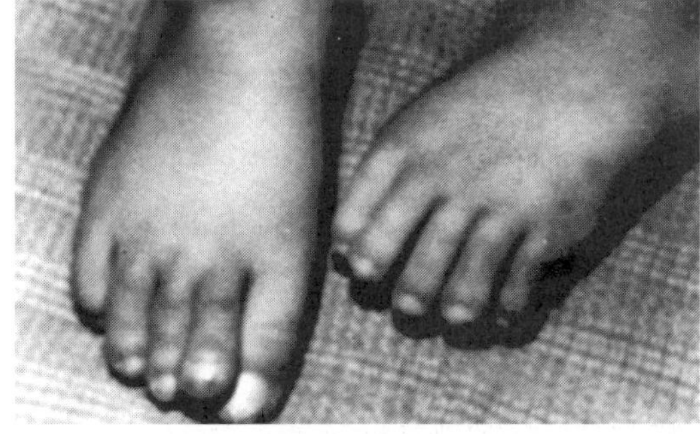

Fig. 23.2 Clinical photograph of a two-year-old child of sickle cell trait with AS pattern showing symmetrical swelling of both feet. Patient had a severe anemia, was in poor general condition, debilitated, dehydrated and was admitted in crisis

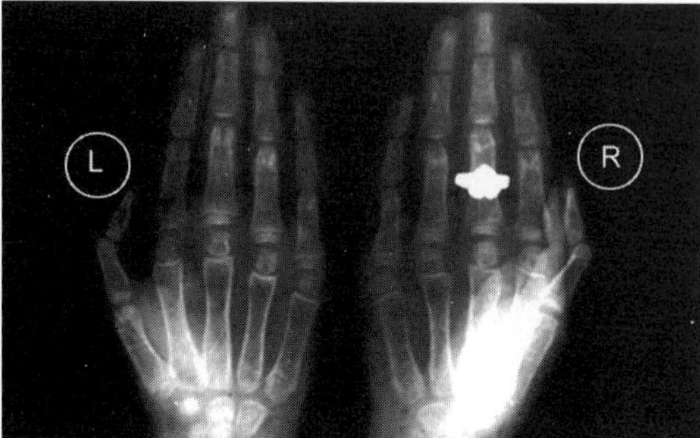

Fig. 23.3 X-ray of both hands showing typical radiological features of hand-foot syndrome. There is cortical thinning of metacarpals, phalanges with areas of intramedullary deposits and rectangular shape of metacarpals

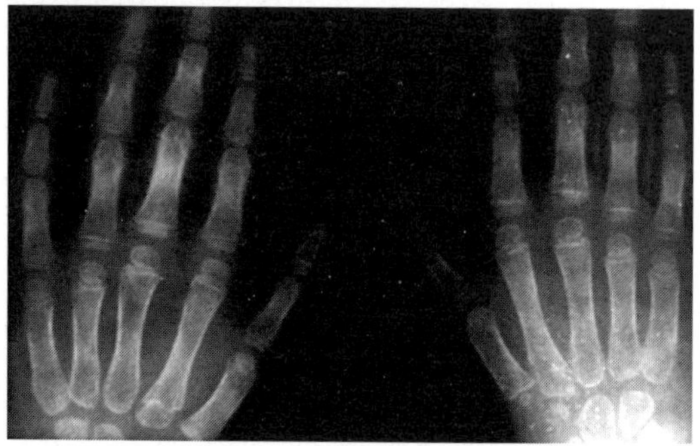

Fig. 23.4 X-ray of both hands showing intramedullary deposits with spotty destruction and cortical thinning

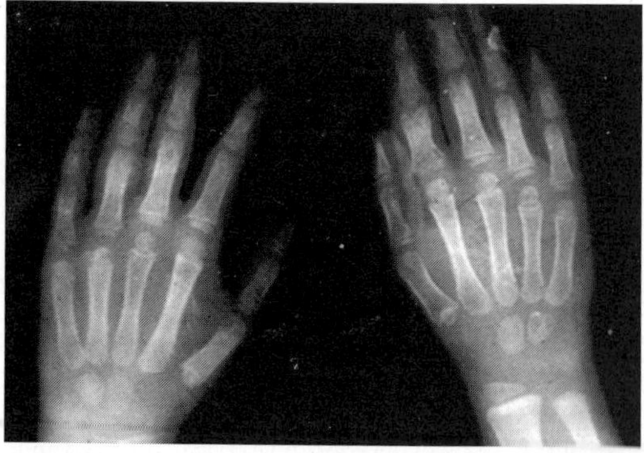

Fig. 23.5 X-ray of both hands showing spotty areas of intramedullary deposits and destruction with subperiosteal new bone formation

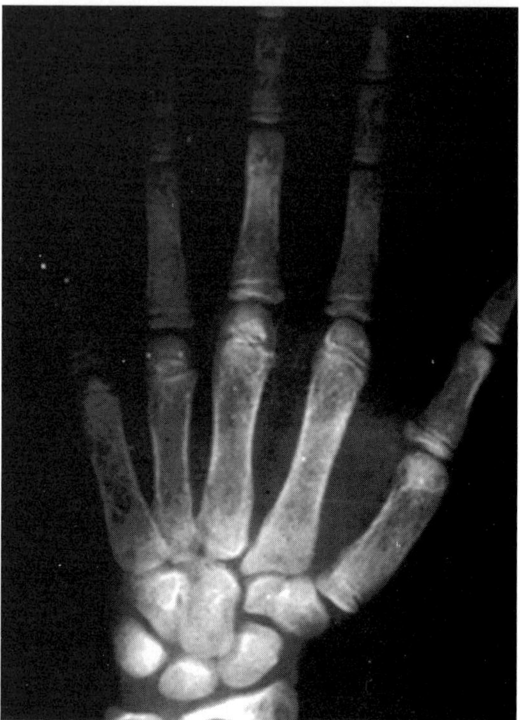

Fig. 23.6 X-ray of the hand showing fine and prominent trabeculations with intramedullary deposits and the moth-eaten appearance

at times symmetrical. The smaller bones of the hands and feet become rectangular in outline and shape. Since, the lesion usually causes periosteal elevation because of subperiosteal new bone formation, radiolucent areas intermingled with areas of increased density it give "moth-eaten" appearance (Fig. 23.6). Hand-foot syndrome presents as mottled, lucent and sclerotic patches seen in shafts of metacarpals, metatarsals, and phalanges with periosteal changes (Figs 23.7 and 23.8).

Watson J, Burco H et al.[3] 1963 designated "Hand-Foot Syndrome" as painful swelling of hands and feet seen in thrombotic crisis in young children. The clinical manifestation described was seen only in children under six years of age. At the onset the child usually had concomitant respiratory infection and fever. There was puffiness of the dorsum of the hands and feet

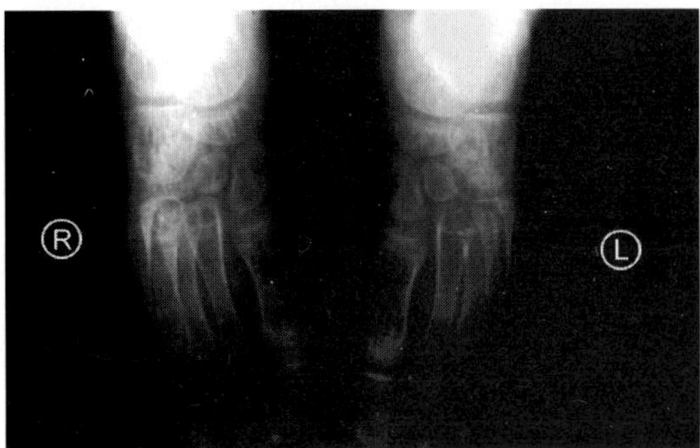

Fig. 23.7 X-ray of both feet in a young two-year-old boy with classical features of hand-foot syndrome showing marked cortical thinning, porosis and prominent trabeculations

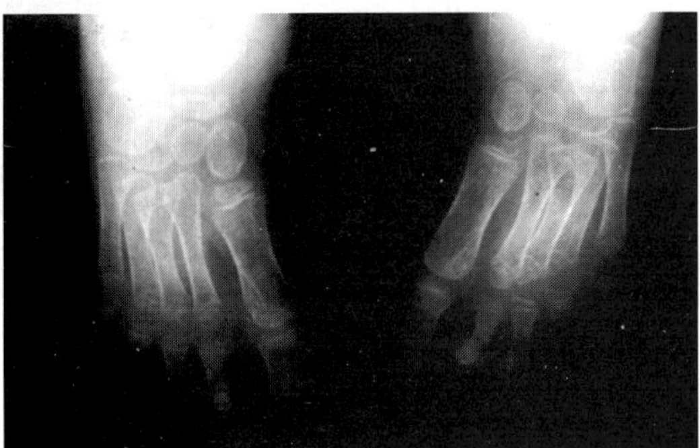

Fig. 23.8 X-ray of both feet in a young child with a SS pattern showing thinning of cortices with areas of intramedullary deposits and spotty destruction

and tender fusiform swelling of phalanges. The first case of dactylitis in a child with sickle cell anemia was reported by Danford and associates[4] in 1941. In 1960, Smith WS[5] used the term "Hand-Foot Syndrome" while describing the acute swelling in the hands and feet of children with sickle cell disease. The lesion is frequently mistaken for acute osteomyelitis.

The true incidence of sickle cell dactylitis is not clear. It occurs in 10 to 20 percent of children with sickle cell disease. Dactylitis occurs most frequently in first four years of life. No instances have been reported in children older than seven years. The onset is usually acute and is characterized by painful

swelling of hands, feet, accompanied by fever, leukocytosis and anemia. The clinical symptoms in this syndrome are self-limiting and spontaneous improvement should be expected without any medical or surgical treatment. The roentgenographic features are usually noted between 7 and 15 days after the onset of clinical symptoms. Initially, there is only soft tissue swelling in the affected extremity. X-ray pictures seem to follow two distinct patterns; the earliest change is appearance of subperiosteal new bone in one or more metacarpals or phalanges. This results in the rectangular outline of the involved bone (Fig. 23.3). The second change is cortical thinning and irregular intra-medullary density in the involved bone (Figs 23.4 and 23.5). The radiological changes are completely reversible within 6 to 20 weeks.

The exact pathological process responsible for this acute syndrome remains somewhat unclear. Cockshott WP[6] 1958, Diggs LW[7] 1965, supported the theory of sickle cell thrombosis from abnormal RBC's with subsequent obstruction of flow and hypoxia resulting in cell death in the metaphyseal area of involved bone, whereas in 1953 Ivy RE and Howard FH,[8] thought that irregular densities within the medullary area of bone is best explained by marrow hyperplasia.

CLINICAL FEATURES

All the patients were admitted in crisis and it was the first manifestation of the disease in 14 cases.[1,2] The presentation was of acute onset with symmetrical swelling of hand and feet. Fever of varying degrees was a constant feature. The children were debilitated, with poor general condition and at times dehydrated. The disease took an average of 21 days to resolve. Hand-foot syndrome was seen in 46 patients (0.62%) in the study of 7380 cases of sickle cell hemoglobinopathy. The maximum number of patients (29) was in the age group of 2 to 3 years of age. All patients were below 5 years of age. There were 27 males and 19 females.

Hemoglobin electrophoresis was "SS" in 12 patients, "As" in 24 and "ASF" in 10 children.

RADIOLOGY

The radiological changes are characteristic and were seen after an average of 10 days after onset of symptoms.[1,2] After the onset of swelling, the earliest change is the appearance of subperiosteal new bone formation in one or multiple bones of the hands or feet. There is cortical thinning and multiple irregular intramedullary deposits, areas of spotty destruction and periosteal new bone formation. Since, the lesion usually causes periosteal elevation and new bone formation, radiolucent areas intermingled with areas of increased density it give a "moth-eaten appearance". The small bones of the hands and feet become rectangular in outline and shape. These changes are seen in association with the classical changes described earlier.

MANAGEMENT

All the patients in this study were treated by conservative means. The drug treatment included analgesics, antibiotics, folic acid, zinc and soda-bicarbonate and supportive treatment with splints. Patients required correction of fluid imbalance and on rare occasions blood transfusions.

DISCUSSION

Danford LW and associates[4] in 1941 reported the first case of dactylitis in a child of sickle cell anemia. Tori G[9] (1954) reported destruction and periosteal reaction in metacarpals of both hands in a patient of sickle cell anemia. Smith WS[5] (1960) used the term 'Hand-Foot Syndrome' to describe the acute swelling in the hands and feet of children with sickle cell disease. Watson J et al.[3](1963) reported hand-foot syndrome as a common initial manifestation of Sickle cell disease usually in children. Since the early reports only few studies have appeared in the literature.[7,8,10–15]

The true incidence of the hand-foot syndrome is not clear. It has been reported to occur in 10 to 20 percent of patients of sickle cell disease with orthopedic manifestations.[2,10,13,14] Most of the patients are below four years of age and it has not been reported after the age of seven years (Watson J et al.[3] 1963).The low incidence in this study may be due to the fact that the patients included were the ones who were treated by the orthopedician. The age distribution observed is comparable to the studies reported earlier. The clinical symptoms in this syndrome are self-limiting, the duration may vary from several days to a month.[3,4,8,14,15] Skeletal changes in sickle cell hemoglobinopathies occur mainly because of hyperplasia of the bone marrow and vascular insufficiency resulting in thrombosis and infarction. Hyperplasia of erythrocytes increases the viscosity of blood leading to stasis and thrombosis in the microcirculation and eventually infarction and secondary infection. The exact pathological process responsible for the hand-foot syndrome remains unclear. Cockshott WP[6] (1958) and Diggs LW[7] (1965) were of the opinion that thrombosis due to sickle cell disease leads to obstruction of microcirculation and hypoxic cell death in the metaphyseal area of the bone. Ivy and Howard[8] (1953) thought that increased density within the medullary area seen in sickle cell disease is explained by marrow hyperplasia. Weinberg and Currarino[16] (1972) reported histopathologic features observed at autopsy of a child with sickle cell dactylitis. The changes observed included extensive infarction of the marrow, medullary trabeculae and inner layers of the cortical bone. This was associated with circumferential periosteal elevation and subperiosteal new bone formation. The radiologic changes of this disease are completely reversible and may take between 6 week to 8 months.[1–4,6,11,17] The clinical and radiological features are characteristic but at times may pose a diagnostic problem. Hand-foot syndrome may be the earliest and the only clinical manifestation of sickle cell hemoglobinopathy. Hand-foot syndrome is a self-limiting condition requiring only supportive treatment and preventive therapy to avoid secondary infection.

CONCLUSION

This study highlights the diagnostic clinical and radiological features of the hand-foot syndrome. The hand-foot syndrome is often misdiagnosed. The importance of this condition lies in the fact that it may be the earliest and the only manifestation of sickle cell disease and may be mistaken for osteomyelitis. It requires only conservative treatment, the changes being completely reversible, since it is a presentation of vascular insult like osteonecrosis which is completely reversible. Hand-foot syndrome is a benign self-limiting condition, usually seen during the period of sickle cell crisis in young children. It is commonly seen during the attack of sickle cell crisis in the age group of two to three years, because of relative avascularity. It was observed between 1 and 5 years of age, commonly in males, and is rarely seen after six years of age. Radiological picture is very classical showing subperiosteal new bone formation in one or multiple bones of hands or feet with cortical thinning and areas of spotty destruction and periosteal new bone formation.

REFERENCES

1. Babhulkar SS, Ketan Pande, Sushrut Babhulkar. Hand foot syndrome in Sickle cell haemoglobinopathy. J Bone Joint Surg Br. 1995; 77B:310-12.

2. Babhulkar Sudhir. Orthopaedic manifestations and bone changes in sickle cell haemoglobinopathy. Monogram by CBS Publishers; 1997. pp.78-93.

3. Watson J, Burco H, Megas H, Robinson M. The Hand Foot Syndrome in Sickle cell disease in young children. Paediatrics. 1963;31:975.

4. Danford LW, Marr R, Elsey E. C-Sickle cell anaemia with unusual bone changes. American J. Roentgen. 1941;45:223.

5. Smith WS. Sickle cell anaemia and *Salmonella* osteomyelitis. Ohio Med J. 1960;49:692.

6. Cockshott WP. Dactylitis and growth disturbances. J Fac Radiologists. 1958;9:211.

7. Diggs LW. Sickle cell crisis. American J Clin Path. 1965;44:1.

8. Ivy RE, Horward FH. Sickle cell anaemia with unusual bone changes. J Paediat. 1953;43:312.

9. Tori G. Clinical and Radiological observations on 102 cases of Sickle cell anaemia. Radiol CIin 1954;23:87.

10. Macht SH, Roman PW. The Radiologic Changes in Sickle cell anaemia. Radiology. 1948;51:697-707.

11. Victor AB, Imperiale LE. The Pulmonary and small bone changes in infants with Sickle cell anaemia. New York State J Med. 1957;57:1403-8.

12. Lambotte C. Hand Foot Syndrome in Sickle cell disease. Am J Dis Child. 1962;104:200-1.

13. Porter FS, Thurman WG. Studies of Sickle cell disease. Diagnosis in infancy. Am J Dis Child 1963;106:35-42.

14. Worrall VT, Butera V. Sickle cell dactilytis. J Bone Joint Surg Am. 1976;58A:1161-3.

15. Rowe CW, Haggard ML. Bone infarcts in Sickle cell anaemia. Radiology. 1957;68:661-8.

16. Weinberg AG, Currarino G. Sickle cell dactilytis. Histopathologic observations. Am J of Clincal Pathology. 1972;58:518-23.

17. Moseley JE. Patterns of Bone Changes in Sickle cell crisis. J Mt Sinai Hosp. 1959;26:424-39.